Neuroimaging Anatomy, Part 2: Head, Neck, and Spine

Editor

TARIK F. MASSOUD

NEUROIMAGING CLINICS OF NORTH AMERICA

www.neuroimaging.theclinics.com

Consulting Editor
SURESH K. MUKHERJI

November 2022 • Volume 32 • Number 4

ELSEVIER

1600 John F. Kennedy Boulevard ● Suite 1800 ● Philadelphia, Pennsylvania, 19103-2899

http://www.neuroimaging.theclinics.com

NEUROIMAGING CLINICS OF NORTH AMERICA Volume 32, Number 4
November 2022 ISSN 1052-5149, ISBN 13: 978-0-323-85003-2

Editor: John Vassallo (j.vassallo@elsevier.com)
Developmental Editor: Karen Solomon

Neuroimaging Clinics of North America (ISSN 1052-5149) is published quarterly by Elsevier Inc., 360 Park Avenue South, New York, NY 10010-1710. Months of issue are February, May, August, and November. Business and editorial offices: 1600 John F. Kennedy Blvd., Suite 1800, Philadelphia, PA 19103-2899. Business and editorial offices: 6277 Sea Harbor Drive, Orlando, FL 32887-4800. Periodicals postage paid at New York, NY, and additional mailing offices. Subscription prices are USD 401 per year for US individuals, USD 932 per year for US institutions, USD 100 per year for US students and residents, USD 469 per year for Canadian individuals, USD 946 per year for Canadian institutions, USD 546 per year for international individuals, USD 946 per year for international institutions, USD 100 per year for Canadian students and residents and USD 260 per year for foreign students and residents. To receive student/resident rate, orders must be accompanied by name of affiliated institution, date of term, and the *signature* of program/residency coordinator on institution letterhead. Orders will be billed at individual rate until proof of status is received. Foreign air speed delivery is included in all *Clinics* subscription prices. All prices are subject to change without notice. POSTMASTER: Send address changes to *Neuroimaging Clinics of North America*, Elsevier Health Sciences Division, Subscription **Customer Service, 3251 Riverport Lane, Maryland Heights, MO 63043. Telephone: 1-800-654-2452 (U.S. and Canada); 314-447-8871 (outside U.S. and Canada). Fax: 314-447-8029. E-mail: journalscustomerservice-usa@elsevier.com (for print support); journalsonlinesupport-usa@elsevier.com (for online support).**

Reprints. For copies of 100 or more of articles in this publication, please contact the Commercial Reprints Department, Elsevier Inc., 360 Park Avenue South, New York, NY 10010-1710. Tel.: 212-633-3874; Fax: 212-633-3820; E-mail: reprints@elsevier.com.

Neuroimaging Clinics of North America is covered by *Excerpta Medical/EMBASE,* the RSNA Index of Imaging Literature, *MEDLINE/PubMed (Index Medicus),* MEDLINE/MEDLARS, SciSearch, Research Alert, and Neuroscience Citation Index.

PROGRAM OBJECTIVE

The goal of *Neuroimaging Clinics of North America* is to keep practicing radiologists and radiology residents up to date with current clinical practice in radiology by providing timely articles reviewing the state of the art in patient care.

TARGET AUDIENCE

Practicing radiologists, radiology residents, and other healthcare professionals who utilize neuroimaging findings to provide patient care.

LEARNING OBJECTIVES

Upon completion of this activity, participants will be able to:

1. Review the anatomy of the head, neck, and spine to detect and identify variants utilizing neuroimaging to assist appropriate treatment decision-making.
2. Discuss the role of conventional and novel neuroimaging techniques in clinical decision making in diagnosing, evaluating, and treating findings during head, neck, and spine imaging.
3. Recognize neuroimaging as a crucial and useful noninvasive method for determining normal and abnormal head, neck, and spine anatomy.

ACCREDITATION

The Elsevier Office of Continuing Medical Education (EOCME) is accredited by the Accreditation Council for Continuing Medical Education (ACCME) to provide continuing medical education for physicians.

The EOCME designates this journal-based CME activity for a maximum of 13 *AMA PRA Category 1 Credit*(s)™. Physicians should claim only the credit commensurate with the extent of their participation in the activity.

All other healthcare professionals requesting continuing education credit for this enduring material will be issued a certificate of participation.

DISCLOSURE OF CONFLICTS OF INTEREST

The EOCME assesses conflict of interest with its instructors, faculty, planners, and other individuals who are in a position to control the content of CME activities. All relevant conflicts of interest that are identified are thoroughly vetted by EOCME for fair balance, scientific objectivity, and patient care recommendations. EOCME is committed to providing its learners with CME activities that promote improvements or quality in healthcare and not a specific proprietary business or a commercial interest.

The planning committee, staff, authors, and editors listed below have identified no financial relationships or relationships to products or devices they or their spouse/life partner have with commercial interest related to the content of this CME activity:

Ayca Akgoz Karaosmanoglu, MD; Yoshimi Anzai, MD; John C. Benson, MD; Mary Beth Cunnane, MD; Akinrinola Famuyide, MD; Lotfi Hacein-Bey, MD, FASFNR; Syed S. Hashmi, MD; David C. Hatcher, DDS, MSc, MRCD; Benjamin Y. Huang, MD, MPH; Jacqueline C. Junn, MD; Pradeep Kuttysankaran; John I. Lane, MD; Tarik Massoud, MD, PhD; Kassie L. McCullagh, MD; Gul Moonis, MD; Carrie D. Norris, MD; Curtis Edward Offiah, BSc MB ChB FRCS FRCR; Burce Ozgen, MD; Osama Raslan, MD; Katherine L. Reinshagen, MD; Kimberly D. Seifert, MD, MS; Rupali N. Shah, MD; Peter M. Som, MD; Doreen Thomas-Payne, MSN, BSN, RN, PMHNP-BC; Sanjay Vaid, MD; Neelam Vaid, MS, DNB(ENT); Eric K. van Staalduinen, DO

UNAPPROVED/OFF-LABEL USE DISCLOSURE

The EOCME requires CME faculty to disclose to the participants:

1. When products or procedures being discussed are off-label, unlabelled, experimental, and/or investigational (not US Food and Drug Administration [FDA] approved); and
2. Any limitations on the information presented, such as data that are preliminary or that represent ongoing research, interim analyses, and/or unsupported opinions. Faculty may discuss information about pharmaceutical agents that is outside of FDA-approved labelling. This information is intended solely for CME and is not intended to promote off-label use of these medications. If you have any questions, contact the medical affairs department of the manufacturer for the most recent prescribing information.

TO ENROLL

To enroll in the *Neuroimaging Clinics of North America* Continuing Medical Education program, call customer service at 1-800-654-2452 or sign up online at http://www.theclinics.com/home/cme. The CME program is available to subscribers for an additional annual fee of USD 265.00.

METHOD OF PARTICIPATION

In order to claim credit, participants must complete the following:

1. Complete enrolment as indicated above.
2. Read the activity.
3. Complete the CME Test and Evaluation. Participants must achieve a score of 70% on the test. All CME Tests and Evaluations must be completed online.

CME INQUIRIES/SPECIAL NEEDS

For all CME inquiries or special needs, please contact elsevierCME@elsevier.com.

NEUROIMAGING CLINICS OF NORTH AMERICA

SERIES OF RELATED INTEREST

Advances in Clinical Radiology
Available at: Advancesinclinicalradiology.com
MRI Clinics of North America
Available at: MRI.theclinics.com
PET Clinics
Available at: https://www.pet.theclinics.com/
Radiologic Clinics of North America
Available at: Radiologic.theclinics.com

THE CLINICS ARE AVAILABLE ONLINE!
Access your subscription at:
www.theclinics.com

Contributors

CONSULTING EDITOR

SURESH K. MUKHERJI, MD, MBA, FACR
Clinical Professor of Radiology and Radiation Oncology, University of Illinois, Peoria, Illinois, USA; Robert Wood Johnson Medical School, Rutgers University, New Brunswick, New Jersey, USA; Faculty, Otolaryngology–Head Neck Surgery, Michigan State University, Farmington Hills, Michigan, USA; National Director of Head and Neck Radiology, ProScan Imaging, Carmel, Indiana, USA

EDITOR

TARIK F. MASSOUD, MD, PhD, FRCR
Professor, Division of Neuroimaging and Neurointervention, Department of Radiology, Stanford University School of Medicine, Stanford Health Care, Director, Stanford Initiative for Multimodality Neuro-Imaging in Translational Anatomy Research (SIMITAR), Center for Academic Medicine, Radiology, Palo Alto, California, USA

AUTHORS

AYCA AKGOZ KARAOSMANOGLU, MD
Associate Professor, Department of Radiology, Hacettepe University Medical School, Ankara, Turkey

YOSHIMI ANZAI, MD, MPH
Professor, Department of Radiology and Imaging Sciences, University of Utah, Salt Lake City, Utah, USA

JOHN C. BENSON, MD
Associate Professor, Department of Radiology, Division of Neuroradiology, Mayo Clinic, Rochester, Minnesota, USA

MARY BETH CUNNANE, MD
Assistant Professor, Chief, Department of Radiology, Massachusetts Eye and Ear, Harvard Medical School, Boston, Massachusetts, USA

AKINRINOLA FAMUYIDE, MD
Columbia University Irving Medical Center, New York, New York, USA

LOTFI HACEIN-BEY, MD, FASFNR
Neuroradiology, Radiology Department, University of California, Davis Medical School of Medicine, Sacramento, California, USA

SYED S. HASHMI, MD
Clinical Assistant Professor, Department of Radiology, Stanford University School of Medicine, Center for Academic Medicine, Palo Alto, California, USA

DAVID C. HATCHER, DDS, MSC, MRCD(C)
Department of Orthodontics, Adjunct Professor, School of Dentistry, University of the Pacific, Clinical Professor, Orofacial Sciences, School of Dentistry, University of California, San Francisco, San Francisco, California, USA; Clinical Professor, School of Dentistry, University of California, Los Angeles, Los Angeles, California, USA; Clinical Professor Volunteer, Department of Surgical and Radiological Sciences, School of Veterinary Medicine, University of California, Davis, Davis, California, USA

BENJAMIN Y. HUANG, MD, MPH
Clinical Professor, Division of Neuroradiology, Department of Radiology, The University of North Carolina at Chapel Hill, Chapel Hill, North Carolina, USA

JACQUELINE C. JUNN, MD
Department of Radiology, The Icahn School of Medicine at Mount Sinai, New York, New York, USA

JOHN I. LANE, MD
Professor, Department of Radiology, Division of Neuroradiology, Mayo Clinic, Rochester, Minnesota, USA

TARIK F. MASSOUD, MD, PhD, FRCR
Professor, Division of Neuroimaging and Neurointervention, Department of Radiology, Stanford University School of Medicine, Stanford Health Care, Director, Stanford Initiative for Multimodality Neuro-Imaging in Translational Anatomy Research (SIMITAR), Center for Academic Medicine, Radiology, Palo Alto, California, USA

KASSIE L. MCCULLAGH, MD
Clinical Assistant Professor, Division of Neuroradiology, Department of Radiology, The University of North Carolina at Chapel Hill, Chapel Hill, North Carolina, USA

GUL MOONIS, MD
NYU Langone Medical Center, New York, New York, USA

CARRIE D. NORRIS, MD
Adjunct Faculty, University of Utah, Department of Radiology and Imaging Sciences, Salt Lake City, Utah, USA

CURTIS EDWARD OFFIAH, BSc, MB, ChB, FRCS, FRCR
Consultant Neuroradiologist, Department of Radiology and Imaging, Royal London Hospital, Barts Health NHS Trust, Whitechapel, London, United Kingdom; Senior Lecturer, William Harvey Research Institute, Barts and The London School of Medicine and Dentistry,

Queen Mary University of London, London, United Kingdom

BURCE OZGEN, MD
Professor of Clinical Radiology, Department of Radiology, University of Illinois at Chicago, University of Illinois Hospital, Chicago, Illinois, USA

OSAMA RASLAN, MD
Neuroradiology, Radiology Department, University of California, Davis School of Medicine, Sacramento, California, USA

KATHERINE L. REINSHAGEN, MD
Assistant Professor, Department of Radiology, Massachusetts Eye and Ear, Harvard Medical School, Boston, Massachusetts, USA

KIMBERLY D. SEIFERT, MD, MS
Clinical Instructor, Department of Radiology, Stanford University School of Medicine, Center for Academic Medicine, Palo Alto, California, USA

RUPALI N. SHAH, MD
Clinical Associate Professor, Division of Voice and Swallowing, Department of Otolaryngology–Head and Neck Surgery, The University of North Carolina at Chapel Hill, Chapel Hill, North Carolina, USA

PETER M. SOM, MD
Departments of Radiology, Otolaryngology, and Radiation Oncology, Icahn School of Medicine at Mount Sinai, New York, New York, USA

NEELAM VAID, MS, DNB (ENT)
Department of Otorhinolaryngology, K.E.M. Hospital, Pune, Maharashtra, India

SANJAY VAID, MD (RADIOLOGY)
Head Neck Imaging Division, Star Imaging and Research Center, Pune, Maharashtra, India

ERIC K. VAN STAALDUINEN, DO
Department of Radiology, Stanford University School of Medicine, Center for Academic Medicine, Palo Alto, California, USA

Contents

Each orbit is a complex structure housing the globe, multiple cranial nerves, muscles, vascular structures, which support the visual sense. Many of these structures have been delineated in careful detail by anatomists but remain beyond the resolution of conventional imaging techniques. With the advances of higher resolution MR, surface coil usage, and thinner section computed tomographic images, the ability to resolve these small structures continues to improve, allowing radiologists to provide more detailed anatomic descriptions for preoperative and pretreatment planning.

It is imperative for all imaging specialists to be familiar with detailed multiplanar computed tomography imaging anatomy of the paranasal sinuses and adjacent structures. This article reviews, in brief, the radiologically relevant embryology of the sinonasal region and discusses the imaging anatomy of the nasal cavity and paranasal sinuses. Radiologists should understand the importance and clinical implications of identifying the numerous anatomic variations encountered in this region and prepare a structured report that provides a surgical road map to the referring clinician.

In this article, we discuss the anatomy and development of the face. One should become familiar with the layers, muscles, vessels, and nerves of the face. Embryologic development of the face and supporting structures is also discussed. Additionally, different clinical manifestation of facial paralysis is highlighted.

Oral behavior encompasses active movement of the oral structures. The range and quality of oral behavior is essential for establishing and maintaining health and well-being. Key oral behaviors include breathing, chewing, swallowing, and speech. Key hard tissue elements involved in oral behavior include the mandible, temporomandibular joints, and dentition. This article will discuss the anatomy and interaction of the hard tissue elements and selected soft tissue elements associated with oral behavior.

Temporal bone anatomy is highly complex, with a complicated configuration of minute anatomic structures housed in a dense osseous structure. Nevertheless, a robust understanding of this anatomy is essential for clinicians, who must accurately diagnose and describe the various pathologies that exist in this region. In this article, we provide a comprehensive overview of temporal bone anatomy, ranging from its large components to its smallest foramina, canals, and clefts.

Knowledge of anatomy is essential to the understanding of disease and conditions of the oral cavity and salivary glands. This article is intended to serve as an overview of the oral cavity, its subsites, and that of the neighboring salivary glands. The authors cover the anatomy of the lips, tongue, floor of mouth, hard palate, teeth, various mucosal areas, and salivary ducts. When appropriate, radiological imaging along with figures serves as a companion to highlight the clinical relevance and practical applications of specific anatomic locations.

The pharynx is a complex muscular structure allowing breathing, swallowing, as well speech through common airspace. The normal imaging appearance of the pharynx and cervical esophagus can be challenging given the numerous interleaved surrounding muscles and numerous connections. This article presents the imaging anatomy of the pharynx and cervical esophagus and also discusses the clinical relevance of selected anatomical structures that have important significance in disease development and extension.

The larynx serves as the gateway between the upper and lower respiratory tracts and is involved in the tasks of phonation, deglutition, and airway protection. Familiarity with the complex anatomy of the larynx is critical for detecting and characterizing disease in the region, especially in cancer staging. In this article, we review the anatomy of the larynx and cervical trachea, including an overview of their cartilages, supporting tissues, muscles, mucosal spaces, neurovascular supply, and lymphatics, followed by correlation to the clinically relevant anatomic sites of the larynx. Imaging techniques for evaluating the larynx and trachea will also be discussed briefly.

Foreword

Neuroimaging Anatomy, Part 2: Head, Neck, and Spine

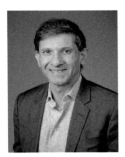

Suresh K. Mukherji, MD, MBA, FACR
Consulting Editor

This is the second half of the wonderful two-part issue of *Neuroimaging Clinics* devoted to Neuroanatomy edited by Dr Tarik Massoud from Stanford University. The first half was devoted to brain and skull base anatomy. This issue is focused on head and neck and spine anatomy and comprises 13 beautifully written and illustrated articles.

Another heartfelt "Thank You" to Dr Massoud for editing this unique and wonderful contribution. As I mentioned in the foreword to the prior issue, Tarik not only accepted the invitation but also took this project to a new level. These wonderful issues would not be possible without the outstanding efforts of the article authors, and I want to personally thank these world-renowned experts for their wonderful contributions to this issue.

This two-part series has far exceeded Dr Massoud's stated goal of presenting anatomic facts of practical value to neuroradiologists, neuroscientists, and their trainees. I will always refer to this two-part series when asked what I feel is the most comprehensive journal for reviewing radiologic neuroanatomy. Many thanks again to Tarik and the wonderful team for this lasting contribution!

Suresh K. Mukherji, MD, MBA, FACR
Marian University, Head and Neck Radiology
ProScan Imaging, Carmel, IN 46074, USA

E-mail address:
sureshmukherji@hotmail.com

Neuroimag Clin N Am 32 (2022) xiii
https://doi.org/10.1016/j.nic.2022.07.026
1052-5149/22/© 2022 Published by Elsevier Inc.

Preface

Neuroimaging Anatomy, Part 2: Head, Neck, and Spine

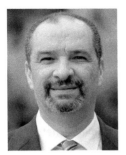

Tarik F. Massoud, MD, PhD, FRCR
Editor

Two wonderful quotations capture the intended essence and objective for compiling this and the previous issue of *Neuroimaging Clinics* on the subject of neuroimaging anatomy: "*Anatomy should rightly be regarded as the firm foundation of the whole art of medicine and its essential preliminary*" (Andreas Vesalius, *De humani corporis fabrica* [1543]), and "*At least half of learning neuroradiology is understanding neuroanatomy*" (Dr Anne G. Osborn).

This issue of *Neuroimaging Clinics* on neuroimaging anatomy of the head, neck, and spine appears after an unusually long interval since some aspects of this topic were last reviewed in a single issue of this series (8:1, Feb 1998, guest editor Lindell Gentry). This was in part dictated by the need to await the steady evolution of neuroimaging techniques we have witnessed over the last two decades that would help us better depict the stunning head, neck, and spine anatomy we encounter in our daily neuroradiologic practice. We believe this *Neuroimaging Clinics* issue covering head, neck, and spine anatomy will help clinical neuroradiologists and specialists in allied fields appreciate the exquisitely detailed anatomy that underlies neuroimaging. We aim to update the reader about the role of current and new advances in imaging techniques that help us visualize and understand this complex anatomy. As such, this issue is not intended to be a formal or exhaustive treatise on anatomy (classical textbooks and atlases are intended for that purpose), but it aims to give an updated anatomic background that would assist clinical practitioners in the diagnosis and treatment of disorders of the head, neck, and spine.

The importance of anatomy in imaging cannot be overstated. As radiologists, we are exceedingly privileged to be able to indirectly see the internal anatomy of our patients. There are many reasons brain neuroanatomy along with head, neck, and spine anatomy are the underpinning of our neuroradiology practice. This is not only because we noninvasively review intricate anatomic structures on images, but also, in practice, we clinically and educationally disseminate the anatomic knowledge we have gained to others. The reasons for the importance of neuroimaging anatomy include the fact that its knowledge is highly relevant to

Neuroimag Clin N Am 32 (2022) xv–xvii
https://doi.org/10.1016/j.nic.2022.07.019
1052-5149/22/© 2022 Published by Elsevier Inc.

the daily work of neuroradiologists in distinguishing normal and variant anatomy from pathologic signs of disease. Thus, to correlate structural and functional neuroimaging findings with the clinical information of patients, to issue radiologic reports, and to communicate meaningfully and on par with referring physicians all require a deep understanding of head, neck, and spine anatomy and the language used to describe it. The central role of these neuroimaging interpretations rooted in knowledge of anatomy has never been stronger for clinical decision making within contemporary clinical care.

As neuroradiology becomes ever more fundamental to clinical pathways and as a hub for decision making in the clinical neurosciences and clinical disciplines pertinent to the head, neck, and spine, an understanding of neuroimaging anatomy is essential to the neuroradiologists of tomorrow. The aim of including anatomy in radiology curricula for residents and fellows in training is not to produce anatomists, but rather, to produce radiologists who will be able to apply anatomic scientific principles, methods, and knowledge to the clinical practice of radiology. I often tell radiology trainees that "radiologists are but applied anatomists." As neuroradiology educators, we must convey to our trainees a sound core knowledge of neuroimaging anatomy. This will form a cornerstone of their future practice and will instill confidence during training by lessening the occurrence of anatomic misinterpretations, defined as errors in identifying the correct anatomic locations of head, neck, and spine pathologic conditions.

The symbiosis of anatomy and radiology is vital to the practice of medicine, and it is also an important element of doctors as scholars and scientists. We therefore also hope that the fine collection of up-to-date reviews contained within this issue will represent a useful foundation of knowledge for neuroradiologists as scientists and physician-investigators aiming to effectively contribute to advancements in the clinical neurosciences as well as clinical disciplines pertinent to the head, neck, and spine. This may entail performance of "reverse translational" neuroimaging anatomy research where clinical problems can be identified and addressed with studies of anatomy and morphometry as depicted on neuroimages. For example, in a manner that answers hypothesis-driven questions, anatomy pertinent to improving safety and efficacy of head, neck, and spine surgical and interventional procedures can be studied using morphometric measurements and statistical analyses of anatomic information seen on MR and CT images, all to the ultimate benefit of our patients.

Until now, no succinct book has been available as a comprehensive updated source of information and knowledge on neuroimaging anatomy of the head, neck, and spine. While the actual anatomy has not changed since the previous *Neuroimaging Clinics* issue on this subject, more recent advances in neuroradiology have enabled new imaging techniques for diagnostic neuroimaging and therapeutic neurointerventions that have rendered some of the older techniques obsolete. These changes as well as advances in clinical neuroscientific knowledge and practice have required revision of all previous articles, with the addition of several new ones and many more illustrations of modern, more informative structural ways to visualize head, neck, and spine anatomy using neuroimaging.

This issue of *Neuroimaging Clinics* consists of 13 articles providing reference material on the latest methods to visualize head, neck, and spine anatomy. This issue is organized to provide a broad core knowledge related to imaging anatomy of the viscerocranium, soft tissues, and organs of the face and neck, and the spine. The contents of this issue are presented as separate review articles, any one of which is complete in itself. Each article is beautifully illustrated with many high-resolution images that present the relevant anatomy in multiple planes.

Of note, we have tried to conform as much as possible to standard anatomic English terminology shown in the *Terminologia Anatomica* (the international standard for human anatomic terminology developed by the International Federation of Associations of Anatomists [IFAA]), with sporadic Latin usage. In the future, neuroradiologists will inevitably need to adhere to the recommendations of this international standard to uniformly adopt more accurate terminology for head, neck, and spine anatomy. As for eponyms, we have for now continued the use of standard, well-known eponyms. However, the use of eponyms is counter to the recommendation of the IFAA to omit all eponyms in the description of anatomic structures. The slow replacement of eponyms in our neuroimaging anatomic language will be uncomfortable for older generations of neuroradiologists, but for future generations, it will be a relief. On the other hand, we did not shy away from presenting common neuroimaging anatomic variants. These may be defined as slight deviations from the accepted standard human anatomy without causing a demonstrable impairment in function. However, an in-depth description of anatomic variations is a vast topic in its own right and beyond the scope of this issue, as there exists an extremely wide range of "normal" in the body.

Finally, this issue has been compiled with the goal of presenting anatomic facts of practical value to clinical neuroradiologists, other clinical neuroscientists, head and neck and spine specialists, and their trainees. We are immensely grateful to each one of the team of expert contributors to this issue who have provided readers with the most up-to-date knowledge on neuroimaging anatomy of the head, neck, and spine. The success of this issue is largely a result of their time, effort, and expertise in preparing their articles.

It has been a privilege and pleasure for me to guest edit this issue. I wish to express my sincere thanks to Dr Suresh Mukherji, Consulting Editor, for his invitation, and to Elsevier for their excellent support throughout the process leading to completion of this issue.

Tarik F. Massoud, MD, PhD, FRCR
Division of Neuroimaging and Neurointervention
Department of Radiology
Stanford University School of Medicine
Stanford Health Care
Stanford Initiative for Multimodality Neuro
Imaging in Translational Anatomy Research
(SIMITAR)
Center for Academic Medicine
Radiology MC: 5659
453 Quarry Road
Palo Alto, CA 94304, USA

E-mail address:
tmassoud@stanford.edu

Anatomy of the Orbit

Katherine L. Reinshagen, MD[a],*, Tarik F. Massoud, MD, PhD[b],
Mary Beth Cunnane, MD[a]

KEYWORDS

• Anatomy • Orbit • CT • MR

KEY POINTS

- The orbit is a complex structure with multiple contributing bones, important foramina, complex neurovascular and muscular anatomy, and a lacrimal apparatus, which all support the visual sense.
- The orbital septum is a continuation of the periorbita and anatomically divides the orbit into preseptal and postseptal compartments, providing a strong barrier to the spread of disease.
- The extraocular rectus muscles originate from the common tendinous ring (annulus of Zinn) and further divide the postseptal orbit into intraconal and extraconal spaces, an important distinction for presurgical planning.

INTRODUCTION

Each orbit is a complex structure housing the globe, multiple cranial nerves, muscles, vascular structures, which support the visual sense. Many of these structures have been delineated in careful detail by anatomists but remain beyond the resolution of conventional imaging techniques. With the advances of higher resolution MR, surface coil usage, and thinner section computed tomographic (CT) images, the ability to resolve these small structures continues to improve, allowing radiologists to provide more detailed anatomic descriptions for preoperative and pretreatment planning.

BONY ORBIT

The bony orbit is cone-shaped and has contributions from 7 bones: the frontal, zygomatic, maxilla, lacrimal, ethmoid, palatine, and sphenoid bones (Fig. 1). The frontal bone forms the anterior roof and superior rim of the orbit. A notch in the superior orbital rim contains the supraorbital nerve (branch of the first division of the trigeminal nerve), supraorbital artery, and supraorbital vein and is termed the supraorbital notch or foramen. The zygomatic bone contributes to the lateral orbital wall, whereas the maxilla forms the anterior floor and inferior rim of the orbit. From posterior to anterior, the groove, canal, and foramen within the floor of the orbit and inferior rim of the orbit are termed the infraorbital groove, canal, and foramen, respectively, and they enclose the infraorbital nerve (branch of the second division of the trigeminal nerve) and infraorbital artery and vein (see Fig. 1; Fig. 2). Posteriorly, a portion of the maxilla forms the inferior margin of the inferior orbital fissure. The lacrimal bone forms the anteromedial portion of the bony orbit and has a crescentic shape forming the fossa of the lacrimal sac. Most of the medial orbital wall is derived from the orbital plate of the ethmoid bone and is particularly thin, giving its name "lamina papyracea," or "paperthin." The anterior and posterior ethmoidal grooves are located within the orbital plate of the ethmoid (see Figs. 1 and 2). Owing to its thin nature, disease from the adjacent air cells can spread into the orbit. The ethmoid bone articulates with the body of the sphenoid bone posteriorly.[1] Posteromedialy, there is a small contribution to the bony orbit from the orbital process of the palatine bone located medial to the superior orbital fissure (see Fig. 1). Most of the posterior orbit, including the 3 major posterior foramina (optic canal, superior orbital fissure, and inferior orbital fissure), is derived from the sphenoid bone (see Fig. 1;

[a] Department of Radiology, Massachusetts Eye and Ear/Harvard Medical School, 243 Charles Street, Boston, MA 02114, USA; [b] Stanford Neuroscience Health Center, 213 Quarry Road, MC 5659, Palo Alto, CA 94304, USA
* Corresponding author.
E-mail address: katherine_reinshagen@meei.harvard.edu

Neuroimag Clin N Am 32 (2022) 699–711
https://doi.org/10.1016/j.nic.2022.07.020
1052-5149/22/© 2022 Elsevier Inc. All rights reserved.

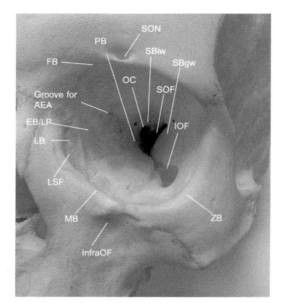

Fig. 1. Frontal view of the left bony orbit in a human skull. EB/LP, ethmoid bone/lamina papyracea; FB, frontal bone; Groove for AEA, groove for the anterior ethmoid artery; InfraOF, infraorbital foramen; IOF, inferior orbital fissure; LB, lacrimal bone; LSF, fossa for the lacrimal sac; MB, maxillary bone; OC, optic canal; PB, palatine bone; SBgw, sphenoid bone greater wing; SBlw, sphenoid bone lesser wing; SOF, superior orbital fissure; ZB, zygomatic bone.

Fig. 3). The greater and lesser wings of the sphenoid bone form part of the orbit. The greater wing of the sphenoid contributes to the posterolateral margin of the orbit and, importantly, forms the

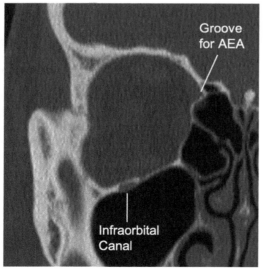

Fig. 2. Coronal noncontrast CT of the right orbit in bone windows demonstrating the groove for the anterior ethmoidal artery (AEA) and the infraorbital canal containing the infraorbital nerve.

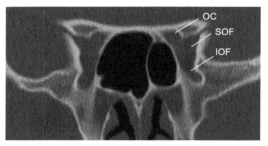

Fig. 3. Coronal noncontrast CT of the orbits in bone windows at the orbital apices demonstrating the posterior foramina. IOF, inferior orbital fissure; OC, optic canal; SOF, superior orbital fissure.

lateral margin of the superior orbital fissure laterally and lateral margin of the inferior orbital fissure. The lesser wing of the sphenoid contributes to the upper medial margin of the superior orbital fissure and also contains the optic canal.

The 3 posterior foramina of the orbit from superior to inferior are the optic canal, superior orbital fissure, and inferior orbital fissure (see Figs. 1 and 3). The optic canal contains the optic nerve and ophthalmic artery. The superior orbital fissure is a comma-shaped opening and contains the nerves to the extraocular muscles (CN III: oculomotor, CN IV: trochlear, CN VI: abducens) as well as the terminal branches (lacrimal, frontal, and nasociliary nerves) of the first division of the trigeminal nerve (V1, ophthalmic nerve) and ophthalmic veins. The inferior orbital fissure, with contribution from the sphenoid and maxilla, transmits the zygomatic nerve branch of the second division of the trigeminal nerve (V2, maxillary nerve) and the infraorbital nerve and vessels. Through the inferior orbital fissure, the orbit communicates with the pterygopalatine fossa.

ORBITAL SEPTUM AND PERIORBITA

The periorbita or periosteum of the orbit is particularly important because it forms part of the structural support of the orbit and is a critical barrier for spread of pathologic condition. It is composed of a fibrous connective tissue that surrounds the bony orbit and is contiguous posteriorly with the dura surrounding the optic nerve near the superior orbital fissure.[1,2] The dura mater contributes to the periosteum of the orbit and continues as the optic nerve sheath. Anteriorly, the periorbita continues as the orbital septum. Here medially, it is thin, separating from the medial palpebral ligament to attach to the lacrimal bone at its posterior crest, whereas laterally, the septum is attached to the orbital margin, about 1.5 mm in front of the lateral orbital tubercle attachment of the lateral palpebral ligament. The septum attaches to the lid superiorly via the levator aponeurosis and inferiorly via the capsulopalpebral fascia, which then thicken and form the superior and inferior tarsal plates within the eyelids (see next section).[2] The contents of the orbit can be divided into preseptal and postseptal compartments by the orbital septum (Figs. 4 and 5). The orbital septum forms a strong barrier, which provides resistance to spread of disease from the preseptal to the postseptal compartments.

PRESEPTAL ORBIT: EYELIDS

The superior and inferior tarsal plates within the upper and lower eyelids, respectively, are thickened continuations of the orbital septum (Fig. 6A). Medially and laterally, the superior and inferior tarsal plates form the medial and lateral palpebral raphe or ligaments, respectively. These attach to the bony orbit, as stated earlier, thus forming the overall structure of the eyelid. The superior transverse ligament of the eye (Whitnall's ligament) extends from the levator palpebrae superioris muscle into the superior tarsus, allowing for superior and inferior movement of the superior tarsus (Fig. 6B). The superior tarsal muscle (Müller's muscle) is a smooth muscle that arises from the levator palpebrae superioris muscle and aponeurosis and attaches to the superior tarsal plate, contributing to lid elevation[3] (see Fig. 4). Inferiorly, the inferior tarsal muscle is more indistinct and in cadaveric studies can be seen wrapped by the capsulopalpebral fascia, which then inserts onto the inferior tarsal plate. The capsulopalpebral fascia extends from the inferior rectus, fuses with the orbital septum and inserts on the inferior tarsal plate.[4,5] The analogous ligament to the superior transverse ligament inferiorly is Lockwood ligament, which extends from the lateral orbital tubercle to the medial canthal ligament.[6] The orbicularis oculi muscle is a ring-like muscle that is superficial to the orbital septum (see Fig. 4). Although distinguishing the fascial layers remains challenging with conventional large field of view MR imaging, use of microscopy coils particularly at 1.5 T[7] or dedicated orbital MR sequences with thin section (2 mm), small field of view imaging at 3T may help delineate the overall structure of the eyelids.

POSTSEPTAL ORBIT

The postseptal orbit can be readily divided into intraconal and extraconal compartments separated by the rectus muscles (superior, inferior, medial, and lateral). The optic nerve and nerve sheath course centrally within the intraconal compartment. The space between the globe,

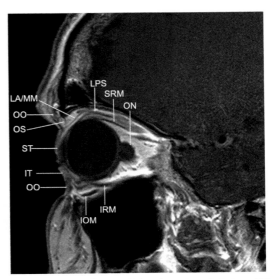

Fig. 4. 3T sagittal T1-weighted post gadolinium MR image of the orbit. IOM, inferior oblique muscle; IRM, inferior rectus muscle; IT, inferior tarsus; LA/MM, levator aponeurosis/Müller muscle; LPS, levator palpebrae superioris muscle; ON, optic nerve; OO, orbicularis oculi muscle; OS, orbital septum; SRM, superior rectus muscle ST, superior tarsus.

extraocular muscles, and vessels and nerves is filled with adipose tissue (the orbital adipose body). This intraorbital fat is of interest owing to several distinctions from body fat by embryology, structure, and function. In adults, intraorbital fat consists of white adipose tissue that differs from body fat by its smaller adipocytes and fat lobules, and denser stroma.[8]

GLOBE AND OPTIC NERVE

The globe can be divided into 2 segments—anterior and posterior (Fig. 7). The anterior segment is substantially smaller and consists of the portion of the

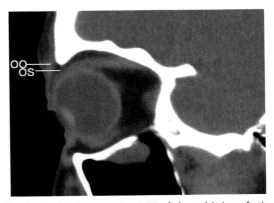

Fig. 5. Sagittal noncontrast CT of the orbit in soft tissue windows. OO, orbicularis oculi muscle; OS, orbital septum.

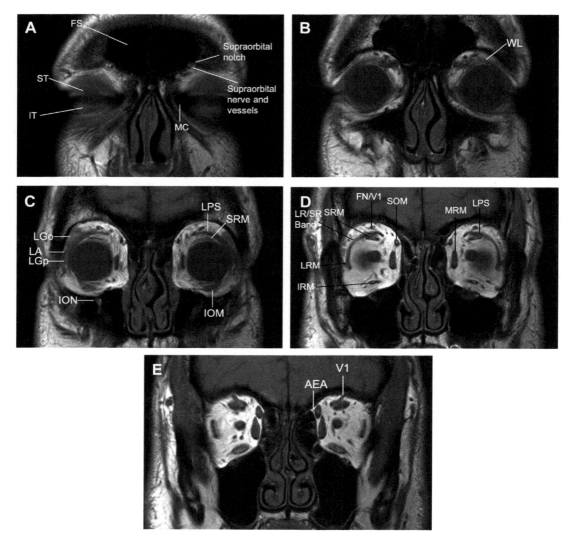

Fig. 6. 3T coronal T1-weighted MR image of the orbits. (*A*) FS, frontal sinus; IT, inferior tarsus; MC, medial canthus; ST, superior tarsus; ; (*B*) WL, Whitnall ligament; (*C*) LGo, lacrimal gland orbital lobe; LA, levator palpe-brae muscle aponeurosis; LGp, lacrimal gland palpebral lobe; LPS, levator palpebrae superioris muscle; SRM, su-perior rectus muscle; IOM, inferior oblique muscle; ION, infraorbital nerve; (*D*) FN/V1, frontal nerve, first division of the trigeminal nerve; IRM, inferior rectus muscle; LR/SR band, lateral rectus/superior rectus band; LRM, lateral rectus muscle; LPS, levator palpebrae superioris muscle; MRM, medial rectus muscle; SRM, superior rectus muscle; SOM, superior oblique muscle; (*E*) AEA, anterior ethmoidal artery; V1, first division of the trigeminal nerve.

globe anterior to the lens. The anterior segment contains aqueous humor and can be further subdi-vided into the anterior and posterior chambers, separated by the iris (see Fig. 7). The posterior segment of the globe consists primarily of the vitre-ous body/humor and contains the important neuro-sensory elements of the retina. Extending through the vitreous is the hyaloid canal, which courses from the posterior aspect of the lens centrally to the optic disc. The hyaloid canal is notable in the fetal stage through which the hyaloid artery passes,

supplying the developing lens. Near birth, the hya-loid artery and canal regress.

The sclera is the tough, white fibrous outer layer of the globe. Owing to its fibrous nature, this can often be seen as a thick dark layer on both T1-weighted and T2-weighted MR imaging[9] (see Fig. 7; Fig. 8). It is contiguous with the optic nerve sheath dural layer and continues to the lateral margin of the cornea. The sclera has many perfo-rations through which long and short posterior ciliary arteries and anterior ciliary arteries pass,

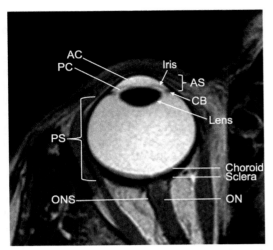

Fig. 7. 3T axial T2-weighted MR image of the right orbit. AC, anterior chamber; AS, anterior segment; CB, ciliary body; PC, posterior chamber; PS, posterior segment; ON, optic nerve; ONS, optic nerve sheath.

the latter of which accompany the extraocular muscle insertions. The optic nerve enters through the sclera through the perforation called the lamina cribrosa. In addition, the central retinal artery and vein pass through an opening in the lamina cribrosa.

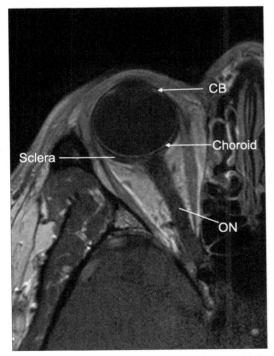

Fig. 8. 3T axial T1-weighted post gadolinium MR image of the right orbit. CB, ciliary body, ON, optic nerve.

The uvea or uveal tract is the layer of the globe between the retina and the sclera. The uvea consists of the choroid, ciliary body, and iris. These are all highly vascular and will avidly enhance on postcontrast MR imaging[9,10] (see Fig. 8). The choroid layer is the layer specifically between the retinal layer and sclera in the posterior globe and provides vascular supply and temperature regulation to the globe.[2,10] Anteriorly, the choroid continues as the ciliary body, which includes a ring-like muscle, the ciliary muscle, and the ciliary stroma and epithelium. The ciliary body contributes to lens accommodation as well as maintenance of the aqueous humor in the anterior segment of the globe. The iris is the ring-like muscle that functions as an aperture and controls the opening of the pupil.

The retina is the innermost, thin neurosensory layer containing the photoreceptors (rods and cones) that transmit light signals to the optic nerve. The macula lutea is a region slightly temporal/lateral to the optic disc and is notable for the fovea centralis, a small depression approximately 3.5 mm temporal to the optic disc with the greatest concentration of cones leading to the most distinct vision. A discussion of the cellular elements of the retina is beyond the scope of this article.

The optic nerve is a continuation of the central nervous system with sensory reception in the retina. The optic nerve has 4 main segments— intraocular, intraorbital, intracanalicular, and intracranial/prechiasmatic. The intraorbital optic nerve is surrounded by the optic nerve sheath, which is a continuation of the dura, arachnoid, and pia mater. The dura mater is composed of collagenous connective tissue forming the outer layer of the optic nerve sheath and fuses anteriorly with the sclera (see Fig. 7). The arachnoid mater is contiguous with the subarachnoid CSF space and terminates at the lamina cribrosa, where the optic nerve fibers enter through the sclera.[2] The pia mater encloses the optic nerve. Because the optic nerve sheath fuses with the periosteum at the optic canal, it is relatively fixed at this location.

The intraorbital optic nerve and its vascular supply from the ophthalmic artery and central retinal artery are slightly tortuous in the intraconal region, allowing some laxity for movement of the globe (see Fig. 8). The optic nerve passes through the annulus of Zinn (the common tendinous ring) before entering the optic canal and continuing intracranially.

Tenon capsule is a fascial sheath that surrounds the posterior globe and forms a fibroelastic socket separating the globe from the intraconal fat and allowing for movement of the globe. It fuses with the sclera and the optic nerve sheath.[2,11]

EXTRAOCULAR MUSCLES AND NERVES

The extraocular muscles comprise the 4 rectus muscles (superior rectus, inferior rectus, medial rectus, and lateral rectus), the 2 oblique muscles (superior and inferior), and the levator palpebrae superioris (Fig. 6C, D). With the exception of the inferior oblique muscle, which originates from the anterior orbital floor, the extraocular muscles originate at the orbital apex from the common tendinous ring known as the annulus of Zinn.

The superior and inferior rectus muscles are termed the vertical rectus muscles because their primary action is to move the globe superiorly and inferiorly along the vertical plane (see Fig. 6D; Fig. 9C, H). The medial and lateral rectus muscles are termed the horizontal rectus muscles because they control abduction and adduction in the horizontal plane (Fig. 9F). Although the primary action of these muscles may be vertical or horizontal movement, the inferior rectus muscle is also involved in external rotation and adduction. The tendons of the extraocular rectus muscles insert on the sclera posterior to the equator of the globe.[12,13]

The medial rectus muscle runs parallel to the medial orbital wall. Because this muscle runs in a plane parallel to the anatomic sagittal plane of the body, the muscle is seen in plane on sagittal images and perpendicular to the plane on standard coronal images of the orbit. The remaining extraocular muscles also run parallel to the orbital walls but because the orbits are conical in shape and directed at an angle to the sagittal plane, they may be best evaluated with imaging that is sagittal and coronal to the orbit rather than the body (Fig. 10). In particular, the width of the lateral rectus muscle is very difficult to accurately evaluate on standard coronal images. Coronal reformats in the plane of the orbit can also be helpful in delineating the relationship of pathologic condition with the optic nerve, which runs *en face* with the reformat.

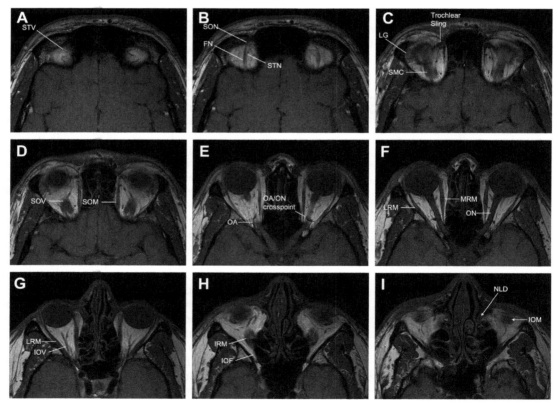

Fig. 9. 3T axial T1-weighted MR image of the orbits. (*A*) STV, supratrochlear vessels; (*B*) SON, supraorbital nerve; STN, supratrochlear nerve; FN, frontal nerve; (*C*) LG, lacrimal gland; SMC, superior muscle complex; (*D*) SOV, superior ophthalmic vein; SOM, superior oblique muscle; (*E*) OA, ophthalmic artery; OA/ON, crossing point of the ophthalmic artery along the medial margin of the optic nerve; (*F*) LRM, lateral rectus muscle; MRM, medial rectus muscle; ON, optic nerve; (*G*) LRM, lateral rectus muscle; IOV, inferior ophthalmic vein; (*H*) IRM, inferior rectus muscle; IOF, inferior orbital fissure; (*I*) NLD, nasolacrimal duct; IOM, inferior oblique muscle.

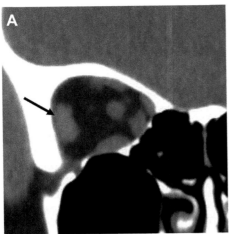
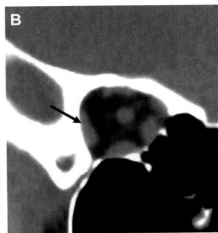

Fig. 10. Noncontrast CT of the right orbit. As the orbit is angled somewhat laterally in the skull, coronal views through the head do not always provide the most accurate view of the orbital structures. In this example, the lateral rectus muscle (*black arrow*) seems enlarged on a coronal view of the head (*A*); however, on an image that is reformatted to be coronal to the orbit (*B*), the lateral rectus muscle is normal in appearance.

The rectus muscles act on the globe via pulleys that are condensations of connective tissue in Tenon capsule and attach to the outer surface of the extraocular muscles.[14] These are not directly visible on MR imaging or CT; however, their presence can be inferred by the lack of change of the posterior muscle bellies during gaze deviation and the sideslip of the muscles anteriorly at the level of the globe insertion, opposite to the direction of gaze.[15]

The superior oblique muscle originates from the annulus of Zinn. The muscle belly parallels the medial orbital wall. It has a long tendon that enters the fibrocartilagenous trochlea (which may calcify in the elderly) before making a sharp turn to insert on the superior aspect of the globe deep to the superior rectus muscle (see Fig. 6D; Fig. 9C, D).[2,16] Its primary action is depression of the globe. The inferior oblique is the shortest of the extraocular muscles (see Fig. 6C; Fig. 9I). It originates anteriorly on the orbital floor at the orbital plate of the maxilla and extends to the postero-inferior globe. Its primary action is elevation of the globe.

The levator palpebrae superioris originates in the posterior orbit and passes superficial to the superior rectus muscle (see Fig. 6C, D). Its primary action is to elevate the lid. Especially on coronal CT and low-resolution MR images, it may seem inseparable from the underlying superior rectus muscle, and together may be referred to as the levator palpebrae superioris/superior rectus complex (see Fig. 9C).

Congenital anomalies of the extraocular muscles are rarely reported. Accessory muscles may be appreciated, however, even in patients without

strabismus. Often, these are vertical muscular bands that connect the lateral margins of the superior and inferior rectus muscles (Fig. 11).[17]

Innervation to the extraocular muscles is provided by the third, fourth, and sixth cranial nerves. The third cranial nerve innervates the superior, medial, and inferior rectus muscles, as well as the levator palpebrae and the inferior oblique muscle. The sixth nerve innervates the lateral rectus muscle, and the fourth nerve innervates the superior oblique muscle. Each of these cranial nerves originates from the brainstem and then travels through the basilar cisterns to enter a dural tunnel or compartment before entering the cavernous sinus. The third nerve enters the oculomotor cistern, the fourth nerve enters the trochlear groove and trochlear cistern, and the sixth nerve enters Dorello canal (Fig. 12). After leaving their respective cisterns, the nerves travel through the cavernous sinus to reach the orbit. The third and fourth nerves are incorporated into the lateral wall of the

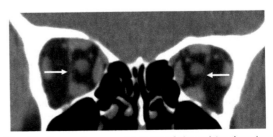

Fig. 11. Coronal noncontrast CT of the orbits showing soft tissue bands representing accessory extra-ocular muscles connect the lateral margins of the superior and inferior rectus muscles bilaterally (*white arrows*).

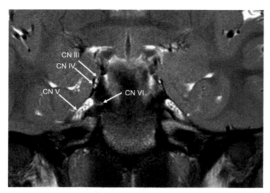

Fig. 12. 3T coronal T2-weighted MR image through the cranial nerve cisterns. After leaving the brainstem and traveling through the basilar cisterns, each cranial nerve to the orbit travels in its own dural canal before entering the cavernous sinus. In this image, the oculomotor cistern (CN III), the trochlear cistern (CN IV), the trigeminal nerve in Meckel cave (CN V) and the abducens nerve in Dorello canal (CN VI) are demonstrated.

cavernous sinus, whereas the sixth nerve is more medially located, contacting the lateral wall of the internal carotid artery (ICA)[18,19] (Fig. 13). They pass into the orbit through the superior

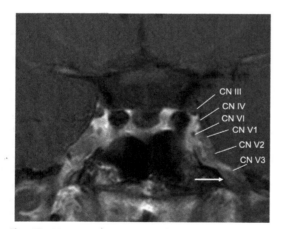

Fig. 13. 3T coronal T1 post gadolinium MR image of the cavernous sinus. After exiting their respective dural canals, the nerves to the orbit enter the cavernous sinus. The oculomotor nerve and the trochlear nerve lie along the lateral margin of the cavernous sinus. The abducens nerve is more medial. The trigeminal nerve gives off V3 through foramen ovale (arrow) while the fibers of V1 and V2 travel along the lateral margin of the cavernous sinus. CN III, oculomotor nerve (third cranial nerve); CN IV, trochlear nerve (fourth cranial nerve); CN VI, abducens nerve (sixth cranial nerve); CN V1, ophthalmic division of the trigeminal nerve (fifth cranial nerve); CN V2, maxillary division of the trigeminal nerve (fifth cranial nerve); CN V3, mandibular division of the trigeminal nerve (fifth cranial nerve).

orbital fissure. The third cranial nerve divides into superior and inferior divisions just before the superior orbital fissure[20] (Fig. 14). The superior division extends to the superior rectus and levator palpebrae muscle, and the inferior division sends branches to the inferior and medial rectus muscles and the inferior oblique. The sixth nerve enters the medial aspect of the lateral rectus muscle.[19]

In addition to the motor innervation of the extraocular muscles, branches of the first and second divisions of the trigeminal nerve pass through the orbit. The first division, or ophthalmic nerve, divides into the nasociliary nerve, the frontal nerve, and the lacrimal nerves. All of these branches enter the orbit through the superior orbital fissure. The nasociliary branch travels in the central sector of the superior orbital fissure within the annulus of Zinn. The frontal and lacrimal branches travel lateral to the annulus in the lateral sector of the superior orbital fissure.[21] The frontal branch of V1 then runs superior to the levator palpebrae muscle (Fig. 6D, E) and divides into the supratrochlear nerve and the supraorbital nerve (Fig. 9B). The supraorbital nerve continues anteriorly along the roof to exit the orbit at the supraorbital notch (see Figs. 1 and 6A).

The second division of the trigeminal nerve travels from the cavernous sinus (see Fig. 13), through foramen rotundum into the pterygopalatine fossa. The infraorbital nerve branch of the second division passes from the pterygopalatine fossa into the inferior orbital fissure (see Fig. 9H) and then enters the infraorbital groove and canal on the floor of the orbit (see Fig. 2). The infraorbital

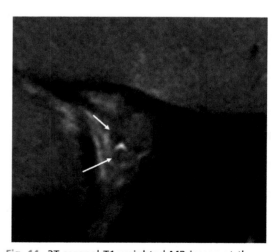

Fig. 14. 3T coronal T1-weighted MR image at the superior orbital fissure. As the right third nerve exits the cavernous sinus, it divides into the superior (short arrow) and inferior (long arrow) divisions of the third nerve before entering the superior orbital fissure.

nerve exits the orbit through the infraorbital foramen (see Fig. 6C).

VASCULAR ANATOMY

The ophthalmic artery typically arises from the supraclinoid internal carotid artery but occasionally originates from the clinoid segment or cavernous segment of the internal carotid artery in 2% to 8% of patients.[22,23] In these variant origins of the ophthalmic artery, the artery may pass through the superior orbital fissure or a foramen in the optic strut, the ophthalmic foramen.[22,24] Very rarely, the ophthalmic artery can originate from the middle meningeal artery.[22,25–27] Although rare, the presence of an aberrant origin of the ophthalmic artery, particularly one arising from the middle meningeal artery, can have important implications during embolization or pterional craniotomies when the middle meningeal artery may be affected. The ophthalmic artery most commonly passes through the optic canal inferolateral to the optic nerve before coursing superiorly around the lateral margin of the optic nerve and medially across the superior aspect of the optic nerve. The superior crossing of the optic nerve by the ophthalmic artery is considered a type 1 ophthalmic artery and is present in 82% to 90% of patients[2,28] (Fig. 15). A type 2 ophthalmic artery occurs in 10% to 17% of patients and crosses the optic nerve inferiorly before coursing superiorly through the medial intraconal space[28] (Fig. 16). The type 2 variant of the ophthalmic artery is important in the setting of endoscopic endonasal approaches to the medial orbit where the medial course of the ophthalmic artery through the medial intraconal space is directly in the path of the endoscopic surgeon.[29] The proximal course of the ophthalmic artery can be readily seen on a contrast-enhanced CT or dedicated CT angiogram. It can also be seen on MR on T1 nonfat suppressed spin echo images as a black flow void[30] (Fig. 9E).

The ophthalmic artery then has several branches within the orbit. These can be classified into 4 sections: ocular, orbital, extraorbital, and dural. Although many of these branches are just beyond the resolution of standard MR and CT, some of the main branches can be appreciated. The central retinal artery is one of the first branches of the ophthalmic artery and main portion of the ocular branch of the ophthalmic artery. The central retinal artery courses along the optic nerve inferiorly to supply the retina (see Fig. 15). Visualization of the central retinal artery is limited by noninvasive imaging techniques; however, it can be consistently visualized using cone beam CT angiography during diagnostic catheter angiograms.[31] Cadaveric studies have shown that the central retinal artery typically penetrates the optic nerve sheath along the inferior surface of the optic nerve sheath and approximately 5 to 18 mm posterior to the globe.[32] The orbital section of the ophthalmic artery consists of the lacrimal artery and muscular branches. The lacrimal artery extending far lateral within the orbit to supply the

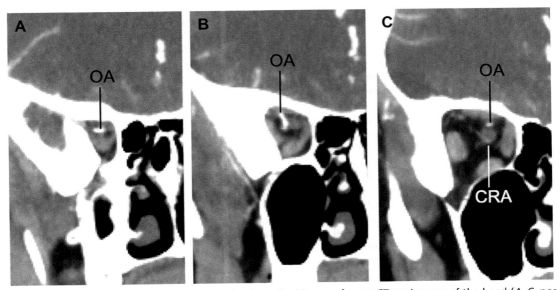

Fig. 15. Maximum intensity projection coronal reformatted images from a CT angiogram of the head (A–C, posterior to anterior). A type 1 course of the right ophthalmic artery (OA) in the right orbit is noted. There is visualization of the central retinal artery (CRA).

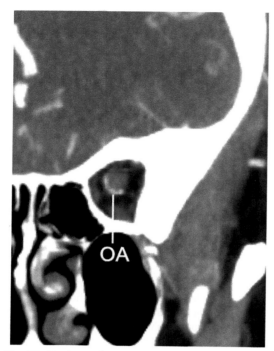

Fig. 16. Maximum intensity projection coronal reformat image from a CT angiogram of the head. A type 2 variant course of the left ophthalmic artery (OA) is noted within the left orbit.

lacrimal gland courses with the lacrimal nerve in the superomedial orbit. The muscular branches supply the extraocular muscles. The inferomedial muscular trunk of the orbital portion of the ophthalmic artery is an important anatomic landmark in endoscopic endonasal approaches of the medial orbit defining the boundaries of the anterior and posterior zones of the medial orbit.[29] Lesions posterior to the inferomedial muscular trunk of the ophthalmic artery are technically more challenging owing to the small space at the orbital apex. Although the inferomedial muscular trunk can be seen intraoperatively, this is not well seen on CT angiogram (CTA) or MR angiogram (MRA). As such, cadaveric studies have shown that a reasonable alternative to the inferomedial muscular trunk of the ophthalmic artery is the location of where the ophthalmic artery crosses the medial border of the optic nerve[30] (see Fig. 9E). The extraorbital branches of the ophthalmic artery comprise of the anterior and posterior ethmoidal arteries, supraorbital, palpebral, dorsal nasal, and supratrochlear arteries. The anterior and posterior ethmoidal arteries supply the ethmoid air cells, nasal cavity, and septum. The anterior ethmoidal artery is typically larger than the posterior ethmoidal artery and courses inferior to the superior oblique muscle and through the anterior

ethmoidal foramen, a groove which can be readily seen on CT and MR (see Figs. 2 and 6E). The posterior ethmoidal artery can be more variable and may not be readily seen on imaging. If present, the posterior ethmoidal artery can course inferior or superior to the superior oblique muscle before passing through the posterior ethmoidal foramen and may also contribute branches to the dura of the anterior cranial fossa. The supraorbital artery exits through the supraorbital foramen/notch in the superior orbital rim and can form an anastomosis with the superficial temporal artery. Terminal branches of the ophthalmic artery include the supratrochlear and dorsal nasal arteries. The supratrochlear artery courses medially and exits the orbit along the medial supraorbital ridge (Fig. 9A). The dorsal nasal artery extends through the orbital septum superior to the medial palpebral ligament and courses along the nose. Dural branches of the ophthalmic artery are beyond the scope of this article.

Venous drainage of the orbit occurs via the superior and inferior ophthalmic veins. The superior ophthalmic vein has contribution from the supraorbital and facial veins and continues to receive contributions, for example, from the central retinal vein and posterior ciliary veins, because it drains posteriorly. The superior ophthalmic vein may also have communication with the inferior ophthalmic vein at the orbital apex. The superior ophthalmic vein exits the orbit through the superior orbital fissure and drains into the cavernous sinus. The typical course of the superior ophthalmic vein is from anterior to posterior: posterolateral to the medial aspect of the superior rectus muscle, superolateral to the optic nerve and inferior to the superior rectus muscle, and posteromedial toward the superior orbital fissure (see Fig. 9D; Fig. 17).[2,28] The inferior ophthlamic vein is more variable and derives contributions from the facial vein. It passes intraconally along the inferior rectus muscle and commonly exits the orbit through the inferior orbital fissure before draining into the pterygoid venous plexus (Fig. 9; see Fig. 17).

LACRIMAL APPARATUS

The main function of lacrimal apparatus is to provide adequate moisturization of the cornea and conjunctiva—this requires a correct balance between inflow and outflow of tears to the lacrimal sac.[33] The lacrimal apparatus therefore consists of secretory and drainage components. The secretory part, consists of the lacrimal gland, small accessory lacrimal glands (up to 50 found in the superior fornix of the conjunctiva, and only 5 or 6 in the inferior fornix), sebaceous glands of Zeiss,

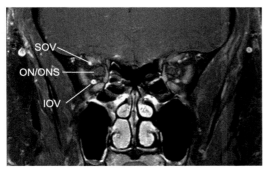

Fig. 17. 3T coronal T1-fat suppressed MR image of the orbits. IOV, inferior ophthalmic vein; ON/ONS, optic nerve and optic nerve sheath; SOV, superior ophthalmic vein.

and meibomian tarsal glands. The drainage part consists of lacrimal pathways that start near the medial angle of the palpebral fissure with 2 lacrimal puncta (upper and lower) located on the summits of the lacrimal papilla. Orbicularis oculi muscle fibers surround this papilla, directing its apex posteriorly and medially. Tears drain through bilateral lacrimal pathways to the inferior nasal meati and then to the nasopharynx.

The lacrimal gland is located in the superolateral part of the orbit, above the lateral angle of the eyelids. The tendon of the levator palpebrae superioris muscle divides the gland into a larger superior (orbital) part, about 20 × 12 mm in size, which lies in the fossa of the lacrimal gland. This is a small depression in the orbital surface of the frontal bone, just under the zygomatic process. The much smaller inferior (palpebral) part is near the superior fornix of the conjunctiva.

Tears secreted by the lacrimal gland spread over the corneal surface during blinking. Some tears evaporate and others drain down from the conjunctival sac to accumulate in the lacrimal lake that surrounds the lacrimal caruncle in the medial angle of the eye. The lacrimal fluid penetrates through lacrimal puncta into the lacrimal drainage system, each formed by upper and lower lacrimal canaliculi that converge into the common canaliculus, lacrimal sac, and nasolacrimal duct (NLD)[34] (Fig. 18). The lower canaliculus is the main route for tear drainage from the conjunctival sac, responsible for 80% to 90% of the total tear fluid drainage. The common canaliculus enters at a sharp angle through a small recess in the lateral wall of the lacrimal sac, known as the sinus of Maier. Lacrimal puncta and canaliculi form the upper lacrimal pathway, lined with stratified cuboidal epithelium. The lacrimal sac and NLD form the lower lacrimal pathway, lined with double-layered columnar epithelium.

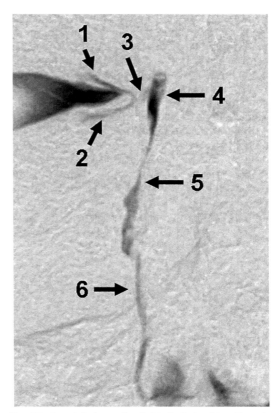

Fig. 18. Frontal view of a right digital subtraction dacrycystogram showing normal anatomic segments (arrows) of the lacrimal drainage pathway outlined by contrast medium. 1, superior canaliculus; 2, inferior canaliculus; 3, common canaliculus; 4, lacrimal sac; 5, nasolacrimal duct; and 6, free spill of contrast medium in the nasal cavity. (From Yedavalli V, Das D, Massoud TF. Eponymous "valves" of the nasolacrimal drainage apparatus. I. A historical review. Clin Anat. 2019 Jan;32(1):41-45.)

The lacrimal sac is located in its fossa within the medial orbital wall. It is separated from the orbit by the orbital septum. The sac is about 12.5 mm in length, 2.5 mm in transverse diameter, and 4 mm in anteroposterior diameter, with a volume of 0.1 mL. The wall of the lacrimal sac is formed by screw-shaped elastic connective tissue. The lower part of the lacrimal sac narrows and continues into the NLD. Here there is a mucous membrane fold, known as the valve of Krause, which separates the sac from the NLD.[35,36]

The NLD divides into 2 parts: an approximately 12 mm upper intraosseous part and an approximately 5 mm lower membranous part. The surrounding bony nasolacrimal canal is approximately 1 mm in diameter. The intraosseous NLD travels posterolaterally through the nasolacrimal canal within the maxillary bone, whereas the membranous part runs within the nasal mucosa, eventually opening into the inferior meatus of the nose under the inferior turbinate. Numerous vascular plexi in the NLD wall play an important role in the tear drainage regulation.

Multiple so-called valves have been named along the lacrimal drainage pathway (Fig. 19). Massoud and colleagues observed these most consistently in the distal NLD when using digital subtraction dacryocystography.[35,36] The distal valve of Hasner (plica lacrimalis) is present in 98.9% of cases. Two other more proximal mucosal folds, the valve of Taillefer (93.5%) and the valve of Krause (79.3%), are less frequent. Many of the other proximal so-called valves represent infrequently observed mounds of mucosa and are unlikely to possess any valvular action.

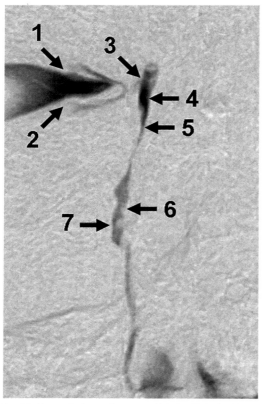

Fig. 19. Frontal view of a normal right digital subtraction dacrycystogram showing the lacrimal drainage pathway outlined by contrast medium and the expected locations (*arrows*) of the eponymous "valves" of the lacrimal drainage pathways: 1, Bochdalek; 2, Foltz; 3, Rosenmüller and Huschke together at the same location; 4, Aubaret; 5, Krause; 6, Taillefer; and 7, Hasner. (*From* Yedavalli V, Das D, Massoud TF. Eponymous "valves" of the nasolacrimal drainage apparatus. I. A historical review. Clin Anat. 2019 Jan;32(1):41-45.)

SUMMARY

Improvements in imaging techniques have allowed for better delineation of the complex internal anatomy of the orbit and cranial nerve pathways. Understanding of these structures and their relationship with each other allows for better preoperative and pretreatment planning.

CLINICS CARE POINTS

- Improvements in imaging, including higher resolution MR, surface coil usage, and thinner section computed tomography, allow visualization of detailed orbital anatomy, which supports preoperative and pretreatment planning.
- Understanding the relationship between the neurovascular structures is critical to providing optimal preoperative planning for novel surgical techniques.
- Direct coronal images through the orbit can be particularly helpful for assessing the extraocular muscles and the relationship of the optic nerve with pathologic condition.

DISCLOSURE

The authors have nothing to disclose.

REFERENCES

1. Martins C, Costa ESIE, Campero A, et al. Microsurgical anatomy of the orbit: the rule of seven. Anat Res Int 2011;2011:468727. https://doi.org/10.1155/2011/468727.
2. Mafee M, Som P. Embryology, Anatomy, and Imaging of the Eye and Orbit. In: Som PM, Curtin HD, editors. Head and Neck imaging. 5 edition. Elsevier; 2011. p. 527–89. chap 8.
3. Beard C. Muller's superior tarsal muscle: anatomy, physiology, and clinical significance. Ann Plast Surg 1985;14(4):324–33.
4. Fink WH. Ligament of Lockwood in relation to surgery of the inferior oblique and inferior rectus muscles. Arch Ophthal 1948;39(3):371–82.
5. Hawes MJ, Dortzbach RK. The microscopic anatomy of the lower eyelid retractors. *Arch Ophthalmol* Aug 1982;100(8):1313–8.
6. Gentry LR. Anatomy of the orbit. *Neuroimaging Clin N Am* Feb 1998;8(1):171–94.
7. Dobbs NW, Budak MJ, White RD, et al. MR-Eye: High-Resolution Microscopy Coil MRI for the Assessment of the Orbit and Periorbital Structures,

Part 1: Technique and Anatomy. AJNR Am J Neuroradiol 2020;41(6):947–50.

8. Bremond-Gignac D, Copin H, Cussenot O, et al. Anatomical histological and mesoscopic study of the adipose tissue of the orbit. Surg Radiol Anat 2004;26(4):297–302.

9. Malhotra A, Minja FJ, Crum A, et al. Ocular anatomy and cross-sectional imaging of the eye. Semin Ultrasound CT MR 2011;32(1):2–13.

10. Mafee MF, Peyman GA. Retinal and choroidal detachments: role of magnetic resonance imaging and computed tomography. Radiol Clin North Am 1987;25(3):487–507.

11. Mafee M, Putterman A, Valvassori G, et al. Orbital space-occupying lesions: role of computed tomography and magnetic resonance imaging. An analysis of 145 cases. Radiologic Clin North America 1987;25(3):529–59.

12. Bron A, Tripathi R, Tripathi B. Wolff's anatomy of the eye and orbit. 8th edition. Chapman & Hall Medical; 1997. p. 107–76. The extra ocular muscles and ocular movements.

13. Haładaj R. Normal anatomy and anomalies of the rectus extraocular muscles in human: a review of the recent data and findings. Biomed Research International 2019;2019.

14. Clark RA, Miller JM, Demer JL. Location and stability of rectus muscle pulleys. Muscle paths as a function of gaze. Invest Ophthalmol Vis Sci 1997;38(1):227–40.

15. Khitri MR, Demer JL. Magnetic resonance imaging of tissues compatible with supernumerary extraocular muscles. Am J Ophthalmol 2010;150(6):925–31.

16. Haladaj R, Tubbs RS, Brzezinski P, et al. Anatomical variations and innervation patterns of the superior oblique muscle. Ann Anat Jul 2020;230:151522. https://doi.org/10.1016/j.aanat.2020.151522.

17. Kightlinger B, Saraf-Lavi E, Sidani C. Anomalous extraocular muscles: a case series of orbital bands connecting the superior rectus to inferior rectus. Neurographics 2017;7(2):88–91.

18. Joo W, Rhoton AL Jr. Microsurgical anatomy of the trochlear nerve. Clin Anat Oct 2015;28(7):857–64.

19. Joo W, Yoshioka F, Funaki T, et al. Microsurgical anatomy of the abducens nerve. Clin Anat 2012; 25(8):1030–42.

20. Park HK, Rha HK, Lee KJ, et al. Microsurgical Anatomy of the Oculomotor Nerve. Clin Anat 2017;30(1): 21–31.

21. Joo W, Yoshioka F, Funaki T, et al. Microsurgical anatomy of the trigeminal nerve. Clin Anat 2014; 27(1):61–88.

22. Perrini P, Cardia A, Fraser K, et al. A microsurgical study of the anatomy and course of the ophthalmic artery and its possibly dangerous anastomoses. J Neurosurg 2007;106(1):142–50.

23. Gibo H, Lenkey C, Rhoton AL Jr. Microsurgical anatomy of the supraclinoid portion of the internal carotid artery. J Neurosurg 1981;55(4):560–74.

24. Rhoton AL, Natori Y. The orbit and sellar region: microsurgical anatomy and operative approaches 1996.

25. Hayreh SS, Dass R. The Ophthalmic Artery: I. Origin and Intra-Cranial and Intra-Canicular Course. Br J Ophthalmol 1962;46(2):65–98.

26. Liu Q, Rhoton AL Jr. Middle meningeal origin of the ophthalmic artery. Neurosurg 2001;49(2):401–6. ; discussion 406-7.

27. Watanabe A, Hirano K, Ishii R. Dural caroticocavernous fistula with both ophthalmic arteries arising from middle meningeal arteries. Neuroradiology 1996;38(8):806–8.

28. Rootman J. Diseases of the orbit : a multidisciplinary approach. Lippincott 1988;628, xxiv.

29. Yao WC, Bleier BS. Endoscopic management of orbital tumors. Curr Opin Otolaryngol Head Neck Surg Feb 2016;24(1):57–62.

30. Jafari A, Lehmann AE, Wolkow N, et al. Radioanatomic Characteristics of the Posteromedial Intraconal Space: Implications for Endoscopic Resection of Orbital Lesions. AJNR Am J Neuroradiol 2020; 41(12):2327–32.

31. Raz E, Shapiro M, Shepherd TM, et al. Central Retinal Artery Visualization with Cone-Beam CT Angiography. Radiol Feb 2022;302(2):419–24.

32. Merriam JC, Casper DS. The entry point of the central retinal artery into the outer meningeal sheath of the optic nerve. Clin Anat 2021;34(4):605–8.

33. Maliborski A, Różycki R. Diagnostic imaging of the nasolacrimal drainage system. Part I. Radiological anatomy of lacrimal pathways. Physiology of tear secretion and tear outflow. Med Sci Monit 2014;20: 628–38.

34. Horsburgh A, Massoud TF. Normative dimensions and symmetry of the lacrimal drainage system on dacryocystography: statistical analysis of morphometric characteristics. Folia Morphol (Warsz) 2013; 72(2):137–41.

35. Yedavalli V, Das D, Massoud TF. Eponymous "valves" of the nasolacrimal drainage apparatus. I. A historical review. Clin Anat 2019;32(1):41–5. PMID: 30260544.

36. Yedavalli V, Das D, Massoud TF. Eponymous "valves" of the nasolacrimal drainage apparatus. II. Frequency of visualization on dacryocystography. Clin Anat 2019;32(1):35–40.

Sinonasal Anatomy

Sanjay Vaid, MD (Radiology)[a],*, Neelam Vaid, MS, DNB (ENT)[b]

KEYWORDS

- Nasal cavity • Paranasal sinuses (PNSs) • Anatomy • Anatomic variants
- Computed tomography (CT)

KEY POINTS

- The radiologist needs to be familiar with the imaging anatomy as visualized by an endoscopic sinus surgeon.
- Multiplanar region-specific reporting and preoperative identification of anatomic variants provide the endoscopic surgeon with a useful intraoperative roadmap and avoid intraoperative complications.
- This article reviews the imaging anatomy of the nasal cavity and paranasal sinuses and discusses the clinical relevance of the anatomic variants in the sinonasal region.

 Video content accompanies this article at http://www.neuroimaging.theclinics.com.

INTRODUCTION

Anatomic concepts of the paranasal sinuses (PNSs) have been known since the late nineteenth and early twentieth centuries.[1] This article reviews the embryology of the PNSs and mentions, in brief, the computed tomography (CT) and MR imaging techniques for imaging this region. CT is the imaging modality of choice for identifying key anatomic features and anatomic variants of the nasal cavity and PNSs.

Imaging Techniques and Protocol

All CT examinations are performed on a multichannel CT scanner and viewed on a workstation to facilitate multiplanar reconstructions in standard orthogonal and nonorthogonal planes. This enables image reconstruction at a submillimeter level (up to 0.34 mms). CT studies should be viewed in all 3 orthogonal planes for optimal visualization of anatomic structures. Three different window level and window width settings should be used for viewing the CT images (PNS, bone, and brain settings) to avoid missing or misinterpreting important findings (Fig. 1). Customized low-dose CT protocols are used while scanning the pediatric population.[2] Use of cone-beam CT is advised, if available, to minimize radiation dose in children and young adults.[3,4] Contrast-enhanced CT or MR imaging examinations are indicated for evaluating intracranial, intraorbital, and nasopharyngeal complications.[5]

Embryology

The embryo develops its first identifiable head and face between the fourth and fifth weeks of gestational age with a central orifice called the stomodeum, which is surrounded by the mandibular, maxillary, and frontonasal prominences. The ethmoid sinuses are present at birth, whereas the other sinuses (frontal, maxillary, and sphenoid) develop owing to pneumatization beyond the confines of the olfactory capsule. Hence the ethmoid sinus is phylogenetically, anatomically, embryologically, and functionally different from the other air-containing PNSs.[6] The further ossification pattern is complex and the reader is referred to numerous excellent texts in the literature for a

[a] Head Neck Imaging Division, Star Imaging and Research Center, Connaught Place (ground floor), Bund Garden Road, Pune 411001, Maharashtra, India; [b] Department of Otorhinolaryngology, K.E.M. Hospital, 489 Rasta Peth, Pune 411001, Maharashtra, India
* Corresponding author.
E-mail address: svaidhn@gmail.com

Neuroimag Clin N Am 32 (2022) 713–734
https://doi.org/10.1016/j.nic.2022.07.007

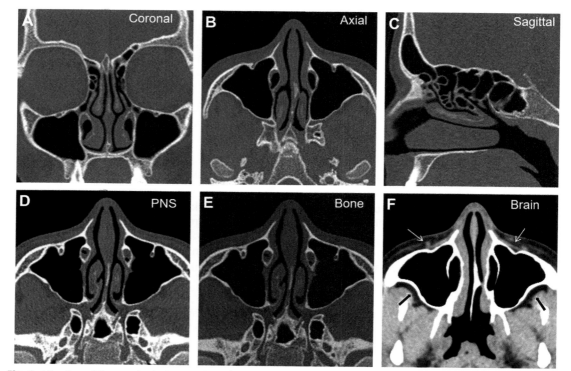

Fig. 1. Viewing planes and window settings for paranasal CT scans. Axial (*A*), Coronal (*B*), and sagittal (*C*) planes for optimal viewing anatomy of the PNSs. Axial CT images in paranasal sinus (*D*), bone (*E*), and brain (*F*) windows showing premaxillary (*white arrows*) and retro-antral (*black arrows*) regions.

more detailed discussion. The pneumatization pattern is unique to each group of sinuses and the continuous change in the size and aeration of the sinus as the child grows has a significant impact on the treatment/surgery of sinus pathologic condition in the pediatric age group.[7] Table 1 outlines the growth pattern of each sinus group and the ostiomeatal complex with the resultant clinical implications. Fig. 2 depicts the childhood development of the PNSs and related structures.

Anatomy Overview of the Sinonasal Region

1. Anterior sinonasal region
   - Nasal cavity: nasal valves, nasal septum, nasal turbinates, and meatuses.
   - Uncinate process.
   - Frontal sinus and the frontal sinus drainage pathway (FSDP) anatomy.
   - Anterior ethmoid sinuses and lamellar anatomy.
   - Maxillary sinus and the ostiomeatal complex.
2. Posterior sinonasal region
   - Posterior sinus group: posterior ethmoid sinus and the sphenoid sinus.
3. Shared anatomic interfaces with adjacent structures

- Anterior skull base: the olfactory fossa and the ethmoidal skull base.
- Lamina papyracea and the anterior ethmoidal artery (AEA).

The Nasal Cavity

The nasal cavities are triangular structures separated by the nasal septum in the midline, limited superiorly by the cribriform plate and inferiorly by the hard palate.

The nasal cycle

The mucosal lining over the nasal septum and the nasal turbinates is influenced by the nasal cycle, which is responsible for alternating changes in the turbinate sizes owing to mucosal engorgement.[8] This cyclical and physiologic enlargement of the turbinates alternates between both nasal cavities every 45 minutes to an hour and should not be mistaken for pathologic condition.

The nasal valves

Most texts discussing nasal cavity imaging anatomy tend to concentrate on the bony posterior three-fourth portion, that is, the nasal septum, septal spurs, and nasal turbinates. The anterior one-fourth is an important but frequently

Table 1
Pneumatization/ossification pattern of paranasal sinuses and related structures

Sr.no	Sinus/Structure	Childhood Development	Clinical Implications
1.	Frontal sinus	Not seen on imaging at birth. Present as a small pit or furrow at birth Slow pneumatization between 1 and 4 y, rapid growth between 4 and 8 y, reaching the orbital roof by 5–7 y of age and attaining adult appearance by 12 y of age Narrower antero-posterior diameter as compared with the adult	Children cannot develop frontal sinusitis before 4 y of age Frontal trephination procedures are contraindicated in an immature frontal sinus (till it reaches the orbital plate) due to the risk of inadvertent intracranial penetration, meningeal trauma, and likely iatrogenic infection
2.	Ethmoid sinus	Present and seen on imaging at birth Rapid pneumatization between 1 and 4 y Slow growth between 4 and 8 y Adult appearance by 12 y of age	Source of sinus/contiguous orbital infection in young children Accessible to both internal and external drainage procedures if required
3.	Maxillary sinus	Not seen on imaging at birth. Present as a shallow rounded sac at birth Rapid pneumatization between 1 and 4 y: floor of the sinus reaches level of the inferior meatus by 7 y of age Adult appearance is attained by 12–14 y when the floor of the sinus reaches level of the nasal cavity floor Slow pneumatization continues till 20 y of age	Height discrepancy between the inferior margins of the sinus and the nasal cavity precludes the use of certain surgical techniques in children. These procedures may damage developing teeth, cause inadvertent injury to lateral sinus wall, or may be ineffective in treating the pathologic condition completely
4.	Sphenoid sinus	Not seen on imaging at birth. Tiny mucosal sac posterior to the nasal capsule at birth Pneumatizes between 1 and 3 y of age. Grows progressively between 7 and 14 y and may continue to pneumatize further into adulthood	Limited clinical significance before the age of 10 y As the posterior ethmoid sinus pneumatizes earlier, it can grow above the developing sphenoid sinus to form the Onodi cell. Location of critical neurovascular structures around the sphenoid sinus depends on the degree of pneumatization of the sinus
5.	The ostiomeatal complex	All components are developed and present in the newborn	All the components of the ostiomeatal complex are packed tightly together leading to a narrow caliber of the infundibulum, which must be appreciated preoperatively. Proximity of the uncinate osseous to the lamina papyracea predisposes to inadvertent intraorbital penetration
6.	Anterior cranial fossa	The midline structures (crista galli, cribriform plates, and perpendicular ethmoid plate) are cartilaginous at birth and ossify by 2 y of age. They represent the "lucent stripe" on CT scans of infants because the surrounding ethmoid bone, vomer, and palate are ossified	The "lucent stripe" should not be misinterpreted as a bony defect, sinus tract, cephalocele, or bony destruction

From Vaid S, Vaid N. Normal Anatomy and Anatomic Variants of the Paranasal Sinuses on Computed Tomography. Neuro-imaging Clin N Am. 2015 Nov;25(4):527 to 48.

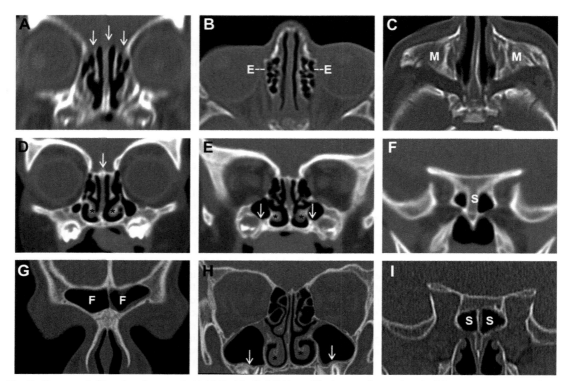

Fig. 2. Paranasal sinus development. At birth (*A–C*): (*A*) Unossified central anterior skull base structures resulting in "lucent stripes" (*arrows*), (*B*) pneumatized ethmoidal labyrinth (E), (*C*) M: nonpneumatized maxillary sinuses. At 1 year (*D–F*): (*D*) Anterior skull base ossification (*arrow*) is complete. (*E*) Partially pneumatized maxillary sinus floor (*arrows*) to level of inferior turbinates (*). (*F*) Early sphenoid sinus (S) pneumatization. At 5 years (*G–I*): (*G*) Frontal sinus (*F*) pneumatized to the orbital roof. (*H*) Maxillary sinus floor (*arrows*) to level of the inferior meatus. (*I*) Progressive sphenoid sinus pneumatization. (*From* Vaid S, Vaid N. Normal Anatomy and Anatomic Variants of the Paranasal Sinuses on Computed Tomography. Neuroimaging Clin N Am. 2015 Nov;25(4):527 to 48.)

neglected anatomic area comprising the external nasal valves (ENVs) and internal nasal valves (INVs) with intervening nasal vestibule (Fig. 3). The ENV is formed by the columella, the nasal floor, and the nasal rim. The INV is the narrowest region in the anterior nose formed by the nasal septum, the upper lateral nasal cartilage, head of the inferior turbinate, and the pyriform aperture soft tissues[9] (see Fig. 3). The cross-sectional area and angle of the INV are measured in a standardized coronal image, anterior to the head of the inferior turbinate (see Fig. 3). The normal range for the INV angle ranges from 10° to 15°,[9] and INV areas range from 0.47 to 0.51 cm². An INV having an area of less than 0.30 cm² on CT suggests the presence of clinically significant nasal airway obstruction.[10]

The nasal septum

The nasal septum consists of an anterior cartilaginous component (the septal cartilage) and a posterior bony component (the bony septum)

comprising of the vomer and the perpendicular plate of the ethmoid.[11]

Anatomic Variations

(Fig. 4) 1. Septal deviation: Seen in 20% to 79% of the population.[12] The septum is commonly deviated in its inferior portion near the chondro-vomeral junction and can also assume an "S"-shaped configuration with deviation to both sides of the midline. Bony septal spurs may be associated with septal deviations and may form adhesions with the adjacent turbinates.

2. Septal pneumatization: Pneumatization can occur anteriorly from the crista galli or posteriorly from the sphenoid sinus.

The Nasal Turbinates and Meatuses (or Meati)

The lateral walls of the nasal cavities are complex structures that support the inferior, middle, and superior nasal turbinates, and occasionally, a fourth turbinate known as the supreme turbinate.

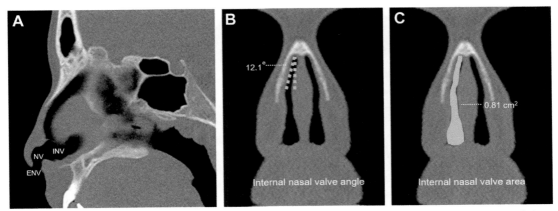

Fig. 3. Anatomy of the nasal valves. Parasagittal image (*A*) showing locations of the ENV and INV with intervening nasal vestibule (NV). Coronal CT images show measured angle (*B*) and measured area (*C*) for the INV.

These turbinates divide the nasal cavity into the superior, middle, and inferior meatuses (or meati) (Fig. 5). The superior meatus drains the posterior ethmoidal air cells and the sphenoid sinus through the spheno-ethmoidal recess. The middle meatus drains the frontal sinus via the FSDP, the maxillary sinus via the maxillary ostium, and the anterior ethmoidal air cells. The inferior meatus drains the

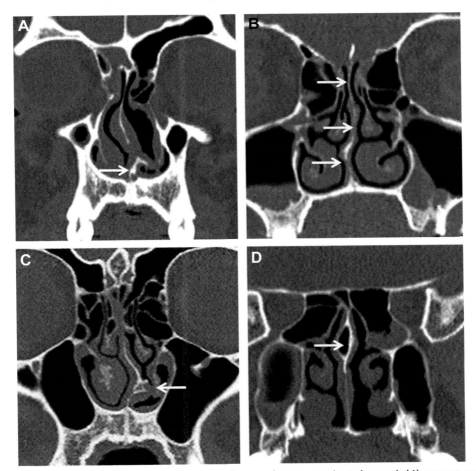

Fig. 4. Nasal septum variants. Coronal CT images showing nasal septum variants (*arrows*): (*A*) vomero-septal junction deviation, (*B*) S-shaped deviation, (*C*) bony septal spur with adhesion to inferior turbinate, and (*D*) posterior septal pneumatization.

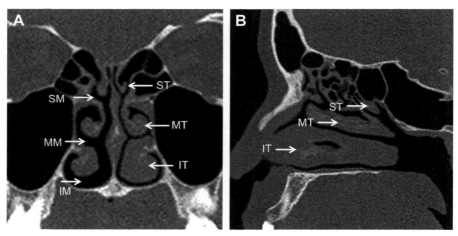

Fig. 5. Nasal turbinates and meatuses. Coronal (*A*) and parasagittal (*B*) images show inferior, middle, and superior nasal turbinates (IT, MT, ST) with corresponding inferior, middle, and superior nasal meatuses (IM, MM, SM).

nasolacrimal apparatus via the nasolacrimal duct.[8] The middle and inferior nasal turbinates usually have a similar shape exhibiting a convex margin medially and a concave margin laterally.

The middle turbinate is a part of the ethmoid bone with attachments in all 3 orthogonal planes.[8] The anterior part of the middle turbinate is oriented vertically, attaching superiorly to the anterior skull base at the lateral border of the cribriform plate. The posterior part attaches to the lamina papyracea and to the medial wall of the maxillary sinus (Video 1: Coronal CT depicting multiplanar attachments of the middle turbinate). The obliquely directed midportion of the middle turbinate is known as the basal lamella marking the division between the anterior and posterior ethmoidal sinuses.[12]

Anatomic Variants

1. Concha bullosa: Pneumatization of the inferior bulbous portion of the middle turbinate occurs in approximately 24% to 55% of the population and is usually bilateral (Fig. 6).[8] If the pneumatization is restricted to the vertical lamella of the turbinate, above the level of the ostiomeatal unit, it is termed as an interlamellar cell of Grunwald, lamellar bulla, or a conchal neck air cell. Pneumatization of the middle turbinate has also been classified in the past as bulbous, lamellar, and extensive by Bolger and colleagues.[13] A new classification has been proposed by Calvo-Henríquez and colleagues[14] according to the degree of pneumatization of the vertical lamella of the middle turbinate.
2. Paradoxic middle turbinate: In 26% of the population, the middle turbinate exhibits a paradoxic lateral convexity (12).

3. Rare anatomic variants: Occasionally, the inferior portion of the middle turbinate curves acutely on itself producing a deep invagination called a turbinate sinus.[8] A bifid turbinate is formed when 2 bony lamellae share the same root.[15]
4. Pneumatized basal lamella may be mistaken for an anterior ethmoidal air cell leading to incomplete exploration of the posterior ethmoid sinuses.

The Uncinate Process

The uncinate process is a thin crescent-shaped bone oriented in a sagittal oblique anterosuperior to a posteroinferior direction. Posteriorly the uncinate has a free concave margin. The superior attachment of the uncinate process may be variable. The ethmoidal infundibulum is located between the uncinate process and the inferomedial wall of the orbit.[16]

Anatomic Variants

1. Variable superior attachments: The uncinate process may attach either to the lamina papyracea, the anterior skull base, or the middle turbinate and may also have multiple attachments to these structures. The pattern of attachment determines the position of the FSDP (Table 2, Fig. 7).
2. The uncinate process may be pneumatized (Fig. 8A) in 4% of the population or everted.[8]
3. An atelectatic uncinate process (Fig. 8B), commonly seen in maxillary sinus hypoplasia and silent sinus syndrome, is closely related to the inferior and medial wall of the ipsilateral orbit.[11] This increases the risk of inadvertent

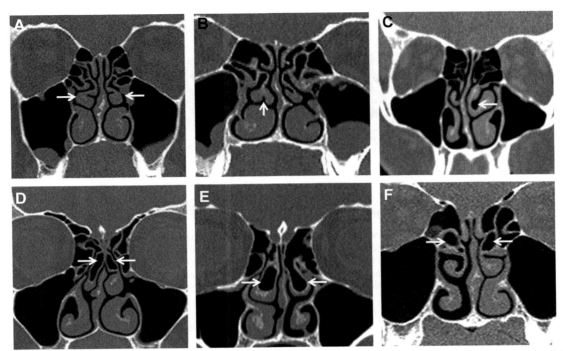

Fig. 6. Coronal CT images showing middle turbinate variants (*arrows*): (*A*) bilateral paradoxic turbinates, (*B*) bifid right middle turbinate, (*C*) left turbinate sinus, (*D*) bilateral interlamellar cells of Grunwald, (*E*) bilateral concha bullosa, and (*F*) bilateral pneumatized basal lamella.

Table 2
Pattern of superior attachment of the uncinate process

Lamina Papyracea	Seen in more than 50% of individuals,[12] resulting in a medial FSDP draining into the middle meatus, creating a blind pouch laterally termed as the recessus terminalis
Anterior skull base	Results in a lateral FSDP opening into the ethmoidal infundibulum increasing chances of retrograde spread of infection into the frontal sinus from the ethmoidal sinus
Middle turbinate	FSDP is displaced posterior to the agger nasi cell, which needs to be fractured to access the FSDP[11]

From Vaid S, Vaid N. Normal Anatomy and Anatomic Variants of the Paranasal Sinuses on Computed Tomography. Neuroimaging Clin N Am. 2015 Nov;25(4):527 to 48.

orbital penetration during functional endoscopic sinus surgery (FESS).

4. Rarely, the uncinate process may be absent[17] as seen in maxillary sinus hypoplasia.

The Frontal Sinus and Frontal Sinus Drainage Pathway

The frontal sinuses develop as extensions from the anterior ethmoidal air cells. They may be absent in 5% and hypoplastic in 4% of the population.[8] Well-pneumatized frontal sinuses show typical scalloped margins with intact internal septa. The frontal beak (frontonasal process of the maxilla) forms an important surgical and imaging landmark in the anatomy of the FSDP.[18] It is identified on both coronal and parasagittal images (Fig. 9) with the frontal sinus superiorly and the FSDP inferiorly. The frontal beak corresponds to the level of the frontal ostium and hence its thickness determines the size of the frontal ostium. The agger nasi cell is the anterior-most extramural ethmoidal air cell, seen in 93% of the population,[8] and lies within the anterior portion of the FSDP. It is best viewed on parasagittal images and serves as an important surgical landmark.[12]

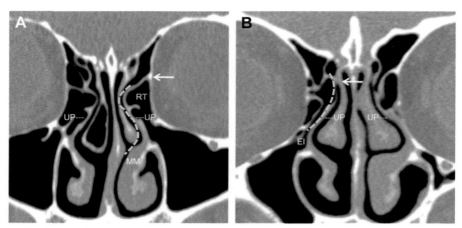

Fig. 7. Coronal CT images showing uncinate process attachments. (A). Left uncinate process (UP) attached to lamina papyracea (*arrow*) with the FSDP (dashed *lines*) draining into the medial meatus (MM), RT: recessus terminalis. (B). Right uncinate process attaching to the middle turbinate (*arrow*) with the FSDP (dashed *lines*) draining into the ethmoidal infundibulum (EI). (*From* Vaid S, Vaid N. Normal Anatomy and Anatomic Variants of the Paranasal Sinuses on Computed Tomography. Neuroimaging Clin N Am. 2015 Nov;25(4):527 to 48.)

Anatomic Variants

1. Fronto-ethmoidal cells: The classification of frontal cells was first described by Kuhn in 1995[8] and modified by Wormald[18] (Table 3, Fig. 10). The authors also refer the readers to the latest classification of fronto-ethmoidal air cells (The International Frontal Sinus Anatomic Classification [2016] by Wormald[19]) used primarily by endoscopic sinus surgeons.
2. The frontal bullar cell arises superior to the bulla ethmoidalis and extends below the floor of the anterior cranial fossa, which forms the posterior border of this anatomic variant (Fig. 11).

ANTERIOR ETHMOID SINUSES AND LAMELLAR ANATOMY

The anterior ethmoid sinuses are located anterior to the basal lamella. The largest cell in this group is the bulla ethmoidalis, which is a key surgical landmark during endoscopic sinus surgery. The cleft between the anterior margin of the bulla and the uncinate process is called the hiatus semilunaris.

Ethmoidal Lamellar Anatomy

Lamellae are organizational plates that develop within the cartilaginous olfactory capsule. They are important surgical landmarks and partition

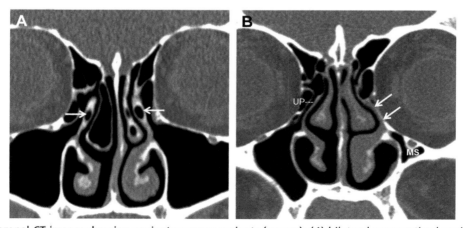

Fig. 8. Coronal CT images showing uncinate process variants (*arrows*): (A) bilateral pneumatized uncinate processes and (B) left atelectatic uncinate process owing to left maxillary sinus hypoplasia (MS). (*From* Vaid S, Vaid N. Normal Anatomy and Anatomic Variants of the Paranasal Sinuses on Computed Tomography. Neuroimaging Clin N Am. 2015 Nov;25(4):527 to 48.)

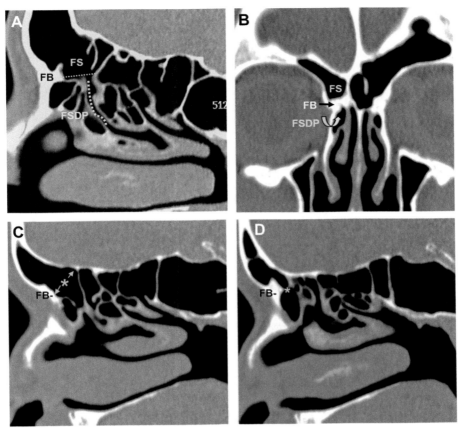

Fig. 9. Parasagittal (*A*) and coronal CT (*B*) showing frontal beak (FB) separating the frontal sinus (FS) above the dotted orange line in (*A*) from the FSDP (dotted yellow *line* in a, curved yellow *arrow* in b) below. Parasagittal CT sections (*C–D*) depict the impact of the frontal beak thickness (*arrow*) on the size of the frontal sinus ostium (green *arrows/asterisk*).

Table 3	
Classification of frontoethmoidal cells	
Type 1 frontal cell	Single cell above the agger nasi and below the frontal beak (below the frontal ostium)
Type 2 frontal cells	Two or more cells above the agger nasi and below the frontal beak (below the frontal ostium)
Type 3 frontal cell	Single cell above the agger nasi with extension through the frontal ostium into the frontal sinus not exceeding 50% of the vertical height of the ipsilateral frontal sinus
Type 4 frontal cell	Single cell above the agger nasi with extension through the frontal ostium into the frontal sinus exceeding 50% of the vertical height of the ipsilateral frontal sinus, or an isolated cell within the frontal sinus
Frontal bullar cell	Single cell extending from the suprabullar region along the undersurface of the anterior skull base into the frontal sinus (anterior margin lies within the frontal sinus)
Interfrontal sinus septal cell	A cell associated with the frontal intersinus septum and may compromise the frontal ostium

From Vaid S, Vaid N. Normal Anatomy and Anatomic Variants of the Paranasal Sinuses on Computed Tomography. Neuroimaging Clin N Am. 2015 Nov;25(4):527 to 48.

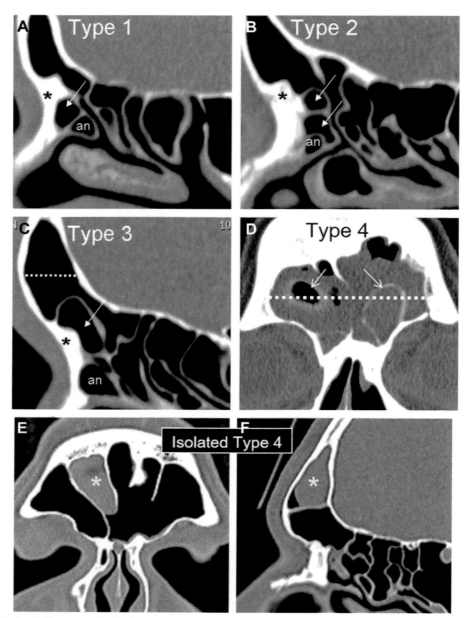

Fig. 10. Sagittal CT images (*A–C*) showing Types 1 to 3 fronto-ethmoidal cells (*arrows*). (*D*) Coronal CT image shows bilateral Type 4 fronto-ethmoidal cells (*arrows*). Frontal beak (*asterisk*); agger nasi (*an*). The dotted white line depicts the midpoint of the height of the ipsilateral frontal sinus. Coronal (*D & E*) and sagittal (*F*) images depict opacified and superiorly located Type 4 fronto-ethmoidal cell.

the sinonasal cavity into well-defined compartments.[12] The lamellae course through the ethmoidal air cells and extend superiorly up to the skull base from the lateral nasal wall. These structures are best seen in the parasagittal planes (Fig. 12) and from anterior to posterior include the uncinate process, anterior margin of the bulla ethmoidalis, lamella of the middle turbinate (basal lamella), lamella of the superior turbinate, and, if present, the lamella of the supreme turbinate. If the supreme turbinate is absent, the anterior face of the sphenoid sinus is considered the fifth lamella.

Anatomic Variants

1. The suprabullar recess lies between the superior wall of the bulla ethmoidalis and the roof

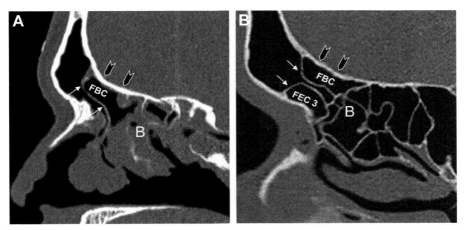

Fig. 11. Parasagittal image (*A*) shows a large frontal bullar cell (FBC), above the bulla ethmoidalis (B) with anterior margin related to the frontal sinus (*arrows*) and posterior margin formed by the anterior skull base (*arrowheads*). Arrows in parasagittal image (*B*) show the difference between the superiorly located FBC and the inferiorly located Type 3 fronto-ethmoidal cell (FEC 3).

of the ethmoid sinus and is best appreciated on a parasagittal image (Fig. 13A). This recess can extend laterally as supraorbital cells (Fig. 13B).

2. Anterior ethmoidal air cells extending along the floor of the orbits, lateral to the sagittal plane of the lamina papyracea are called Haller cells (Fig. 14A), reported in 10% to 45% of the patients.[8] The inferomedial strut line of the orbit is a useful anatomic structure to differentiate between bulla ethmoidalis cell (above the line) and Haller cells (below the line; Fig. 14B, C).[20] Haller cells narrow the maxillary sinus ostium.

The Maxillary Sinus and Ostiomeatal Complex

The maxillary sinus or antrum occupies the body of the maxillary bone. The roof is formed by the orbital floor, and the floor is formed by the alveolar process of the maxilla. The infraorbital nerve (a branch of the maxillary division of the trigeminal nerve) runs in a bony canal along the roof of the maxillary sinus. The maxillary ostium is located along the superior aspect of the medial wall of the sinus and drains into the base of the ethmoidal infundibulum.[12] The components of the ostiomeatal complex or unit as identified on coronal CT (Fig. 15) comprise the maxillary ostium, the middle

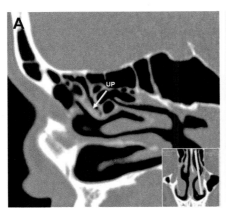
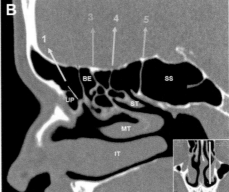

Fig. 12. Sagittal oblique (*A*) and sagittal (*B*) CT images showing lamellar anatomy: 1: uncinate process (UP: *white arrow* in a). 2: anterior margin of bulla ethmoidalis (BE). 3: basal lamella MT: middle turbinate. 4: lamella of the superior turbinate (ST). 5: anterior margin of the sphenoid sinus (SS). IT: inferior turbinate. (*From* Vaid S, Vaid N. Normal Anatomy and Anatomic Variants of the Paranasal Sinuses on Computed Tomography. Neuroimaging Clin N Am. 2015 Nov;25(4):527 to 48.)

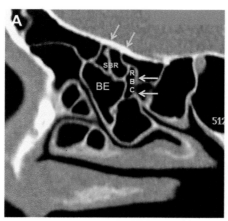
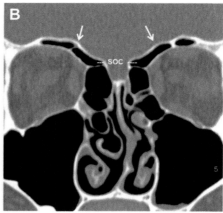

Fig. 13. Sagittal CT image (*A*) shows the suprabullar recess (SBR) and the retro-bullar cleft (RBC). Coronal CT image (*B*) shows bilateral supraorbital cells (*arrows*).

meatus, the ethmoidal infundibulum, the bulla ethmoidalis, the uncinate process, and the hiatus semilunaris.[12]

Anatomic Variants

1. Reduced size of the maxillary sinus is seen in hypoplasia (in up to 10% of the population), silent sinus syndrome and following trauma/surgery (Fig. 16). The congenitally small maxillary sinus is associated with posterior and inferior displacement of the globe. The lamina papyracea in such cases is also lateralized with an increase in the retro-antral fat and thickening of the bony walls (increase in the height of the alveolar process).[21]
2. In hyperpneumatized maxillary sinuses, there is a thin mucosal lining between the maxillary antrum and the dental roots, which can protrude into the sinus. This can predispose to recurrent sinusitis from dental infections and to oroantral fistulas following dental extraction.[22]

3. Septa within the maxillary sinuses are common and may be fibrous or bony. They usually extend from the infraorbital nerve canal to the lateral wall and can affect the drainage of the maxillary sinuses.[12] Bony margins of the infraorbital nerve canal may be dehiscent in up to 14% of cases.[8]
4. Accessory ostia are seen in 10% to 25% of the population, located within the region of the posterior fontanelle, behind the natural ostia.[8] The posterior fontanelle is a bony defect in the lateral nasal wall (medial wall of the maxillary sinus) located superior to the insertion of the inferior turbinate.

The Lamina Papyracea and Anterior Ethmoidal Artery

The lamina papyracea form the lateral walls of the ethmoid sinuses separating them from the adjacent orbits. Focal corticated defects in the lamina papyracea are seen in up to 0.5% to 10% of the population and are not clinically significant.[12]

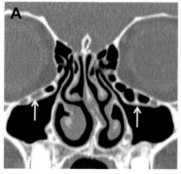
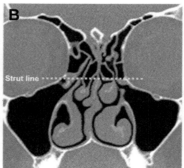
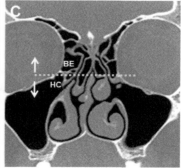

Fig. 14. Haller cells (*arrows* in *A*). The inferomedial strut line of the orbit (dotted orange *line* in *B* and *C*) is a useful anatomic structure to differentiate between the bulla ethmoidalis (BE) and Haller cells (HC).

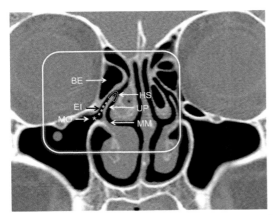

Fig. 15. Coronal CT image showing components of the OMC. MO: maxillary ostium (*asterisk*); EI: ethmoidal infundibulum (*dotted line*); BE: bulla ethmoidalis; MM: middle meatus; UP: uncinate process; HS: hiatus semilunaris (curved block).

Larger defects (congenital, posttraumatic, or postoperative) in the lamina (Fig. 17) need preoperative documentation to avoid inadvertent orbital injury. Defects in the posterior lamina papyracea are more significant because there is a relatively thinner fat pad between the medial rectus muscle and the lamina papyracea with increased chances of orbital injury.[23]

The ethmoidal segment of the AEA (branch of the ophthalmic artery) enters the ethmoid sinus through the olfactory floor and passes superiorly into the anterior skull base. Cadaveric and live dissection studies have shown that the AEA is most often located between the second (anterior margin of the bulla ethmoidalis) and the third lamella (lamella of the middle turbinate; basal lamella).[24] It courses in a bony canal (anterior ethmoidal canal [AEC]) through the upper one-third of the lamina papyracea. This canal can be best identified on coronal CT by a beak-like projection of the medial orbital wall behind the bulla ethmoidalis. Two parallel hyperdense lines extending into the adjacent ethmoid sinus mark the precise location of the AEA (Fig. 18A).[8] The AEC together with the AEA is also well visualized on parasagittal images (Fig. 18C–E) and can be graded based on the location with respect to the skull base.[25]

a. Grade I AEC: located within the ethmoidal roof.
b. Grade II AEC: located under the roof.
c. Grade III AEC: located distant from the ethmoidal roof.

Anatomic Variant

Normal bony covering of the anterior ethmoidal artery may be absent and the canal may be dehiscent inferiorly into the anterior ethmoidal air cells in up to 66% of cases.[24,25] In these cases, the artery is suspended on a mucous membrane mesentery below the skull base, and is prone to injury during surgery, especially if the bony canal is deficient (Fig. 18B, F).

The Anterior Skull Base: Olfactory Fossa and Height of the Ethmoid Skull Base

The olfactory fossa

The olfactory fossa, containing the olfactory bulbs, is formed by the crista galli medially, medial lamella of the cribriform plate inferiorly, and lateral lamella of the cribriform plate laterally. Three types of olfactory fossae were described by Keros[26] based on the length of the lateral lamella of the cribriform plate (Table 4, Fig. 19A–C). The lateral lamella of the cribriform plate is structurally the thinnest bone in the anterior skull base and dehiscent in up to 14% of patients.[8]

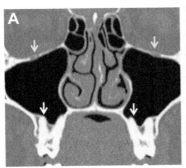
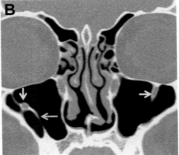
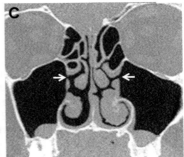

Fig. 16. Coronal CT images showing maxillary sinus variants (*arrows*): (*A*) maxillary dental roots protruding into the sinus floor, normal infraorbital nerve canals (yellow *arrows*). (*B*) bilateral dehiscent infraorbital nerve canals (yellow *arrows*) with an intrasinus septum (orange *arrow*) attaching to the dehiscent canal on the right side. (*C*) bilateral accessory ostia.

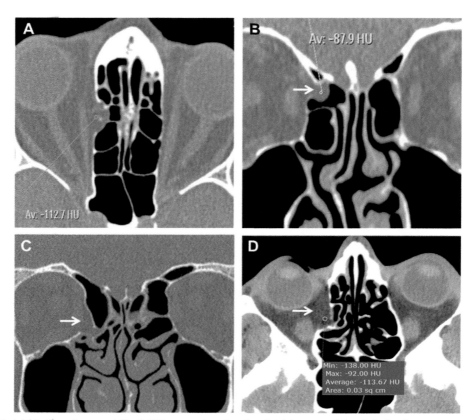

Fig. 17. Axial (*A, D*) and coronal (*B, C*) CT images showing focal dehiscence of the right lamina papyracea (*arrow*). Intraorbital fat herniates through the defect into the ethmoid sinuses.

Anatomic Variant

Asymmetry in the level of the olfactory fossa occurs in up to 10% to 30% of the population (Fig. 19D). The angle between the medial and lateral lamella of the cribriform plate is also variable.[12] Bates and Massoud[27] propose changes in the nomenclature surrounding the term "olfactory" for improved uniformity and accuracy. Fig. 20 depicts the olfactory groove, olfactory recess, olfactory vestibule, and the olfactory cleft as proposed by these authors.

Height of the Ethmoid Skull Base

The roof of the anterior ethmoid sinus is formed by the fovea ethmoidalis laterally and the cribriform plate medially. The height of the ethmoid skull base (ESB) can be assessed by 2 methods proposed by Myers and Valvasorri[28] and more recently by Rudmik and Smith[29] (Table 5, Fig. 21).

Anatomic Variant

A low ESB indicates a dangerously low lying and medially sloping anterior skull base with higher chances of intraoperative intracranial penetration.[29]

The Posterior Sinus Group: Posterior Ethmoid Sinus and Sphenoid Sinus

The posterior ethmoid sinus

The posterior ethmoidal air cells are located between the basal lamella and the sphenoid sinus and are fewer in number than the anterior ethmoidal cells. The lamina papyracea lies laterally and the superior turbinate forms the medial boundary of this sinus group that drains into the superior meatus.

Anatomic Variant

Spheno-ethmoidal cell (Onodi cell): As the posterior ethmoidal cells pneumatize before the sphenoid sinus, they have a high propensity to grow above and lateral to the developing sphenoid sinus forming the Onodi cell. This is seen in 3.4% to 14% of the general population.[8] An Onodi cell should be suspected on coronal CT images that show an obliquely oriented or horizontal septum within the sphenoid sinus (Fig. 22A & B). Some

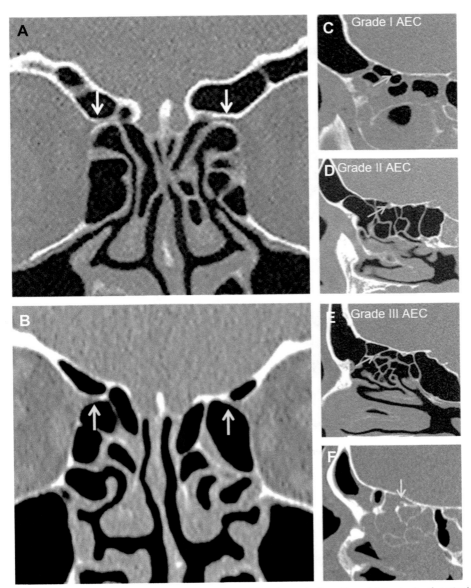

Fig. 18. Coronal CT images showing (*A*) normal bony canal for the anterior ethmoidal arteries (vertical *white arrows*) and (*B*) both arteries suspended in a mesentery without bone cover (vertical yellow *arrows*). Parasagittal images (*C–E*) depict grades of the AEC with respect to the skull base (oblique orange *arrows*). Short vertical yellow arrow in (*F*) depicts a focal defect in the bony canal for the AEA.

Table 4 Keros classification of the olfactory fossa	
Type 1	Length of the lateral lamella is 1–3 mm indicating a shallow or flat olfactory fossa seen in 30% of cases
Type 2	Length of the lateral lamella is 4–7 mm indicating a moderately deep olfactory fossa seen in 49% of cases
Type 3	The lateral lamella is longer measuring 8–16 mm with a resultant deep olfactory fossa seen in 21% of cases[16]

From Vaid S, Vaid N. Normal Anatomy and Anatomic Variants of the Paranasal Sinuses on Computed Tomography. Neuroimaging Clin N Am. 2015 Nov;25(4):527 to 48.

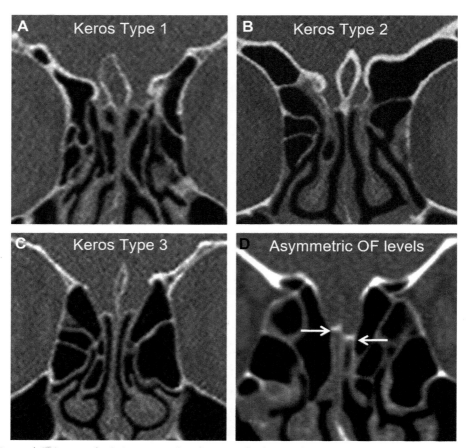

Fig. 19. Coronal CT images depicting Keros classification of olfactory fossae (*A–C*). Asymmetrical levels of the olfactory fossae (*arrows* in *D*).

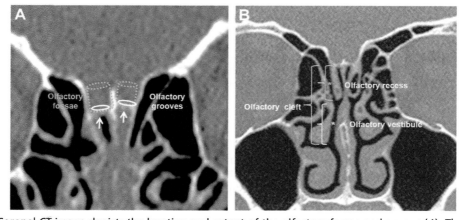

Fig. 20. Coronal CT image depicts the location and extent of the olfactory fossae and groove (*A*). The olfactory recess (medial lamella of the cribriform plate down to the basal lamella of the middle turbinate), the olfactory vestibule (basal lamella down to the lower margin of the middle turbinate), and the olfactory cleft (olfactory recess and vestibule together) are depicted in (*B*).

Table 5
Estimation of the height of the ethmoidal skull base

Authors	Methodology	Interpretation
Myers and Valvasorri[28] 1998	The vertical height of the orbit is divided into 3 equal sections. The position of the ESB is documented in reference to upper, middle, or lower one-third of the vertical orbital height	If the ESB passes above the upper one-third of the vertical height of the ipsilateral orbit it indicates a normal and hence a surgically safe ESB. An ESB passing through or below the midorbital plane is considered a low ESB
Rudmik and Smith29 2012	The vertical distance between the height of the ESB and the midorbital plane is measured in a coronal CT image showing the canal for the anterior ethmoidal artery	In their study, the mean height of the ESB was found to be 8.5 mms. A vertical height of more than 8.5 mms was considered a safe and high ESB, a measurement between 4 and 7 mms was considered as a moderately safe ESB and a height less than 4 mms was deemed as a low and surgically unsafe ESB with high chances of inadvertent intracranial penetration

From Vaid S, Vaid N. Normal Anatomy and Anatomic Variants of the Paranasal Sinuses on Computed Tomography. Neuroimaging Clin N Am. 2015 Nov;25(4):527 to 48.

authors have proposed a "cruciform sign" to diagnose bilateral Onodi cells (Fig. 22C), in which a coronal CT image at the level of the posterior choana demonstrates the sphenoid air cell showing cruciform septation.[11] Important critical relationships of the sphenoid sinus, namely the optic nerves and internal carotid arteries are directly related to the posterior ethmoid sinuses in the presence of Onodi cells.

The Sphenoid Sinus

The sphenoid sinus develops in the body of the sphenoid bone and is generally bilateral although asymmetric in size.[8] The sphenoid sinus is classified into 4 types depending on the degree of pneumatization[30] (Table 6, Fig. 23). Several bony canals and foramina transmit critical neurovascular structures related to the sphenoid sinus (Table 7). The anterior clinoid processes may be

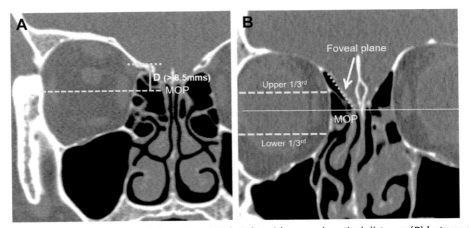

Fig. 21. ESB height. Coronal CT image (*A*) showing ESB height with normal vertical distance (*D*) between the mid-orbital plane (MOP, dashed *line*) and the anterior skull base (*dotted line*) (see Table 5). Coronal CT image (*B*) showing a low-lying foveal plane (dotted orange *line/arrow*) reaching the mid-orbital plane (horizontal white *line*). The dashed yellow lines depict the division of the vertical height of the orbit as reference planes (see table 5). (*From* Vaid S, Vaid N. Normal Anatomy and Anatomic Variants of the Paranasal Sinuses on Computed Tomography. Neuroimaging Clin N Am. 2015 Nov;25(4):527 to 48.)

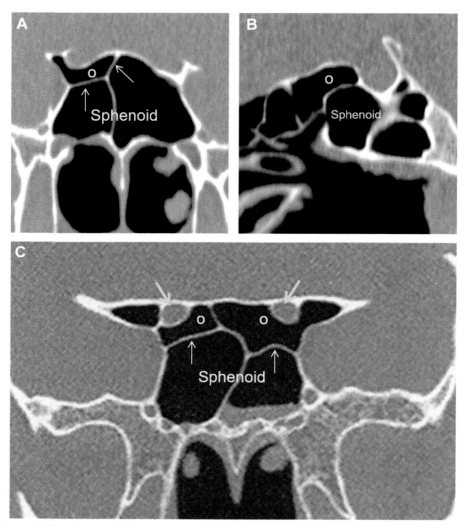

Fig. 22. Coronal (*A*) and sagittal (*B*) CT images showing a right Onodi cell (*O*) with obliquely oriented intrasinus septa (*arrows*). Coronal image (*C*) shows the "cruciform sign" seen with bilateral Onodi cells (*O*). Both optic nerves course through these cells (*arrows*).

Table 6	
Classification of type of sphenoid sinus	
Sphenoid sinus Agenesis	A nonpneumatized sphenoid sinus seen in <0.7% of individuals
Conchal sphenoid sinus	A small rudimentary air cavity within the sphenoid bone not reaching up to the anterior wall of the sella tursica seen in 1%–4% of the population
Presellar sphenoid sinus	The posterior sinus wall extends up to the anterior wall of the sella tursica seen in 35%–40% of the population
Sellar sphenoid sinus	The sinus cavity extends beyond the anterior wall of the sella tursica below the pituitary fossa seen in 55%–60% of the population. Wang J and others[30] further classified this type of sphenoid sinus more recently based on the direction of pneumatization into sphenoid body, lateral clivus, lesser sphenoid wing, anterior rostral, and the combined variety

From Vaid S, Vaid N. Normal Anatomy and Anatomic Variants of the Paranasal Sinuses on Computed Tomography. Neuro-imaging Clin N Am. 2015 Nov;25(4):527 to 48.

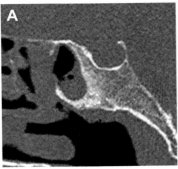 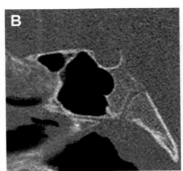 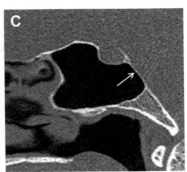

Fig. 23. Sagittal CT images show (*A*) conchal, (*B*) presellar, and (*C*) sellar variants of sphenoid sinus pneumatization. The sellar variant may have a thin posterior bony margin (*arrow*) with a potential risk of intraoperative skull base trauma.

pneumatized in up to 6% to 13% of cases[8] forming the carotico-optic recess between the optic nerve above and the internal carotid artery below.

Anatomic Variants

1. Intrasinus septa attached to the bony walls of the internal carotid artery and optic nerve need preoperative identification because excessive traction on these septa may lead to an avulsion of the bony walls and catastrophic complications (Fig. 24).
2. The position of the neurovascular structures around the sphenoid sinus is determined by the degree of pneumatization. Occasionally, the structures are exposed within the sinus cavity and connected to the sinus walls by bony stalks.
3. Persistence of the lateral craniopharyngeal canal in association with sphenoid hyperpneumatization and raised intracranial pressure may lead to the formation of a spontaneous lateral sphenoid meningoencephalocele and spontaneous cerebrospinal fluid leak.
4. In approximately 80% of cases of anterior clinoid process pneumatization, the optic nerve will be dehiscent into the superolateral aspect of the sphenoid sinus.[31]

Table 7 Critical neurovascular/congenital channels related to the sphenoid sinus	
Optic nerve canals	Related to the roof of the sphenoid sinus. Bony walls can be dehiscent in up to 24% of cases.[8] Delano et al classified the optic nerves into 4 categories based on the relationship of the nerve with the sphenoid and posterior ethmoid sinuses (31)
The internal carotid artery canals	Located along the posterolateral wall of the sphenoid sinus and the bony coverings may be dehiscent in up to 25% of cases[8]
The pterygoid canals (vidian canals)	Along the inferior sinus walls that transmit the combined great petrosal and deep petrosal nerve complex as well as the artery and vein of the pterygoid canal
Foramen rotundum	Along the lateral sinus walls which transmit the maxillary division of the trigeminal nerve, artery of the foramen rotundum, and an emissary vein
Lateral craniopharyngeal canal (Sternberg's canal)	Represents a congenital bony defect in the lateral wall of the sphenoid sinus situated further lateral to the maxillary nerve

From Vaid S, Vaid N. Normal Anatomy and Anatomic Variants of the Paranasal Sinuses on Computed Tomography. Neuroimaging Clin N Am. 2015 Nov;25(4):527-48.

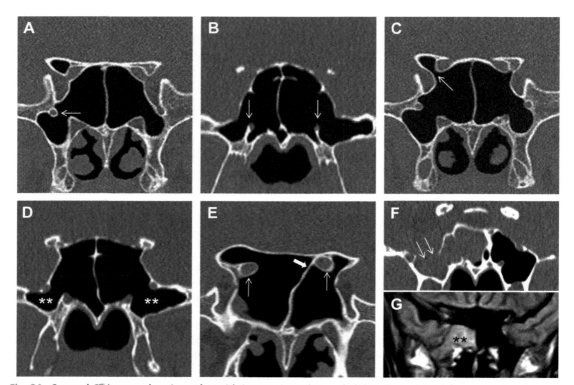

Fig. 24. Coronal CT images showing sphenoid sinus variants (*arrows*). (*A*) Endosinal right foramen rotundum and endosinal vidian canals (*B*). Right carotico-optic recess (*C*) and prominent lateral recesses (** in *D*). Bilateral optic nerve dehiscence (*E*) with intrasinus septum attaching to left optic nerve canal (block *arrow*). Widened lateral craniopharyngeal canal on the right side (*F*) with coronal T1W MR image (*G*) showing an associated meningoencephalocele (**).

SUMMARY

A structured approach to CT scans of the PNSs using multiplanar imaging enables a better understanding of the complex anatomy of this region and its numerous anatomic variants. Radiologists need to be aware of the critical clinical implications of identifying these anatomic variations.

in diagnosis. Sinus pathologic conditions in children aged younger than 4 years are uncommon except in the ethmoid sinuses because these are the only sinuses, which are pneumatized at birth.

CLINICS CARE POINT 1

Multiplanar CT evaluation of PNSs in orthogonal and nonorthogonal planes is important to outline the anatomy and identify surgically important anatomic variants.

Pre-FESS CT examinations of the PNSs are usually noncontrast-enhanced studies. Contrast examinations are reserved for evaluating specific pathologic conditions (aggressive infections, neoplasm, and vascular lesions) and for assessing extension into orbit, intracranial compartment, and surrounding soft tissues.

Knowledge of relevant embryologic events in paranasal sinus development can avoid pitfalls

CLINICS CARE POINT 2

Important nerves and vessels related to the PNSs include the following:

- Infraorbital nerves along the roof of the maxillary sinus.
- Optic nerves.
- Internal carotid arteries.
- Pterygoid artery and vein and the great petrosal-deep petrosal nerve complex in the vidian canal.
- Maxillary division of the trigeminal nerve in the foramen rotundum.

CLINICS CARE POINT 3

The use of the mnemonic "CLOSE" enables the radiologist to identify and report important and surgically relevant sinonasal anatomical variants.[32]

C: Cribriform plate anatomy.

L: Lamina papyracea integrity.

O: Optic nerve anatomy

S: Sphenoid sinus anatomy, internal carotid artery (ICA) anatomy, and presence of the Onodi cell

E: Ethmoidal (anterior) artery anatomy

DISCLOSURE

The authors state that there are no commercial or financial conflicts of interest and no funding sources to declare.

SUPPLEMENTARY DATA

Supplementary data related to this article can be found online at https://doi.org/10.1016/j.nic.2022.07.007.

REFERENCES

1. Ónodi A, Thomson SC. The anatomy of the nasal cavity and its accessory sinuses: an atlas for practitioners and students. London: H.K. Lewis; 1895.

2. Aksoy EA, Özden SU, Karaarslan E, et al. Reliability of high-pitch ultra-low-dose paranasal sinus computed tomography for evaluating paranasal sinus anatomy and sinus disease. J Craniofac Surg 2014;25(5):1801–4.

3. Dahmani-Causse M, Marx M, Deguine O, et al. Morphologic examination of the temporal bone by cone-beam computed tomography: comparison with multislice helical computed tomography. Eur Ann Otorhinolaryngol Head Neck Dis 2011;128:230–5.

4. Bremke M, Leppek R, Werner JA. Digital volume tomography in ENT medicine. HNO 2010;58(8):823–32.

5. Wormald PJ. Imaging in Endoscopic Sinus Surgery. In: Wormald PJ, editor. Endoscopic sinus surgery: anatomy, three-dimensional reconstruction, and surgical technique. 3rd edition. New York, NY: Thieme Medical Publishers; 2013. p. 13–8.

6. Marquez S, Tessema B, Clement PA, et al. Development of the ethmoid sinus and extramural migration: the anatomical basis of this paranasal sinus. Anat Rec (Hoboken) 2008;291(11):1535–53.

7. Goldman-Yassen AE, Meda K, Kadom N. Paranasal sinus development and implications for imaging. Pediatr Radiol 2021;51(7):1134–48.

8. Vaid S, Vaid N. Normal Anatomy and Anatomic Variants of the Paranasal Sinuses on Computed Tomography. Neuroimaging Clin N Am 2015;25(4):527–48.

9. Shafik AG, Rabie TM, Alkady HA, et al. Evaluation of the Internal Nasal Valve using Computed Tomography Pre and Post Rhinoplasty and Its Correlation to Symptomatic Improvement. Egypt J Hosp Med 2018;72(5):4486–9.

10. Moche JA, Cohen JC, Pearlman SJ. Axial computed tomography evaluation of the internal nasal valve correlates with clinical valve narrowing and patient complaint. Int Forum Allergy rhinology 2012;3(7):592–7.

11. Beale TJ, Madani G, Morley SJ. Imaging of the paranasal sinuses and nasal cavity: normal anatomy and clinically relevant anatomical variants. Semin Ultrasound CT MR 2009;30(1):2–16.

12. Vaid S, Vaid N, Rawat S, et al. An imaging checklist for pre-FESS CT: framing a surgically relevant report. Clin Radiol 2011;66(5):459–70.

13. Bolger WE, Butzin CA, Parsons DS. Paranasal sinus bony anatomic variations and mucosal abnormalities: CT analysis for endoscopic sinus surgery. Laryngoscope 1991;101:56–64.

14. Calvo-Henríquez C, Ruano-Ravina A, Martinez-Capoccioni G, et al. The lamellar cell: a radiological study and a new classification proposal. Eur Arch Otorhinolaryngol 2018;275(11):2713–7.

15. Cellina M, Gibelli D, Cappella A, et al. Nasal cavities and the nasal septum: Anatomical variants and assessment of features with computed tomography. Neuroradiol J 2020;33(4):340–7.

16. Lund VJ, Stammberger H, Fokkens WJ, et al. European position paper on the anatomical terminology of the internal nose and paranasal sinuses. Rhinol Suppl 2014;24:1–34.

17. Bolger WE, Woodruff WW, Morehead J, et al. Maxillary sinus hypoplasia: classification and description of associated uncinate process hypoplasia. Otolaryngol Head Neck Surg 1990;103(5):759–65.

18. Wormald PJ. Anatomy of the frontal recess and frontal sinus with three-dimensional reconstruction. In: Wormald PJ, editor. Endoscopic sinus surgery: anatomy, three-dimensional reconstruction, and surgical technique. 4th edition. New York: Thieme Medical Publishers; 2018. p. 52–88.

19. Wormald PJ, Hoseman W, Callejas C, et al. The International Frontal Sinus Anatomy Classification (IFAC) and Classification of the Extent of Endoscopic Frontal Sinus Surgery (EFSS). Int Forum Allergy Rhinol 2016;6(7):677–96.

20. Kim JW, Goldberg Robert A, Shorr N. The Inferomedial Orbital Strut An Anatomic and Radiographic Study. Ophthalmic Plast Reconstr Surg 2002;18(5):355–64.

21. Whyte A, Boeddinghaus R. The maxillary sinus: physiology, development and imaging anatomy. Dentomaxillofac Radiol 2019;48(8):20190205. Erratum in: Dentomaxillofac Radiol. 2019:10.1259: 20190205c.

22. Whyte A, Boeddinghaus R. Imaging of odontogenic sinusitis. Clin Radiol 2019;74(7):503–16.

23. Bhatti MT, Schmalfuss IM, Mancuso AA. Orbital complications of functional endoscopic sinus surgery: MR and CT findings. Clin Radiol 2005;60:894–904.

24. Guarnizo A, Nguyen TB, Glikstein R, et al. Computed tomography assessment of anterior ethmoidal canal dehiscence: An interobserver agreement study and review of the literature. Neuroradiol J 2020;33(2):145–51.

25. Lannoy-Penisson L, Schultz P, Riehm S, et al. The anterior ethmoidal artery: radio anatomical comparison and its application in endonasal surgery. Acta Otolaryngol 2007;127:618–22.

26. Keros P. On the practical value of differences in the level of the lamina cribrosa of the ethmoid. Z Laryngol Rhinol Otol 1962;41:809–13.

27. Bates NS, Massoud TF. Ambiguous "olfactory" terms for anatomic spaces adjacent to the cribriform plate: A publication database analysis and quest for uniformity. Clin Anat 2021;34(8):1186–95.

28. Meyers RM, Valvassori G. Interpretation of anatomic variations of computed tomography scans of the sinuses: a surgeon's perspective. Laryngoscope 1998;108:422–5.

29. Rudmik L, Smith TL. Evaluation of the Ethmoid Skull Base Height Prior to Endoscopic Sinus Surgery: A Preoperative CT Evaluation Technique. Int Forum Allergy Rhinol 2012;2(2):151–4.

30. Wang J, Bidari S, Inoue K, et al. Extensions of the sphenoid sinus: a new classification. Neurosurgery 2010;66(4):797–816.

31. Delano MC, Fun FY, Zinreich SJ. Relationship of the optic nerve to the posterior paranasal sinuses: a CT anatomic study. Am 1996;17(4):669–75.

32. O'Brien WT, Sr., Hamelin S and Weitzel EK, The Preoperative Sinus CT: Avoiding a "CLOSE" Call with Surgical Complications. Radiology 2016;281(1):10–21. doi:10.1148/radiol.2016152230.

Maxillofacial Skeleton and Facial Anatomy

Jacqueline C. Junn, MD[a],*, Peter M. Som, MD[a,b,c]

KEYWORDS

- Superficial musculoaponeurotic system • Superficial fat pads • Arterial anatomy of the face
- Venous anatomy of the face • Facial muscles • Facial bone nomenclature

KEY POINTS

- Normal facial proportions and facial surface landmarks.
- Superficial musculoaponeurotic systems function to connect the skin and the mimic muscles.
- Facial muscle development occurs between the third and eighth weeks of embryogenesis.
- Forty-two facial muscles include the mimic muscles, masseter, and temporalis.

INTRODUCTION

This article will discuss the anatomy of the face. Specifically, the face is divided into 6 layers which include[1]: the skin,[2] the subcutaneous fat,[3] the superficial musculoaponeurotic system (SMAS),[4] the superficial facial muscles,[5] the deep fascia and fat, and[6] the ligaments anchoring the above structures to the facial bones.[1]

Normal Facial Proportions and the Landmarks of the Facial Surface

Although beauty is "in the eye of the beholder," there are proportions of a face that are generally accepted as being the normal. Namely, one-third of the facial height is from the brow to the tip of the nasion, one-third is from the nasion to the tip of the nose, and one-third is from the tip of the nose to the chin. From medial to lateral: one-third is from the outer to inner canthus of each eye and one-third is from one medial canthus to the other medial canthus. From a functional point of view, the face can be divided into upper, middle, and lower regions. The normal facial landmarks are shown in **Fig. 1**.

Superficial Musculoaponeurotic System

SMAS is a fibroadipose network that lies beneath the skin and connects the skin and the mimic (facial) musculatures (**Fig. 2**). The facial muscles are relatively small. Thus, when they contract, there is little overall movement; it is the SMAS that magnifies these muscle movements on the skin allowing nonverbal expressions.[2,3] However, since its first description in the cheek by Mitz and Peyronie,[4] its anatomic definition and architecture have been exhaustively debated. Additionally, there is an ongoing controversy regarding the boundaries of the SMAS and whether or not they are distinct from or integrated with the temporoparietal and parotid fasciae.

Various classifications and types of SMAS have been proposed without consensus. Previously, 2 types of SMA architectures were described: type I, which is lateral to the nasolabial fold, and type II, which is medial to the nasolabial fold.[1] Subsequently, a new classification was proposed by Sandulescu and colleagues[3] that incorporated its functions, including its interactions with the mimic muscle, facial folds, and creases. Type I SMAS is located lateral to the nasolabial fold and also

Funding Information: None.

Disclosures: None.

[a] Department of Radiology, The Icahn School of Medicine at Mount Sinai, One Gustave Levy Place, Box 1234, New York, NY 10029, USA; [b] Department of Otolaryngology, The Icahn School of Medicine at Mount Sinai, One Gustave Levy Place, Box 1234, New York, NY 10029, USA; [c] Department of Radiation Oncology, The Icahn School of Medicine at Mount Sinai, One Gustave Levy Place, Box 1234, New York, NY 10029, USA

* Corresponding author.

E-mail address: Jacqueline.Junn@mountsinai.org

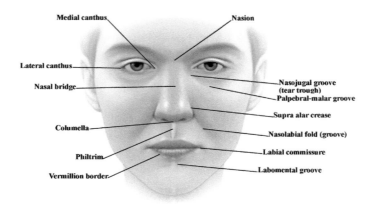

Fig. 1. Frontal drawing of a face indicating the skin landmarks of a normal face.

includes the infraorbital, supraorbital, and the forehead regions. It is composed of fibrous septa in parallel orientation. Type II SMAS overlies the upper and lower lip areas. It is more condensed and has irregular meshwork of connective tissues and short fibrous septa. Type III SMAS is made up of loose connective tissues over the lower and upper eyelids.[5] It connects orbicularis oculi to the skin. Distinctively, Type III SMAS does not contain fat. Finally, Type IV SMAS overlies the parotid and midfacial areas.[3] Type IV comprises parallel fibrous septa extending to the skin and anchors the skin to the parotid fascia. Clinically, understanding different types of SMAS is important for determining surgical procedures, such as the rhytidectomies (facial plastic procedures), and their outcome. In essence, the SMAS acts like a lever that magnifies the small facial muscle contractions into larger facial skin movements.

On imaging, the different types of SMAS are not discretely identified. Based on a cadaveric MR imaging study of the face by Ghassemi and colleagues[1] and Som and colleagues,[6] the SMAS was located below the dermis, within the subcutaneous fat, and superficial to the facial musculature over the cheek region. The peripheral margins were bounded by the lateral aspect of the orbit and the anterior portion of the temporalis, laterally. Because it descended posteriorly and inferiorly from the zygomatic arch and lateral maxilla, it merged with the superficial parotid fascia. Additionally, it continued and blended with the platysma at the caudal most margin. Medially, it was seen anterior to the maxilla and blended

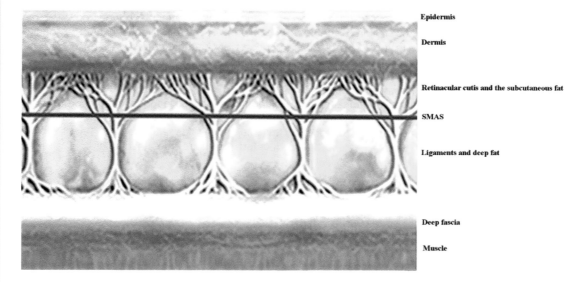

Fig. 2. Cross-sectional drawing of the skin and subcutaneous tissues shows the position of the SMAS and the retinacular cutis fibers that act as levels to magnify the movement of the facial muscles on the skin.

Table 1
Development of the facial muscles from each facial nerve lamina

Lamina	Derived Facial Muscles
Temporal lamina	Superior auricular
Occipital lamina	Occipital belly of the occipitofrontalis, posterior auricular
Cervical lamina	Cervical portion of the platysma and the SMAS
Mandibular lamina	Mandibular portion of the platysma, depressor labii inferioris, mentalis, risorius, depressor anguli oris, levator anguli oris, orbicularis oris inferior fibers
Infraorbital lamina	Zygomaticus major and minor, levator labii superioris, levator labii superioris alaeque nasi, orbicularis oris superior fibers, orbicularis oculi, frontal belly of occipitofrontalis, procerus, corrugator supercilii

with the lateral nasal margin. The SMAS does not have bone or skin attachments.

Embryology of the Facial Muscles and Bones

Development of the face is a complex topic, and it is beyond the scope of this review. The pivotal research was undertaken by Gasser in 1967. The face is developed mostly between the 4th and 89th weeks of gestation. This process includes the formation of the face and oral cavity from the head ectoderm as well as the first branchial arch and its derivatives from the neural crest mesenchyme. By the fifth week, olfactory portion of the nasal sac develops with the maxillary processes growing medially, which results in medial displacement of the nasal sacs. By the seventh week, each nasal cavity develops and each nostril forms.

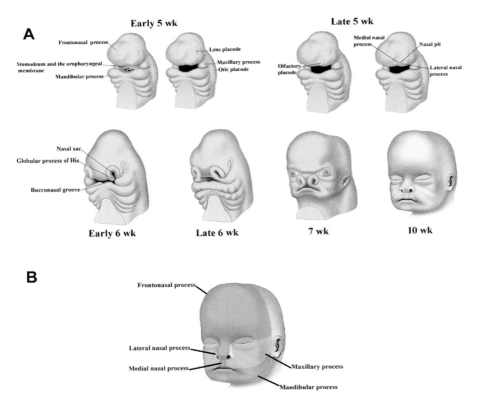

Fig. 3. (A)Serial drawings in the left anterior oblique view of the developing face shows the progressive fusion of the facial processes. (B). A summary drawing of the face in the anterior left oblique view showing the contributions of the facial processes that form the final facial anatomy.

The facial muscles develop between the third and eighth weeks as the second branchial arch mesoderm thickens. By the sixth embryonic week, there is a condensation of mesenchymal cells along the upper surface of the second branchial arch, along the first branchial cleft. By the sixth week, focal extensions, referred to as lamina, develop from these mesenchymal cells, and by the ninth fetal week, there are 5 laminae from which all of the facial muscles develop. Of particular interest to this review is the cervical lamina as the platysma muscle develops from its caudal region, whereas the SMAS develops from its cranial margin (Table 1).

The facial bones develop from the fusion of a number of facial processes each of which is covered with ectoderm and filled with mesoderm. It is the incomplete or lack of fusion of these various processes that results in facial clefts. Fig. 3A illustrates the fusion process between the fifth and tenth week of gestation, and Fig. 3B shows the components that form from each facial process.

Facial Muscles

As previously noted, the facial muscles facilitate facial expression and enable nonverbal communications. There are 42 facial muscles, which include the mimic muscles, masseter, and temporalis muscles. The memetic muscles are innervated by the facial nerve, whereas the masseter and temporalis are innervated by the mandibular branch of the trigeminal nerve. Unlike other muscles in the body that are separated and enveloped by fascial layers, most of these mimic muscles originate from the bone and insert into the dermis through the SMAS.[1] There are 3 muscles that do not originate from the facial bones: the frontalis, risorius, and malaris muscles.[6,7] The risorius muscle typically originates from the fascia overlying the masseter and drapes over the lateral cheek. The malaris muscle originates from the inferior margin of the orbicularis oculi and descends medially toward the nasolabial fold and the outer third of the upper lip as it intertwines with the orbicularis oris muscle fibers. The frontalis (epicranius) muscle has its origin in the galea aponeurosis, and it inserts on the orbicularis muscles.

Although the facial muscles allow nonverbal facial expressions, they cannot be directly seen. However, the movement of the skin can be seen and cataloged. The Facial Action Coding System catalogs these facial movements, assigning an action unit (AU) to each distinct movement.[8] Unfortunately, the imaging identification of the individual facial muscles is challenging owing to their small

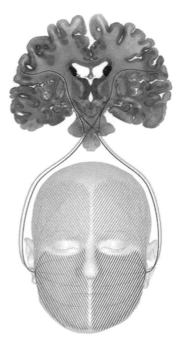

Fig. 4. The facial nerve innervation of the facial muscles. Note that the upper facial muscles are innervated bilaterally while the lower facial muscles are innervated by the contralateral facial nerve.

Table 2 The branches of the facial nerve that innervate the facial muscles	
Facial Muscles	Innervating Branch of Facial Nerve
Frontali Procerus Depressor supercilii Corrugator supercilii	Temporal branch
Orbicularis oculi	Temporal and zygomatic branches
Zygomaticus major Zygomaticus minor Levator labii superioris aleque nasi Levator anguli oris	Zygomatic and buccal branches
Buccinator Risorius	Buccal branch
Oribularis oris	Marginal mandibular and buccal branches
Depressor anguli oris Depressor labii inferioris Mentalis	Marginal mandibular branch
Platysma	Cervical branch

Table 3
MR imaging of the face

Muscle	Origin	Insertion	Imaging on MR
Scalp and Orbital Group			
Orbicularis oculi (Bilateral)	• Orbital part from medial orbital margin • Palpebral part from palpebral ligament • Lacrimal part from lacrimal bone	• Orbital fibers about upper lid to lower palpebral ligament. Palpebral fibers to lateral raphe • Lacrimal part to upper and lower eyelids	Most margins are well seen, but blends with adjacent fascia and muscles
Corrugator supercilii (bilateral)	• Medial part of supraorbital margin	• Skin of medial half of eyebrow	Faintly seen, merges with corrugators supercilii and depressor supercilii
Occipitofrontalis (epicranius) (bilateral)	• Occipital bellies from lateral two-thirds of the superior nuchal line • Frontal bellies from epicranial aponeurosis near coronal suture	• Skin of occipital region, skin of frontal region and galea aponeurosis	Poorly seen, too thin
Depressor supercilii (bilateral)	• Medial orbital rim near lacrimal bone	• Medial aspect of bony orbit	Poorly seen, merges with corrugators supercilii and orbicularis oculi
Procerus (pyramidalis nasi) (midline)	• Fascia over lower nasal and lateral nasal cartilages	• Skin between and above eyebrows	Well seen
Nose and Midface Group			
Nasalis (compressor naris) (midline)	• Canine eminence above and lateral to incisive fossa	• Aponeurosis on nasal cartilages	Fairly well seen but thin
Levator labii superioris alaeque nasi (bilateral)	• Upper frontal process of maxilla	• Skin of lateral nostril and upper lip	Well seen
Levator anguli oris (caninus) (bilateral)	• Canine fossa of maxilla below infraorbital foramen	• Angle of mouth, mixes with orbicularis oris, depressor anguli oris and zygomaticus	Well seen
Levator labii superioris (bilateral)	• From margin of orbit above infraorbital foramen and malar bone	• Muscular substance of skin of nose & lateral upper lip skin of nasolabial groove and upper lip	Well seen
Zygomaticus minor (bilateral)	• Malar bone	• Oral commissure	Poorly seen, stringy or thin
Zygomaticus major (bilateral)	• Zygomatic portion of zygomatic arch	• Angle of mouth. Mingles with orbicularis oris, levator anguli oris, and depressor anguli oris	Well seen

(continued on next page)

Table 3
(continued)

Muscle	Origin	Insertion	Imaging on MR
Depressor sept nasi (bilateral)	• Incisive fossa of maxilla and nasal ala	• Septum and back of nasal cartilages	Poorly seen, too small and blends with adjacent structures
Mouth and Chin Group			
Orbicularis oris (midline)	• Sphincter muscle of mouth.	• Has its own fibers and contributions. from buccinators, levator anguli oris, depressor anguli oris, levator labii superioris, zygomaticus major and minor, depressor labii inferioris	Well seen, but blends with adjacent muscles
Risorius (bilateral)	• Fascia over masseter superficial to playsma	• Skin at angle of mandible	Poorly seen, often wispy
Platysma (bilateral)	• Fascia upper pectoral and deltoid region	• Anterior fiber to chin and mix with depressor labii inferioris and depressor anguli oris. Posterior fibers to mandible and lower face and muscles at angle of mouth and lower mouth.	Well seen, but blends with adjacent muscles
Mentalis (bilateral)	• Incisive fossa of mandible	• Skin of chin	Well seen
Depressor labii inferioris (quadratus labii inferioris) (bilateral)	• Lateral surface of mandible between symphysis and mental foramen	• Skin of lower lip, mixes with orbicularis oris. Medial fibers join those of other side	Fairly well seen
Depressor anguli oris (triangularis) (bilateral)	• Continuous with platysma on oblique line of mandible	• Angle of mouth into orbicularis oris and skin	Fairly well seen
Muscles Not Identified in Atlas			
Dilatator naris (bilateral)	• Margin of nasal notch and lesser alar cartilage	• Skin near margin of nostril	Merges with nasal cartilages
Malaris (bilateral if present)	• Lower margin of orbicularis oculi	• Skin near nasolabial ridge, angle of mouth and upper lip	Inconsistent and very thin

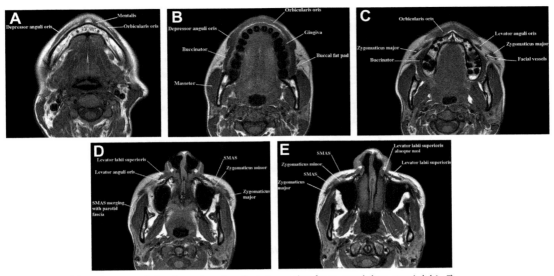

Fig. 5. MR Axial T1 images of the face showing facial muscles from caudal to cranial (*A–E*).

caliber, close proximity, and overlapping anatomy. However, it is the interworking of these muscles that gives rise to the complex facial expressions.

There are few upper facial muscles and many overlapping and interrelated midface and lower facial muscles. This disparity of muscle distribution allows limited eyebrow movement and wrinkling of the forehead in the upper face but numerous movements of the midface and lower (mouth) face. The upper facial muscles are innervated by both the left and right motor nuclei, whereas the lower facial muscles are innervated

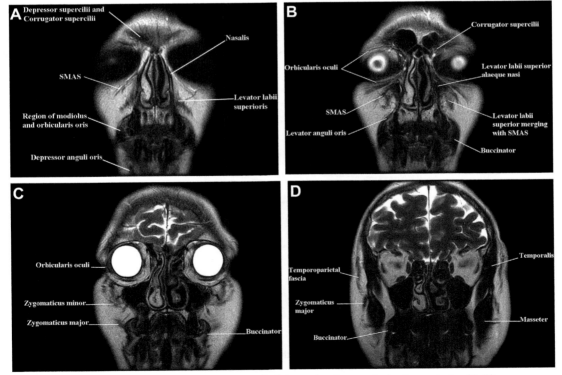

Fig. 6. MR Coronal T2 images of the face showing facial muscles from anterior to posterior (*A–D*).

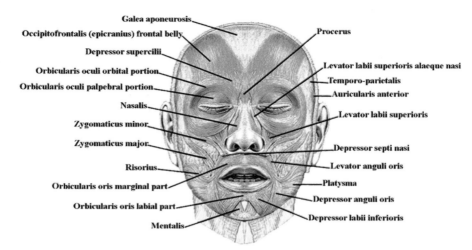

Fig. 7. Frontal drawing of the facial muscles. Paulsen, Waschke, Sobotta Atlas of Human Anatomy, 16th Edition 2018 © Elsevier GmbH, Urban & Fischer, Munich.

by the contralateral motor nucleus (Fig. 4). This innervation pattern allows independent lower facial movement. Further, in the process of recognizing a person's face, the brain appears to interpret the upper face separately from the lower face. Table 2 shows which branches of the facial nerve innervate which facial muscles.

Table 3 shows the origins, insertions, and how well each muscle can be seen on MR imaging of the face (Figs. 5 and 6). Fig. 7 shows an illustration of the facial muscles. Note the relative paucity of muscles in the upper face and the larger number of overlapping muscles in the lower face.

Ligamental Compartments and the Facial Fat Pads

The facial ligaments, mentioned in "Superficial Musculoaponeurotic System" section, form the boundaries of discrete compartments that enclose the various facial fat pads. These facial fat pads include the central and middle forehead compartments, superior, inferior, and lateral orbital

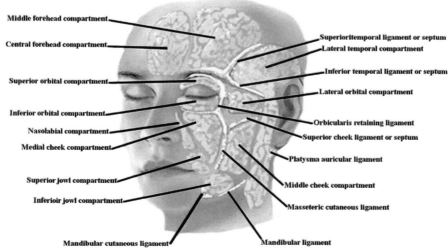

Fig. 8. Frontal oblique drawing of the face showing the ligaments and septi that contain the facial fat pads. (*Modified from* Alghoul M, Codner MA. Retaining ligaments of the face: review of anatomy and clinical applications. Aesthet Surg J. 2013 Aug 1;33(6):769-82.)

compartments, nasolabial compartment, medial cheek compartment, superior and inferior jowl compartments, lateral temporal compartment, and the middle cheek compartment. Notable facial ligaments include the superior temporal ligament/septum, inferior temporal ligament, orbicularis retaining ligament, superior cheek ligament/septum, masseteric cutaneous ligament, mandibular cutaneous ligament, mandibular ligament, and platysma auricular ligament. Fig. 8 summarizes the major ligaments and the enclosed fat pads.

These fat pads play an important role in aging because over time they atrophy and descend in response to gravity. As an example, the dark rings that develop under each eye are the orbicularis oculi muscles showing through the skin, no longer covered by the malar (medial cheek) fat pad.

The Facial Arteries and Veins

The arteries that supply the face come from the branches of the external carotid artery. Similarly, the veins that drain the facial areas are tributaries of the external jugular vein. The facial artery arises at the level of the greater cornu of the hyoid bone and ascends under the posterior belly of the digastric and stylohyoid muscle. The facial artery and its branches supply the lower third of the face, parotidomassetric regions and the buccal, orbital, infraorbital, and nasal regions.[9] The superficial temporal artery originates deep within the parotid gland and travels cranially. It gives off smaller branches including the transverse facial artery and middle temporal artery with frontal and parietal branches. The superficial temporal artery predominantly supplies the superior and lateral face including the forehead, the parotid gland, and temporalis. Additionally, the maxillary artery comes off the external carotid artery to course within the infratemporal fossa. It is responsible for supplying the deep face, nasal, and oral cavities. The internal carotid artery also contributes to the face via the ophthalmic artery, which supplies the eyes, nose, and portions of the forehead.

The venous drainage of the face is complex and shows many variations. The facial vein is the major vein that drains the superior part of the face. The superficial temporal vein and maxillary vein join to form the retromandibular vein. It is also important to note that superficial facial veins have connections to the cavernous sinus. The angular vein has bidirectional flow. It can flow into the facial

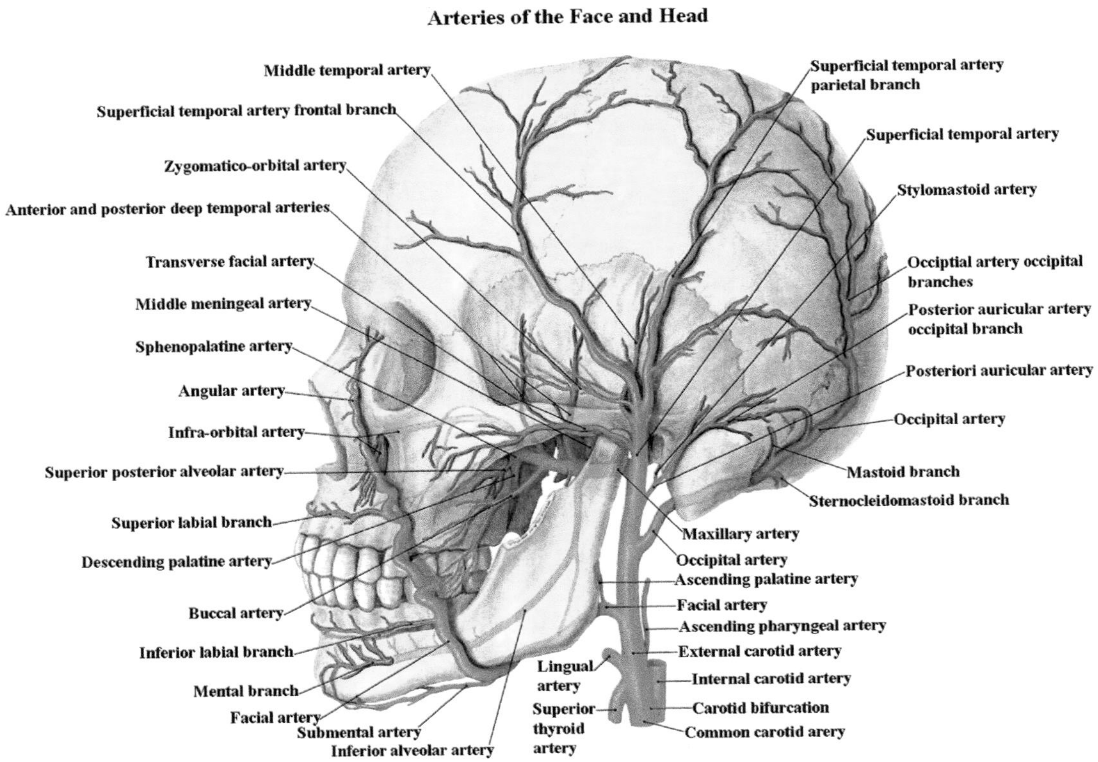

Arteries of the Face and Head

Middle temporal artery
Superficial temporal artery frontal branch
Zygomatico-orbital artery
Anterior and posterior deep temporal arteries
Transverse facial artery
Middle meningeal artery
Sphenopalatine artery
Angular artery
Infra-orbital artery
Superior posterior alveolar artery
Superior labial branch
Descending palatine artery
Buccal artery
Inferior labial branch
Mental branch
Facial artery
Submental artery
Inferior alveolar artery

Superficial temporal artery parietal branch
Superficial temporal artery
Stylomastoid artery
Occiptial artery occipital branches
Posterior auricular artery occipital branch
Posteriori auricular artery
Occipital artery
Mastoid branch
Sternocleidomastoid branch
Maxillary artery
Occipital artery
Ascending palatine artery
Facial artery
Ascending pharyngeal artery
External carotid artery
Internal carotid artery
Carotid bifurcation
Common carotid arery

Lingual artery
Superior thyroid artery

Fig. 9. Lateral drawing of the facial bones showing the branches of the external carotid artery. Paulsen, Waschke, Sobotta Atlas of Human Anatomy, 16th Edition 2018 © Elsevier GmbH, Urban & Fischer, Munich.

Veins of the Face and Head

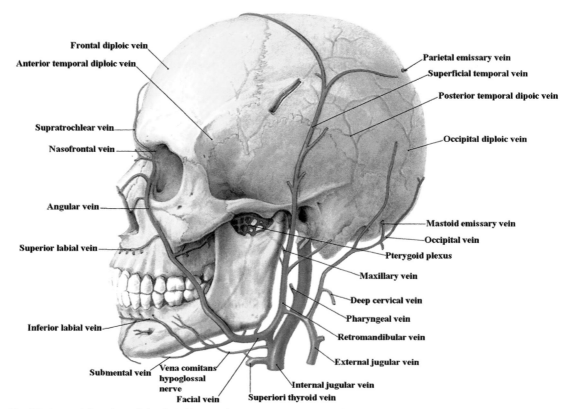

Fig. 10. Lateral drawing of the facial bones showing the branches of the jugular veins. Paulsen, Waschke, Sobotta Atlas of Human Anatomy, 16th Edition 2018 © Elsevier GmbH, Urban & Fischer, Munich.

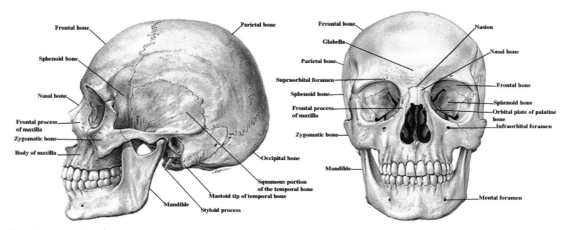

Fig. 11. Lateral and frontal drawings of the facial bones. Paulsen, Waschke, Sobotta Atlas of Human Anatomy, 16th Edition 2018 © Elsevier GmbH, Urban & Fischer, Munich.

vein or ophthalmic vein, which then drains into the cavernous sinus. Additionally, supraorbital, supra-trochlear, superior ophthalmic, deep facial, inferior ophthalmic veins, and the pterygoid plexus can all drain into the cavernous sinus. Therefore, facial infection can extend intracranially via venous hematogenous spread.[10] **Figs. 9** and **10** show facial arterial supplies and venous drainage, respectively.

Adult Facial Bones

The facial bones are made of 14 midline and paired bones that are collectively called the viscerocranium/splanchnocranium. They are made of paired palatine, nasal, lacrimal, inferior nasal concha, zygoma, and maxilla. There are 14 including the paired bone and the four midline bones (sphenoid, ethmoid, vomer, and mandible). The adult facial and skull bones are illustrated in **Fig. 11**. Each of these bones can be clearly identified on imaging studies (**Figs. 12** and **13**). Interestingly, the facial skeleton does not remain the same throughout

life. There are recognized alterations that occur, and these include oblique widening of the orbits, regression of the midface (maxilla), widening of the nasal aperture, and regression of the mandible. These changes are shown in **Fig. 14**.

The facial skeleton can be thought of as a system of vertical and horizontal buttresses.[11,12] The vertical buttresses consist of the paired nasomaxillary (NM), zygomaticomaxillary (ZM), and pterygomaxillary (PM) midfacial buttresses as well as the ramus of the mandible. These buttresses define the vertical height of the face and provide the bony support required for mastication. Each NM buttress is mainly created by the maxilla with contributions from the nasal bone and nasal process of the frontal bone. The PM buttress is mainly created by the pterygoid plates and to a lesser extent the posterior maxilla. The ZM buttress begins in the area above the first molar and continues up the lateral maxilla through the zygomatic bone along the lateral orbital rim, through the frontal process of the zygoma and then through the zygomatic process of the frontal bone. The ZM

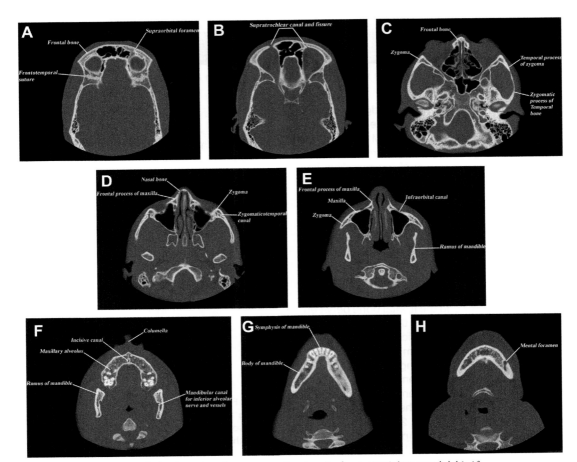

Fig. 12. CT Axial images of the face showing osseous landmarks from cranial to caudal (*A–H*).

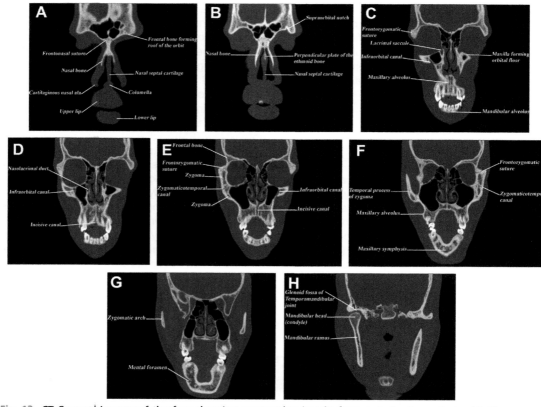

Fig. 13. CT Coronal images of the face showing osseous landmarks from anterior to posterior (A–H).

buttresses (also called the key ridges) transfer most of the masticatory forces. Some of the masticatory forces transmitted to the ZM buttress are dissipated through the zygomatic arch as well as the frontal bone. The ramus of the mandible imparts some force directly to the skull base through the condylar head and glenoid fossa but it serves mainly to transfer masticatory forces to the maxilla.[11]

The horizontal facial buttresses are less well known. However, they act to stabilize the facial skeleton and define the anteroposterior and horizontal dimensions of the face. The superior horizontal buttress is the frontal bar, made of the superior orbital rims and the frontal bone between them. The middle buttress is the most important one, made of the zygomatic arch, zygomatic bone, and inferior orbital rim. This buttress is extremely important in defining the anteroposterior position of the malar eminence, which is crucial for symmetric facial form. The arch of the hard palate and the arch of the mandible (angle, body, and symphysis) form 2 lower horizontal facial buttresses that are important in defining the width of the lower third of the face and occlusal arch.[11]

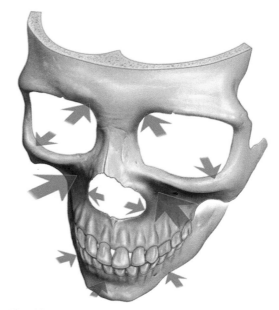

Fig. 14. Frontal left oblique view of the face bones showing the growth changes of the face with age. Mendelson B, Wong CH. Changes in the facial skeleton with aging: implications and clinical applications in facial rejuvenation. Aesthetic Plast Surg. 2012 Aug;36(4):753-60.

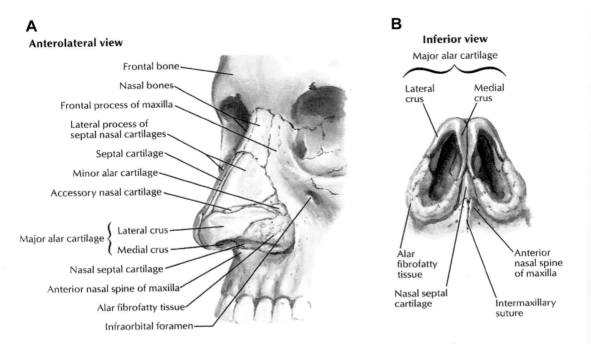

Fig. 15. Left anterior lateral view (*A*) and an inferior view (*B*) of the nasal cartilages and soft tissues. (*Modified from* Frank H. Netter, MD. Atlas of Human Anatomy, 5th edition Saunders Elsevier 2011, Philadelphia. Plate 35.)

The nose is the most protruding part of the face that is part of the respiratory system. The nose is made of the nasal bones as well as the cartilages. The osseous construct of the nose is provided primarily by the maxilla and frontal bones. The nasal part of the frontal bone creates the superior aspect of the nose. Paired nasal bones articulate with the nasal part of the frontal bone on each side superiorly and the frontal process of the maxilla and the lacrimal bones laterally. The nose is also made up of cartilages, mainly contributed by the septal, lateral, major, and minor alar cartilages. Fig. 15 shows the nasal cartilages and bones in detail. The major alar cartilage assists in forming the nasal vestibule, which is bounded laterally by the ala, medially by the columella and the septum.

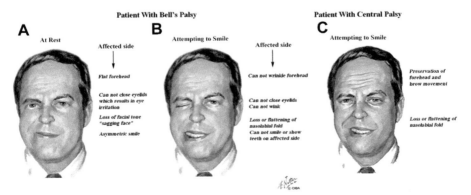

Fig. 16. Frontal drawings of a patient with a Bell's palsy both at rest (*A*) and when attempting to smile (*B*). In (*C*), the drawing shows the preservation of the forehead and brow movement in a central facial palsy due to the bilateral innervation of the upper face. *From* Netter's Clinical Anatomy. Edited by Hansen JT and Lambert DR. Icon Learning Systems, Carlstadt, New Jersey. 2005, figure 555.

Facial Paralysis

Because the innervation of upper face is bilateral while the innervation of the lower face is from the contralateral motor center, when there is a peripheral facial nerve dysfunction, the ipsilateral face is paralyzed. However, when there is a central facial nerve dysfunction, the forehead and brow movements are preserved. These findings are summarized in Fig. 16.

CLINICS CARE POINTS

- Unlike other muscles in the body that are separated and enveloped by fascial layers, most of these mimic muscles originate from the bone and insert into the dermis through the superficial musculoaponeurotic system.
- Three facial muscles do not originate from the facial bones: the frontalis, risorius, and malaris muscles.
- The Facial Action Coding System catalogs these facial movements, assigning an action unit to each distinct movement.

REFERENCES

1. Ghassemi A, Prescher A, Riediger D, et al. Anatomy of the SMAS revisited. Aesthetic Plast Surg 2003; 27(4):258–64.
2. Macchi V, Porionato A, Stecco C, et al. Hidtotpographic study of the fibroadipose connectivecheek system. CellsTissue Organs 2010;191(1):47–56.
3. Sandulescu T, Buechner H, Rauscher D, et al. e. Histological, SEM and three-dimensional Analysis ofthe Midfacial SMAS-New Morphological Soft Tissue. Ann Anat 2019;222:70–8.
4. Mitz V, Peyronie M. The superficial musculo-aponeurotic system (SMAS) in the parotid and cheek area. Plast Reconstr Surg 1976;58:80–8.
5. Sandulescu T, Blaurock-Sandulescu T, Buechner H, et al. Three-dimensional reconstruction of the suborbicularis oculi fat and the infraorbital soft tissue. JPRAS open 2018;16:6–19.
6. Som P, Stuchen C, CY T, et al. The MR Imaging Identification of the Facial Muscles and the Subcutaneous Musculoaponeurotic System. Neurographics 2012;2:35–43.
7. Bentsianov B, Blitzer A. Facial anatomy. Clin Dermatol 2004;22(1):3–13.
8. Siemionow M, Sonmez E. Face as an organ:the functional anatomy of the face. In: Siemionow M, editor. The know-how of the face transplantation. London: Saunders; 2011. p. 3–11.
9. Greco J, Skvarka C. Surgical anatomy of the head ands neck. In: Vidimos A, Ammirati C, Poblete-Lopez C, editors. Dermatologic suregery: requisites in dermatology. Philadelphia: Saunders; 2009. p. 1040.
10. Maruer T, Tuna Y, Demirci S. Facial anatomy. Clin Dermatol 2014;32:14–23.
11. Funk J. Applied facial anatomy. Bony buttresses of the facial skeleton. Available at: https://medicine.uiowa.edu/iowaprotocols/facial-fracture-management-handbook-applied-anatomy. Accessed July 16, 2022.
12. Dreizin D, Nam AJ, Diaconu SC, et al. , Bodanapally UK, Munera F. Radiographics. Multidetector CT Midfacial Fractures: Classification Syst Principles Reduction, Common Complications 2018;38(1): 248–74. https://doi.org/10.1148/rg.2018170074.

Anatomy of the Mandible, Temporomandibular Joint, and Dentition

David C. Hatcher, DDS, MSc, MRCD(C)[a,b,c,d,]*

KEYWORDS

- Tempormandibular joint • TMJ and mandibular biomechanics • Dentition • Mandible
- Masticatory muscles

KEY POINTS

- Functional interactions between teeth, mandible, and tempormandibular joints (TMJs).
- TMJ hard and soft tissue spatial relationships.
- TM Joint capsule and ligaments supply functional stability for the TMJ.

INTRODUCTION

Oral behavior encompasses active movement of the oral structures. The range and quality of oral behavior is essential for establishing and maintaining health and well-being. Key oral behaviors include breathing, chewing, swallowing, and speech. Key hard tissue elements involved in oral behavior include the mandible, temporomandibular joints (TMJs), and dentition. This article will discuss the interaction of the hard tissue elements and selected soft tissue elements associated with oral behavior (Fig. 1).

The craniofacial structures are composed of a series of interconnected anatomic elements, including the mandible, teeth, TMJs, muscles, and central nervous system (see Fig. 1). Numerical modeling has shown that the functional interaction of the anatomic elements generates and propagates stresses and strains throughout craniofacial structures.[1–3] These stresses and resulting strains provide functional signals that can modulate tissue differentiation, growth, development, modeling, remodeling, and tissue breakdown.[4–6] Variability of neuromuscular interactions and genetic and epigenetic influences on facial growth may contribute to a range of morphologic outcomes. Intramembranous ossification occurs at the subperiosteal bony surfaces and endochondral bone formation occurs at the articular surfaces of the TMJs in response to functional stresses. These ossification phenomena are associated with size and shape changes of the mandible and the articular tissues. The changes in skeletal features that occur during growth, development, and aging are referred to as skeletal ontogeny.

MANDIBULAR ANATOMY

The mandible is the largest bone in the human skull, has a parabolic shape, houses the lower teeth, and articulates with the maxillary teeth and temporal bone. Imaging goals for the mandible include visualizing the osseous and dental structures in planes aligned to the mandible's parabolic shape.

Muscle, ligament, and tendon insertions into the mandible create ridges, depressions and

a Arthur A Dugoni School of Dentistry, University of the Pacific, Orthodontic Department, 155 5th Street, San Francisco, CA 94103-2919, USA; b Orofacial Sciences, School of Dentistry, University of California, 707 Parnassus Avenue, San Francisco, CA 94143, USA; c School of Dentistry, University of California, Department of Oral and Maxillofacial Radiology, 10833 Le Conte Avenue, Los Angeles, CA 90095, USA; d Department of Surgical & Radiological Sciences, School of Veterinary Medicine, University of California, 1 Garrod Drive, Davis, CA 95616, USA
* Corresponding author. 99 Scripps Drive, Suite 101, Sacramento, CA 95825.
E-mail address: David@ddicenters.com

Neuroimag Clin N Am 32 (2022) 749–761
https://doi.org/10.1016/j.nic.2022.07.009

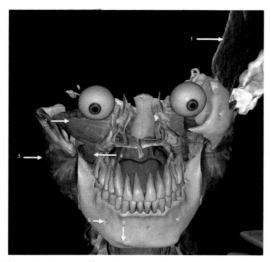

Fig. 1. Human male cadaver rendered to visualize the relative positions of selected muscles of mastication, mandible, temporomandibular joint, and dentition: (1) left temporalis muscle, (2) right lateral pterygoid muscle, (3) right superficial masseter muscle, (4) right medial pterygoid muscle, (5) right mental foramen, and (6) right mental protuberance. (*Courtesy of* Anatomage anatomy table, San Jose, CA.)

prominences including the coronoid processes, genial tubercles, mylohyoid ridge, gonial angles, antegonial notches, mental tubercles, pterygoid fovea, digastric fossa, and lingula (see Fig. 1; Figs. 2–4).[7] The temporalis muscle has a broad

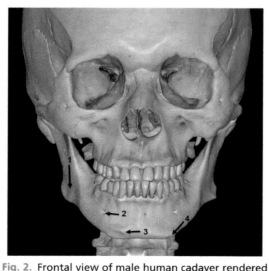

Fig. 2. Frontal view of male human cadaver rendered to visualize the skeleton and selected anatomic structures: (1) shallow depression is attachment site of the right superficial masseter muscle, (2) right mental foramen, (3) right mental turbercle, and (4) left mental tubercle. (*Courtesy of* Anatomage anatomy table, San Jose, CA.)

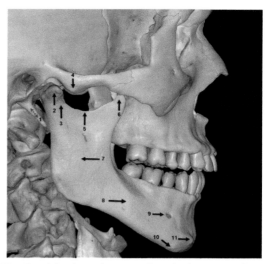

Fig. 3. Right lateral view of male human cadaver rendered to visualize the skeleton and selected anatomic structures: (1) styloid process, (2) lateral pole of condyle, (3) neck of mandible, (4) articular tubercle, (5) sigmoid notch, (6) coronoid process, (7) mandibular ramus, (8) mandibular body, (9) mental foramen, (10) right mental tubercle, and (11) mental protuberance. (*Courtesy of* Anatomage anatomy table, San Jose, CA.)

attachment around the coronoid process and the deep and superficial masseter muscles attach laterally along the gonial angle, antegonial notch, and ramus (Figs. 5 and 6). The medial pterygoid muscle attaches along the medial surface of the ramus and closely mirrors the position of the masseter muscles (see Fig. 6). The inferior and most of the superior lateral pterygoid muscle fibers attach to the condylar fovea located along the anteromedial region of the condyle (Fig. 7). The superior portion of the lateral pterygoid muscle attaches to the fovea region of the condyle superior to the inferior portion of the lateral pterygoid. Some fibers of the superior lateral pterygoid muscle insert into the capsule and/or articular disc.

The mandible has an outer cortical border and internally contains cancellous bone. The mandibular canal contains the inferior alveolar nerve (IAN) and blood vessels. The proximal end of the IAN passes through foramen ovale and enters the mandible through the mandibular foramen located on the medial side of the midramus region of the mandible (see Fig. 4). The IAN is the third division of fifth cranial nerve (V_3) and contains sensory fibers that innervate the mandible, teeth, and adjacent soft tissues. The mental foramen transmits the distal end of the intra-bony segment of the IAN and is typically located on the lateral

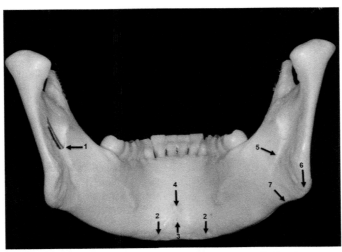

Fig. 4. A posterior photograph of an adult human mandible: (1) Mandibular foramen, (2) digastric fossa, (3) genial turbercles, (4) lingual foramen, (5) mylohyoid ridge, (6) medial side of mandibular angle and attachment site of the medial pterygoid muscle, and (7) antegonial notch.

surface of the mandible inferior to the roots of the bicuspid teeth (Fig. 8). At the mental foramen, the IAN bifurcates into the mental and incisive branches. The mental branch extends through the mental foramen and the incisive branch extends anteriorly inferior to the root apices of the teeth. The alveolar bone is defined as the bone superior to the mandibular canal and the basal bone is inferior to the mandibular canal. The alveolar bone supports the teeth and may contain remnants of tooth germs namely enamel organ, dental

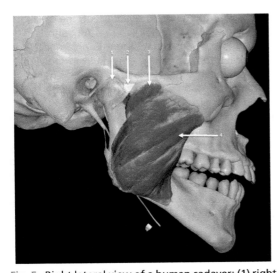

Fig. 5. Right lateral view of a human cadaver: (1) right TMJ capsule, (2) temporomandibular ligament, (3) deep masseter muscle, and (4) superficial masseter muscle. (*Courtesy of* Anatomage anatomy table, San Jose, CA.)

papilla, and dental sac or follicle. The tooth germ cells are derived from the ectoderm of the first pharyngeal arch and the ectomesenchyme of the neural crest and give rise to the teeth. Tooth germ remnants may give rise to odontogenic cysts and tumors.

Mandibular Form

The mandible is derived from embryonic mesenchyme formed in the neural crest cells following migration into the mandibular arch. Omnivores and herbivores have complex mandibular motions including mandibular protrusion, laterotrusion, and posteroinferior rotation of the mandibular symphysis. The occlusal plane in omnivores and herbivores is positioned inferior to the TMJs, and this facilitates the functional movements (see Fig. 5). Carnivores are limited to a downward rotation of the mandibular symphysis around the coupled TMJ rotation axis. The occlusal plane of carnivores is approximately at the same vertical level as the TMJs. The shape of the mandible is likely associated with the biomechanical functional requirements. When compared with carnivores, omnivores including humans have relatively long rami and condylar processes, short coronoid processes, and shallow antegonial notches (Fig. 9). The human mandible has a parabolic shape.

The transverse dimension between the center of the condyles in adults is approximately 100 mm, and the transverse dimensions of the mandible progressively narrow anteriorly. Selected congenital and developmental articular disorders may influence the size and shape of the mandible. The

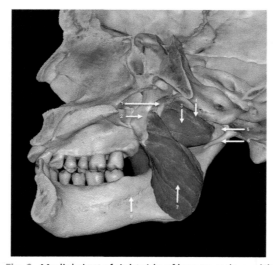

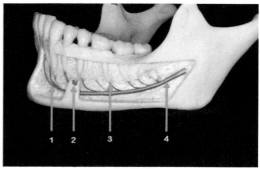

Fig. 8. Lateral view of human mandible demonstrating the neurovascular blood supply and branches of the mandibular canal: (1) incisive branch to supply the anterior mandible, (2) mental branch exiting the mental foramen, (3) dental branches entering the apical foramen of each tooth root, and (4) mandibular canal. The bone superior to the mandibular canal is designated alveolar bone while bone inferior to the mandibular canal is basal bone. (*Courtesy of* Anatomage anatomy table, San Jose, CA.)

Fig. 6. Medial view of right side of human cadaver: (1) lateral pterygoid plate of the sphenoid bone, (2) medial pterygoid plate of the sphenoid bone, (3) inferior lateral pterygoid muscle, (4) superior lateral pterygoid muscle, (5) right condyle, (6) right styloid process, (7) right medial pterygoid muscle, and (8) mylohyoid ridge. (*Courtesy of* Anatomage anatomy table, San Jose, CA.)

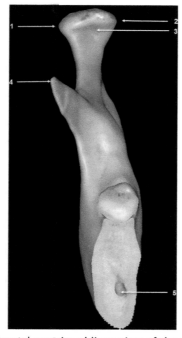

Fig. 7. Frontal superior oblique view of the posterior portion of the right side of the mandible: (1) lateral pole of the condyle, (2) medial pole of the condyle, (3) pterygoid fovea, (4) tip of right coronoid process, and (5) mandibular canal.

initiation of an asymmetrical mandible can begin with TMJ anomalies responsible for the enlargement or reduction in size of the osseous TMJ components. The regional expression of an asymmetry of an underdeveloped side can be described by the following features: small condylar process (condyle and neck), short ascending ramus, vertical shortening of the body of the mandible, diminished lateral development of the mandible, change in mandibular posture, elevation of the occlusal plane on the ipsilateral side, steepening of the mandibular plane, and shifting of the osseous midline of the mandible to the short side (Fig. 10).[8–14] Conversely, there is enlargement of the ipsilateral half of the mandible in individuals with condylar hyperplasia (Fig. 11).[8,9] There is a continuum of shape changes associated with mandibular size. In general, the convexity of the lower and posterior borders of the mandible are directly proportional to the size of the mandible. The antegonial notch will be exceptionally concave in individuals with a small mandible and less concave or convex in individuals with very large mandibles. Similarly, in small mandibles, there is a tendency toward steep mandibular plane angles (MPAs) and obtuse gonial angles (Fig. 12).[8,9]

The vertical dimensions of the anterior region of the mandible in individuals with a steep mandibular plane are large while the labiolingual dimensions of the alveolar bone are small. The osseous midline of an asymmetrical mandible is shifted to the short side.

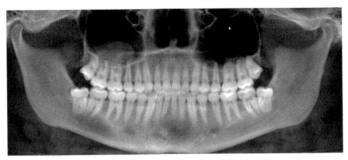

Fig. 9. A panoramic view reconstructed from a cone beam CT (CBCT) scan for an adult woman. All 32 teeth are present but teeth #s 16 (maxillary left third molar), 17 (mandibular left third molar), and 32 (mandibular right third) molar are impacted. A CBCT reconstructed panoramic projection is a curved slab that encompasses the full thickness of the osseous components of the mandible. One advantage of this projection is the simultaneous visualization of the opposing teeth in occlusion and the condyles within the fossa.

Patterns of Mandibular Growth

Mandibular growth uses both endochondral and intramembranous bone formation. Growth and adaptation occur through periosteal stimulated modeling of the cortical bone. Although under function sagittal, transverse and torsional flexion create high subperiosteal regions of strain through compression or tension. Subperiosteal compression, tension, and torsion induce mesenchymal cells to differentiate producing osteoblasts and result in modeling changes to the size and shape of the mandible to achieve optimum strain. The mandible may increase its dimension in a vector aligned with the bending direction to resist the stresses. The cross-sectional dimension of the mandible may adapt to form a circular shape to resist torsional forces.[3]

Facial growth or skeletal growth patterns can be classified using the MPA. The MPA is created by forming an angle between the mandibular plane (Gonion-Menton) and Sella-Nasion. There is a continuum of MPAs that are divided into 3 basic classifications. An average MPA is 30° to 38°, a low angle is less than or equal to 29° and a high angle is greater than 39°. The naming conventions for MPA are brachyfacial for low angle (hypodivergent), mesiofacial for average (normodivergent), and dolichofacial for steep MPAs (hyperdivergent). The right-side lateral view of mesiofacial and brachyfacial individuals show a counterclockwise facial growth pattern (chin has an anterosuperior vector of growth), whereas the dolichofacial individual has a clockwise facial growth pattern (chin has a posteroinferior growth vector; see **Fig. 12**). Individuals with a dolichofacial growth have a greater probability of having an associated TMJ anomaly, anterior open bite, large anterior face height, anteroposterior narrowing of the oropharyngeal airway, and labiolingual thinning of the alveolar bone supporting the mandibular anterior teeth.

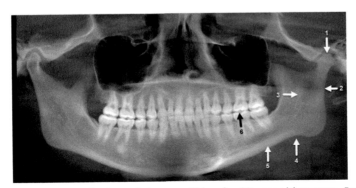

Fig. 10. CBCT reconstructed panoramic view of the mandible of a 30-year-old woman. Patient had a developmental onset of a degenerative disorder involving the left TMJ. The regional effects include alterations of the size and shape of the left half of the mandible: (1) small left condyle and neck, (2) exaggerated concavity of posterior border of mandible, (3) short ramus, (4) deep antegonial notch, (5) thickened lower border cortex and short vertical dimension of the body, and (6) elevated occlusal plane.[8,9,19]

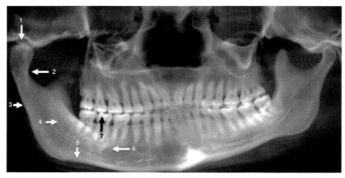

Fig. 11. CBCT reconstructed panoramic view of the mandible in an adult woman with a right-sided condylar hyperplasia (also known as hemimandibular hyperplasia). The key features include (1) large right condyle relative to the contralateral condyle and ipsilateral fossa, (2) elongated neck, (3) flattening of the posterior surface concavity, (4) elongated ramus, (5) shallowing of the antegonial notch, (6) increased vertical dimension of the body, and (7) depressed occlusal plane.[8,20]

TEMPOROMANDIBULAR JOINT

Diagnostic imaging goals for the TMJs include the assessment of the size, shape, quality and open/closed mouth spatial relationships of the osseous and soft tissues of TMJ components. The TMJ is anatomically and biomechanically complex and can influence the growth of the mandible and other craniofacial structures.[15] TMJ function includes essential participation in breathing, chewing, swallowing, speech, and all oral behavior such as lip licking, coughing, and sneezing. The TMJ is one of the most frequently used joints in the human body and the incidence of degenerative disorders is comparable to the knee. TMJ dysfunction causes pain and disability in 20% to 25% of adults.[16]

Temporomandibular Joint Anatomy

Similar to the knee, the TMJ is an arthrodial hinge joint with 2 articulating noncommunicating joint compartments separated by an articular disc.[16] The mandibular condyle translates in an anteroinferior direction during function. There is a mutual but not necessarily symmetric kinematic action between the right and left condyles during function.

In axial view, the condyle has an ellipsoid shape and the mediolateral dimension is approximately 18 to 23 mm, whereas the anteroposterior dimension is approximately 8 to 10 mm. A normal condylar shape in a coronal or coronal oblique view may be convex, flat, angular, or round (Figs. 13 and 14). The anteromedial surface of the condyle inferior to the articular cartilage is mildly concave and is called the pterygoid fovea (see Fig. 7). The superior and inferior lateral pterygoid muscles insert into the pterygoid fovea. The mediolateral long axis of the condyle has an internal rotation angle (lateral pole anterior to medial pole) of approximately 20° to 25°. The internal rotation angle often steepens in individuals with small condyles. The glenoid fossa (mandibular fossa) is the site of the condylar articulation and is an ovoid depression in the inferior surface of the squamous portion of the temporal bone. The

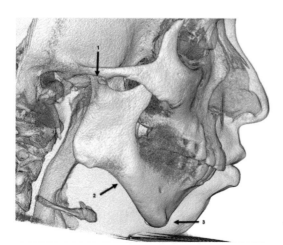

Fig. 12. Volume-rendered CBCT showing a lateral view of the craniofacial skeleton. Patient is a 28-year-old man with juvenile idiopathic arthritis. The mandible is small in all dimensions. (1) Small condyle and neck. The opposing eminence is flat and forms a horizontal incline. The condyle is anteriorly positioned on the skull base. (2) The mandibular plane is steep (dolichofacial). (3) The chin is posterior and inferior to the normal position indicating a clockwise facial growth pattern.[8,21]

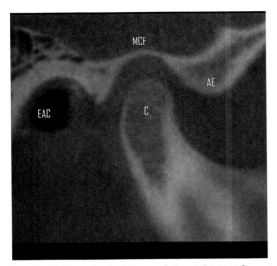

Fig. 13. CBCT sagittal oblique of the right TMJ from a young man. AE, articular eminence crest; C, condyle; EAC, external auditory canal; MCF, middle cranial fossa. This is a normal TMJ demonstrating that the osseous components are smooth, rounded, and without evidence of subchondral defects. The condyle is relatively centered within the glenoid fossa and the resultant joint space is within normal limits.

long axis of the fossa is oriented in an oblique mediolateral direction.

The glenoid fossa is immediately anterior to the external auditory meatus. The roof of the glenoid fossa is a thin layer of cortical bone that separates it from the middle cranial fossa. The roof and portions of the posterior wall of the glenoid fossa are

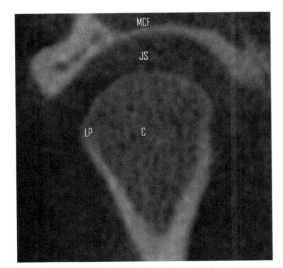

Fig. 14. CBCT coronal oblique for of the right TMJ from a young man. C, condyle; JS, joint space; LP, lateral pole of condyle; MCF, middle cranial fossa. The osseous components are normal.

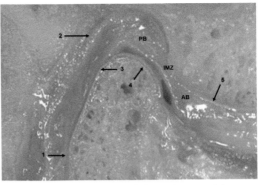

Fig. 15. A cadaver section of the right TMJ: (1) Posteroinferior anatomic boundary of the right TMJ. The inferior lamina and capsule attach at this site. (2) Superior lamina of the bilaminar zone, (3) Inferior lamina, (4) Condylar articular fibrocartilage (5) Eminence fibrocartilage, (PB) Posterior band of the disc, (IMZ) Intermediate zone of the disc, (AB) anterior band of the disc. Image courtesy of Dr. Terry Tanaka, Chula Vista, Ca

lined by periosteum. The articular eminence is a convex prominence that forms the anterior limit of the glenoid fossa. The posterior slope and crest of the articular eminence are lined by articular

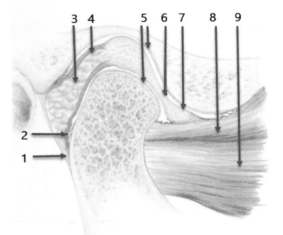

Fig. 17. Figure 16. Sagittal graphic of the right TMJ demonstrating the osseous and soft tissues: (1) Posteroinferior margin of the TMJ shows convergence of the capsule, inferior lamina and the condyle. (2) Synovium (3) Neural vascular tissues in the bilaminar zone, (4) superior lamina, (5) articular fibrocartilage lining the articular regions of the condyle and eminence, (6) Intermediate zone of the articular disc, (7) Anterior band of the articular disc, (8) Super lateral pterygoid muscle, (9) Inferior lateral pterygoid muscle. The disc is normally positioned between the condylar and temporal components of the TMJ.

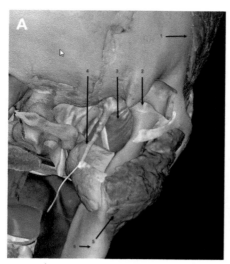
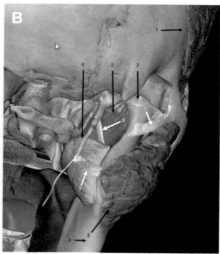

Fig. 17. Posterior oblique view of female cadaver rendered to visualize the skeleton and selected anatomic structures. Figure A: (1) Temporalis muscle (2) Posterior view of left TMJ capsule, (3) Inferior lateral pterygoid muscle shown in blue near the attachment to the condyle, (4) Medial Pterygoid muscle shown in green (5) Superficial masseter muscle, (6) inferior border of mandible. Figure B: Ligaments: (7) Temporomandibular ligament, (8) Sphenomandibular ligament, (9) Stylomandibular ligament. Image courtesy of Anatomage anatomy table, San Jose, Ca)

fibrocartilage, and they brace the condyle during functional movements. The articular tubercle is a small inferior projecting prominence extending from the lateral side of the eminence crest (Figs.

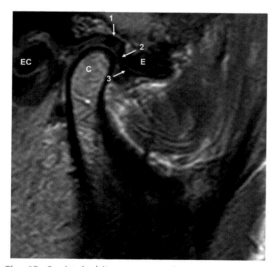

Fig. 18. Sagittal oblique proton density MR imaging of the right TMJ in closed position. (1) Posterior band of the disc located near the 12 o'clock position of the adjacent condyle, (2) intermediate zone of disc, (3) anterior band of the disc, ear canal (EC), condyle (C). The osseous components of the mandible are smooth, rounded with a normal low signal rim and subchondral bone marrow signal. The disc is normally positioned so that the functional portion of the condyle is opposing the intermediate zone of the disc.

15 and 16). The temporomandibular ligament attaches to the articular tubercle (see Fig. 16). The squamotympanic fissure extends posterosuperiorly from the posterior region of the glenoid fossa. The temporosphenoid fissure extends mediosuperiorly from the medial region of the glenoid fossa. The petrotympanic fissure extends posterosuperiorly from the medial region of the glenoid fossa toward the middle ear.

Tempormandibular Joint Capsule and Mandibular Ligaments

Joint stability and protection are aided by the joint capsule and surrounding ligaments. The capsule is a nonelastic fibrous membrane surrounding the TMJ that limits inferior displacement of the mandible.

The temporomandibular, sphenomandibular, stylomandibular ligaments and the joint capsule limit, and guide condylar and mandibular movements (Fig. 17). The temporomandibular ligament is located along the lateral side of the joint capsule and extends anterosuperiorly from the posterior portion of the condylar neck to the eminence tubercle. The temporomandibular ligament prevents inferior and posterior displacement of the condyle and guides the condyle during arcuate translation along the posterior slope of the eminence.

The origin site of the sphenomandibular ligament is the spine of sphenoid bone and the insertion site is the lingula located superior to the mandibular foramen. The sphenomandibular ligament's role is shielding or protecting the nerves and blood vessels entering the mandibular foramen.

The stylomandibular ligament arises from the styloid process and inserts into the angle of the mandible. The stylomandibular ligament limits anterior protrusion of the mandible.

The discomalleolar ligament extends from the malleus and attaches to the disc and retrodiscal tissues near the region of the petrotympanic fissure. The corda tympani nerve passes through the petrotympanic fissure.

TMJ dynamic loading consists of a complex pattern of compressive, shear, and tensile forces.[15,17] The TMJ disc is biconcave in shape and creates congruity between the mobile condyle and the kinematically stable fossa/eminence. It aids in load dissipation, joint lubrication, nutrition, and smooth and nearly frictionless movements. The disc is centered over the superior and anterior surfaces of the condyle (see **Figs. 15 16** and **18**). The condyle rotates against the inferior surface of the intermediate zone during minor vertical opening motions of the mandible but with wider opening, the disc and condyle translate along a mutually coordinated path (**Figs.** 19 and 20).

The disc is attached to the condyle inferior to the medial and lateral condylar poles by the collateral

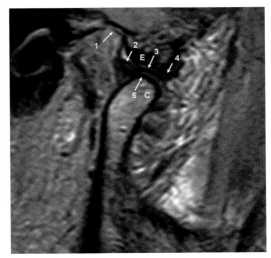

Fig. 20. Sagittal oblique proton density MR imaging of the right TMJ in open position. (1) Superior lamina, (2) posterior band, eminence (E), (3) intermediate zone of disc, (4) anterior band of the disc, (5) low signal rim along the superior surface of the condyle is composed of cortex and articular fibrocartilage, condyle (C). The condyle translated to the crest of the articular eminence with the intermediate zone of the disc interposed between the condyle and eminence.

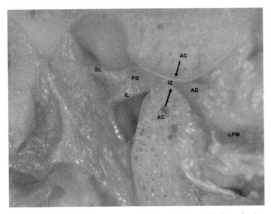

Fig. 19. A cadaver section of the right TMJ simulating an open position of the mandible. AB, anterior band of the disc; AC, articular fibrocartilage lining the surface of the condyle and eminence; IL, inferior lamina of bilaminar zone; IZ, intermediate zone of the disc; LPM, lateral pterygoid muscle; PB, posterior band of the disc; SL, superior lamina of bilaminar zone. In maximum opening, the condyle typically translates the crest of the articular eminence with the intermediate zone of the disc being interposed between the condyle and opposing eminence. Note that the anterior range of PB disc motion lags behind the condylar range of motion. (*Courtesy of* T Tanaka, DDS, Chula Vista, CA.)

ligaments (**Fig. 21**). The attachment points of the medial and lateral collateral ligaments allow the disc to have a "bucket handle" type motion by anteroposteriorly directed pivoting around the attachment points.

In wide opening, the disc anteroposteriorly translates because it is dragged along by the condylar attachments but lags slightly behind the condyle because of the "bucket handle" movements. If tracking the position of the posterior band of the disc (right lateral view), in the closed position, it may be located superior to the 11 to 12 o'clock position of the adjacent condyle, and during maximum opening, the posterior band is posterior to the condyle.

Typically, the kinematic loading path of the condyle along the inferior surface of the disc is in an anteroposterior direction with a mild shift from medial to lateral.

Macroscopic and microscopic anatomy of the disc adapts to meet the biomechanical functional requirements.[15] The collagen fibers in the intermediate zone have an anteroposterior orientation, whereas the collagen fibers in the ring-like bands at the perimeter of the disc, including the anterior and posterior bands, are aligned along the long axis of the band. The collagen fibers are principally aligned in a tensile direction. The ring of collagen at the

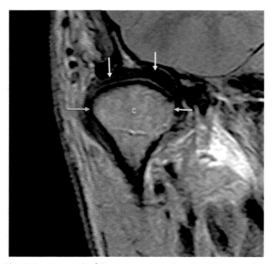

Fig. 21. Coronal oblique proton density MR imaging of the right TMJ in the closed position. The disc (*White arrows*) is mediolaterally centered on the superior surface of the condyle (C). The disc attached inferior to the lateral pole (*orange arrow*) and medial pole (*yellow arrow*) by the collateral ligaments to form a "bucket handle" attachment.

periphery forming the bands of the disc is thought to allow the disc to endure radial and circumferential stresses during condylar rotation and translation. The disc has viscoelastic type properties and is principally comprising collagen, elastin, proteoglycans, glycosaminoglycans, and water (66%–80%). The disc is avascular and aneural.

The posterior attachment to the disc is innervated by the auriculotemporal nerve and vascularized by branches of the superficial temporal and internal maxillary arteries. In addition, the medullary spaces of the condyle are vascularized by branches of the inferior alveolar artery. The disc and disc attachments create separate fluid tight superior and inferior joint compartments. The

posterior and anterior recesses of these compartments are lined by a synovial membrane (see Fig. 15). The posterior attachment to the disc is also referred to as the bilaminar zone owing to the presence of a superior and inferior lamina at the margins. The superior lamina contains fibroelastic tissues and extends from the squamotympanic fissure to the posterosuperior margin of the disc. The inferior lamina is composed of collagen and extends from the posteroinferior margin of the disc to the attachment junction of the capsule with the neck of the condyle. During condylar translation, blood shunts in and out of the loose connective tissues sandwiched between the superior and inferior lamina.

Temporomandibular Joint Biomechanics

Numerical modeling of the jaws has validated the presence of joint loads at all times. The articular surfaces the TMJs are designed for load bearing, whereas the appendicular joints are designed for weight-bearing. The fibrocartilage articular surfaces of the TMJ contain type I and type II collagen and possess the ability to withstand compressive, shear and tensile forces needed during translational motions of the condyle.[15]

The appendicular synovial joints are covered by hyaline or type II cartilage that is most suited to compressive or weight-bearing forces. The geometry of the jaws, masticatory muscles, and dentition coupled with the dynamic function creates unique TM joint loads and load vectors. The peak loads and accumulated history of repetitive loads initiates and maintain TMJ anatomic morphologic changes. The growth (size and shape) of the condyle and opposing articular eminence are driven by the dynamic joint loading patterns. The joint loads are derived from an interactive collaboration between the central nervous system, masticatory muscles, jaw size, jaw shape, tooth

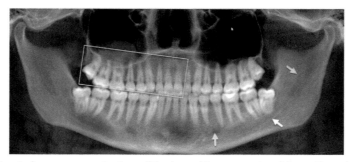

Fig. 22. CBCT reconstructed as a panoramic view of the jaws. (*Orange rectangle*) maxillary right quadrant displaying teeth #s 1 (third molar) to tooth # 8 (central incisor). The left mandibular canal (*white arrow*) and the proximal and distal foramina are indicated with an orange arrow for the mandibular foramen and yellow arrow for the mental foramen.

position, disc position, dental articulation, and the TMJs. The TMJ is a growth site that can enlarge and maintain an ideal size and shape through endochondral bone formation. The endochondral growth allows for the preservation under function of the articular tissues along the anterosuperior surfaces of the condyle and the posterior slope of the articular eminence.

TMJ degenerative disorders involve the loss of articular tissues and occur when the adaptive capacity of the articular tissues is exceeded by the functional demands. Disc disease is a precursor to degenerative joint disease (DJD).[8,9,14] In individuals with displaced discs the shear and tensile forces are different than in individuals with a normal disc position.

In the normal position of the disc while the opposing teeth are maximally interdigitated, the posterior margin of the disc, on a right lateral view, is located opposite the 11 or 12 o'clock position of the adjacent condyle (see Figs. 16–18), mediolaterally centered on the condyle (see Fig. 21) and the intermediate zone of the disc is interposed between the functional portion of the condyle (anterosuperior) and opposing eminence.

It is extremely rare to have a posteriorly displaced disc but the disc can partially or totally displace in anterior, lateral, medial, or combinatorial direction, such as, anteromedial and anterolateral directions. Before and following a displaced disc, there are soft tissue changes associated with the disc attachments and to the disc itself. When a disc totally displaces in an anterior direction, the posterior attachment of the disc is repositioned and the functional loading site is shifted from the disc to the disc attachment. Trauma, degenerative disorders, disc displacement, and inflammatory disorders of the TMJ occurring during the period of somatic growth can inhibit growth of the ipsilateral half of the mandible.[9–14] The growth reduction is, in part, related to the damage experienced by the articular cartilage and a change in fate of the undifferentiated mesenchyme.

TEETH

The nomenclature to depict anatomy and locations in the region of the dentition is different than elsewhere in the body. Teeth can be referred to by name or number. There are 32 teeth in the permanent dentition and 20 in the primary dentition.

The dentition is divided into 4 quadrants. Quadrant I is the maxillary right, quadrant II is the maxillary left, quadrant III is mandibular left, and quadrant IV is mandibular right (Fig. 22). Each quadrant contains the same type and number of teeth. Both the primary and permanent dentition

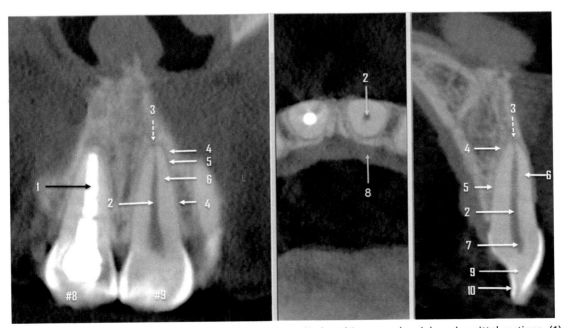

Fig. 23. CBCT of maxillary right and left maxillary incisors displayed in coronal, axial, and sagittal sections. (1) Root canal fill material in tooth #8, (2) unfilled root canal in tooth # 9, (3) apical foramen for tooth # 9, (4) lamina dura, (5) periodontal ligament space, (6) dentin, (7) pulp chamber located in clinical crown region of # 9, (8) palatal soft tissues, (9) dentin located in the coronal region of tooth, (10) enamel.

have a central incisor, lateral incisor, and canine in each quadrant. In addition, the primary dentition has a first and second molar in each quadrant, whereas in the permanent dentition, there is a first and second bicuspid and a first, second, and third molar.

There are 2 systems for numbering teeth: one is the Federation Dentaire International system and the other is the universal system adopted by the United States and will be presented here. In the Universal system, the primary teeth can be indicated with an alphabet letter (A–T) beginning with the maxillary right second molar (Tooth A) and continuing to the maxillary left second molar (tooth J). The mandibular left second molar is tooth K, and the lettering is continuous to the mandibular right second molar (tooth T). In the universal system, the permanent teeth are indicated by a number from 1 to 32 with # 1 being the maxillary right third molar and numbering continues along the maxillary arch to #16 the maxillary right third molar. Tooth # 17 is the mandibular left third molar and the counting continues along the arch to #32 the mandibular right third molar.

Common nomenclature to indicate tooth surfaces are facial/lingual, mesial/distal, and occlusal/incisal. The interproximal surface of a tooth closest to the midline is called the mesial surface, whereas the interproximal surface of a tooth away from the midline is called the distal surface. The lingual tooth surface faces the tongue, whereas the labial or buccal surface faces the lips/cheek. The occlusal surface of a tooth is the articulating surface of the posterior teeth, whereas incisal is the articulating surface of the anterior teeth.

Tooth Anatomy

Each tooth comprises 4 types of dental tissues named enamel, dentin, cementum, and pulp (Fig. 23).[18] Pulpal tissue (pulp chamber and root canal) contains soft tissues and has the lowest attenuation value within the tooth and is located in the central region of the tooth root and crown. The pulp and root canals supply the sensory and blood supply to each tooth.

The neurovascular supply for each tooth enters the root through a small foramen located at the root apex (see Fig. 8). Dentin and cementum have a similar attenuation value while enamel has the highest.

Enamel is the outer tooth layer and surrounds the crown of the tooth, whereas cementum is the outer tooth layer surrounding the root. The anatomic crown is the portion of the tooth that is covered by enamel, whereas the clinical crown is clinically visible portion of the enamel.

Dentin is the inner layer sandwiched between the enamel or cementum and the pulpal tissues. The inferior margin of the enamel abuts the cementum and is referred to as the cementoenamel junction. Similarly, the site where the enamel abuts the dentin is referred to as the dentinoenamel junction.

Periodontium comprises the gingiva, alveolar bone, and uniformly thin periodontal ligament (PDL) that surround the tooth roots. The PDL contains fibers that attach the root to the surface of alveolar socket. The inner surface of the socket has a thin layer of dense bone called the lamina dura. The PDL and lamina dura are anatomic indicators often involved in disease adjacent to a tooth.

Tooth Development and Eruption

Tooth development begins at approximately 20 weeks in utero. The tooth germ (embryonic cells) differentiates into cells that produce dental tissues. The enamel organ produces enamel, the dental papilla contains cells that produce dentin and pulpal tissues, and the dental follicle produces cementoblasts, osteoblasts, and fibroblasts that form cementum, alveolar bone, and the PDL. Tooth formation and eruption are 2 separate events. The primary teeth sequentially erupt with the primary incisors erupting into the mouth between the ages of 6 to 12 months postnatally. All primary teeth are normally erupted with completed root development by the age of 3. Teeth normally erupt into the mouth before the completion of root formation. In the permanent dentition, the root apices fully complete formation approximately 3 years following eruption into the mouth.

CLINICS CARE POINTS

- Mandibular asymmetry may be associated with a temporomandibular joint (TMJ) anomaly
- Steep mandibular plane may be associated with a TMJ anomaly

DISCLOSURE

The author has nothing to disclose.

REFERENCES

1. Hatcher DC, Faulkner MG, Hay A. Development of mechanical and mathematic models to study temporomandibular joint loading. J Prosthet Dent 1986;89: 377.

2. Faulkner MG, Hatcher DC, Hay A. A three dimensional investigation of temporomandibular joint loading. J Biomech 1987;20:997.

3. Korioth TW, Hannam AG. Effect of bilateral asymmetric tooth clenching on load distribution at the mandibular condyles. J Pros Dent 1990;64:62–73.

4. Sommerfeldt DW. Rubin CT Biology of bone and how it orchestrates the form and the function of the skeleton. Eur Spine J 2001;10:S86–95.

5. Carter DR, Beaupre GS. Skeletal Function and Form: Mechanobiology of Skeletal Development, Aging, and Regeneration. New York: Cambridge University Press; 2007. p. 1–31. From and Function.

6. Carter DR, Beaupre GS. Skeletal Function and Form: Mechanobiology of Skeletal Development, Aging, and Regeneration. New York: Cambridge University Press; 2007. p. 31–52. Skeletal Tissue Histomorphology and Mechanics.

7. Tamimi D. Mandible, Specialty Imaging: Temporomandibular Joint. In: Tamimi D, editor. Skeletal Function and Form. Hatcher DC: Elsevier/Amirsys Publishing; 2016. p. 10–37.

8. Tamimi D, Jalali E, Hatcher DC. Temporomandibular Joint Imaging. Radiol Clin North Am 2017;65(a): 157–75.

9. Hatcher DC. Progressive Condylar Resorption: Pathologic Processes and Imaging Considerations. Semin Orthod 2013;19:97–105.

10. Bryndahl F, Legrell PE, Eriksson L, et al. Bilateral TMJ disk displacement induces mandibular retrognathia. J Dent Res 2006;1118–23.

11. Pirttiniemi P, Peltomaki T, Muller L, et al. Abnormal mandibular growth and condylar cartilage. Eur J Orthod 2009;31:1–11.

12. Legrell PE, Isberg A. Mandibular length and midline asymmetry after experimentally induced temporomandibular joint disk displacement in rabbits. Am J Orthod Dentofacial Orthop 1999;115:280–5.

13. Legrell PE, Isberg A. Mandibular height asymmetry following experimentally induced temporomandibular joint disk displacement in rabbits. Oral Surg Oral Med Oral Pathol Oral Radiol Endod 1998;86: 280–5.

14. Legrell PE, Reibel J, Nylander K, et al. Temporomandibular joint condyle changes after surgically induced non-reducing disk displacement in rabbits: a macroscopic study. Acta Odontol Scan 1999;57: 290–300.

15. Huwe LW, Cissel D, Hu J. TMJ Biomechanics and Structure of the Mandibular Condyle. In: Tamimi D, Hatcher DC, editors. Specialty Imaging: Temporomandibular Joint. Philadelphia: Elsevier; 2016. p. 46–9.

16. Bielajew BJ, Donahue RP, Espinosa G, et al. Knee orthopaedics as a template for the temporomandibular joint: pathologies, products, and interventions. Cell Rep Med 2021. https://doi.org/10.1016/j.xcrm. 2021.100241.

17. Katzberg R, Hatcher D, Tamimi D. Fine Structural Details of Disc and Posterior Attachment. In: Tamimi D, Hatcher DC, editors. Specialty imaging: temporomandibular joint. Elsevier/Amirsys Publishing; 2016. p. 486–9.

18. Tamimi D. Teeth. In: Tamimi D, Hatcher DC, editors. Specialty Imaging: Temporomandibular Joint. Philadelphia: Elsevier; 2016.

19. Kasper Dahl Kristensen A, Bjarke Schmidt B, Peter Stoustrup C, Thomas Klit Pedersen D. Idiopathic condylar resorptions: 3-dimensional condylar bony deformation, signs and symptoms. Am J Orthod Dentofacial Orthop 2017;152(2):214–23.

20. Hatcher DC, Koenig LJ. Condylar Hyperplasia. In: Tamimi D, Hatcher DC, editors. Specialty imaging: temporomandibular joint. Elsevier/Amirsys Publishing; 2016. p. 418–23.

21. Shah LM, Hatcher DC. Juvenile Idiopathic Arthritis, Specialty Imaging: Temporomandibular Joint. In: Tamimi D, Hatcher DC, editors. Elsevier/Amirsys Publishing; 2016.

Temporal Bone Anatomy

John C. Benson, MD*, John I. Lane, MD

KEYWORDS

• Temporal bone • Anatomy • CT • MRI

KEY POINTS

- Interpretation of temporal bone imaging requires extensive knowledge of its anatomy across multiple imaging modalities.
- Recent advances in CT and MRI imaging have improved our ability to visualize anatomic details.
- This article highlights the essential anatomy of the temporal bone region, including the osseous landmarks, labyrinthine structures, and transversing nerves and vessels.

INTRODUCTION

Temporal bone anatomy is highly complex and a common source of consternation for radiologists and clinicians alike. Continued advances in high-resolution CT and MR imaging compound the difficulty in mastering the anatomy, as even smaller structures become visible on imaging. More than ever, interpretation of temporal bone imaging requires a thorough knowledge of the three-dimensional relationships between the osseous, nervous, muscular, and vasculature structures that comprise the temporal bone. In this review, we discuss the anatomic features of the temporal bone, with particular attention to the radiologically important structures.

OVERVIEW OF OSSEOUS ANATOMY
Temporal Bone Components

Each of the paired temporal bones is divided into five parts: tympanic, squamous, mastoid, petrous, and styloid. The largest portion is the squamous component, a flat-shaped portion that is the superior-most part of the temporal bone (**Fig. 1**). The squamous component forms the lateral wall of the middle cranial fossa, the roof of the external auditory canal (EAC), and contributes to the glenoid fossa of the temporomandibular joint.[1] From the anteroinferior aspect of the squamous portion

projects the zygomatic process, which articulates with the zygomatic bone.

Just inferior to the squamosal part of the temporal bone is its tympanic component. It forms most of the EAC as well as the posterior surface of the glenoid fossa. The mastoid part, described in greater detail below, is posteroinferior to the squamous portion and more directly posterior to the tympanic part. The groove of the sigmoid sinus identifies the posteromedial aspect of the mastoid portion.

The petrous part of the temporal bone is a pyramidal-shaped ridge, with its wider base near the squamosal and mastoid portions of the bone and its smaller apex located anteromedially. It forms the posterior and anterior portions of the middle and posterior cranial fossae, respectively. The styloid process, a thin osseous structure that serves as the attachment site for multiple tongue and laryngeal muscles, protrudes from the petrous part.

Sutures and Fissures

Numerous sutures run between the temporal bone and adjacent bones of the calvarium. A detailed understanding of this anatomy is important, both because some sutures serve as anatomic landmarks for other structures (eg, the exit pathway of certain nerves) and because the sutures can be confused for acute fractures.[2] Between the

FUNDING INFORMATION: None.

Department of Radiology, Division of Neuroradiology, Mayo Clinic, 723 6th Street, South West, Rochester, MN 55902, USA

* Corresponding author. 723 6th Street. South West, Rochester, MN 55902.

E-mail address: benson.john3@mayo.edu

Neuroimag Clin N Am 32 (2022) 763–775
https://doi.org/10.1016/j.nic.2022.07.010

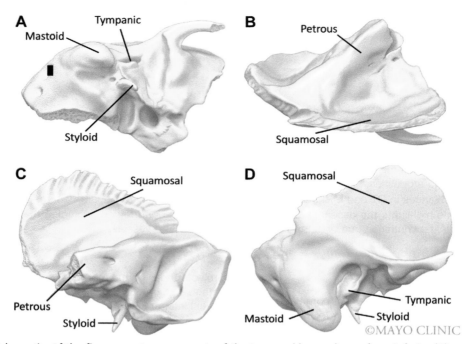

Fig. 1. Schematics of the five separate components of the temporal bone, shown from inferior (*A*), superior (*B*), medial (*C*), and lateral (*D*) views.

temporal bone and adjacent bones lie the occipitomastoid, petrooccipital, zygomaticotemporal, sphenosquamosal, and sphenopetrosal sutures (Fig. 2).

Within the temporal bone, too, there are numerous fissures that are located between the separate parts of the bone. The petrotympanic fissure, for example, connects the tympanic cavity with the infratemporal fossa and is a passageway for the chorda tympani nerve and anterior tympanic artery. On its posterolateral aspect, the petrotympanic fissure continues as the tympanosquamosal fissure anterior to the EAC. The petrosquamosal fissure is continuous with the Koerner septum and appears as a thin partition in the tegmen tympani on coronal images. The tympanomastoid fissure lies just posterior to the EAC and contains a distal segment of Arnold's nerve.[3]

The sphenopetrosal suture and petrotympanic fissure are located relatively close to one another. The osseous proximal aspect of the Eustachian tube is a helpful landmark for distinguishing these structures: the sphenopetrosal suture is located anterior and medial to the Eustachian tube, while the petrotympanic fissure is located lateral to the Eustachian tube. The petrooccipital suture, too, is in relatively close proximity to these structures, but is located most medially and opens into the jugular foramen.

EXTERNAL AUDITORY CANAL AND TYMPANIC MEMBRANE

The EAC is an S-shaped tube that extends from the pinna to the tympanic membrane. Its makeup is mixed: the lateral third is cartilaginous and covered with thicker skin, and the medial two-thirds is osseous. Microscopic openings—not visible on imaging—exist along the anterior portion of the cartilaginous portion, called fissures of Santorini, which permit bidirectional spread of tumor and infection between the EAC and adjacent parotid gland.[4] The anterior EAC wall also forms the posterior part of the glenoid fossa.

The tympanic membrane is a thin, obliquely oriented membrane, typically measuring approximately 10 mm in diameter.[5] It is composed of two parts: the larger pars tensa (located anteroinferiorly) and the smaller pars flaccida (located postero-superiorly). The pars flaccida is composed of a middle layer of loose collagen fibers sandwiched between an external epidermal layer and a mucosal internal layer, while the middle layer of the of the pars tensa is made up of fibrous material. Thus, the aptly named pars tensa and flaccida have differences in robustness, with the tensa being stiffer, and the flaccida relatively fragile.[6] Though the distinction between these regions is not discernible on imaging, the pars flaccida is notably susceptible to perforation, which may lead to the formation of acquired cholesteatomas.

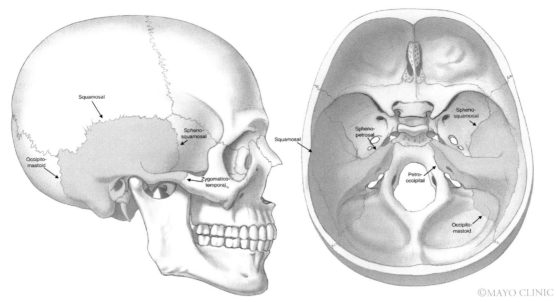

©MAYO CLINIC

Fig. 2. Schematic of the sutures between the temporal bone and adjacent osseous structures.

The tympanic annulus is a fibrocartilaginous thickening of the pars tensa that is anchored at the temporal bone's so-called tympanic sulcus. Superiorly, the pars flaccida attaches to the scutum.[7] The tympanic membrane also connects to the manubrium of the malleus, which pulls the tympanic membrane inward, creating a natural middle ear concavity called the umbo.

MIDDLE EAR AND MASTOID
Tympanic Cavity

The middle ear, also known as the tympanic cavity, is an irregularly shaped air-filled structure located between the EAC and inner ear. It is bound laterally by the tympanic membrane, superiorly by the tegmen tympani, and inferiorly by the jugular wall (also known as the middle ear floor). Its medial wall is made up of different components of the inner ear, including the round and oval windows and the promontory—a convex projection created by the first turn of the cochlea. The middle ear is divided into at least three anatomically distinct compartments, which are defined by their relationship with the tympanic membrane. The hypotympanum, mesotympanum, and epitympanum (also known as the attic) are defined as being inferior to, directly medial to, or superior to the tympanic membrane, respectively (Fig. 3). Some authors also refer to two other compartments: a protympanum—located anterior to the tympanic membrane—and a retrotympanum—located posterior to it. As such, besides the tympanic membrane

and promontory, the mesotympanum is not bound by physical walls.

The epitympanum, or attic, is set immediately above the mesotympanum. Its roof is made up of the tegmen tympani, a fine osseous structure between the tympanic cavity and the overlying middle cranial fossa. The tegmen extends laterally as the tegmen mastoideum, which separates the middle cranial fossa from the mastoid segment of the temporal bone. The anterior aspect of the epitympanum is a distinct region called the anterior epitympanic recess, or supratubal recess. This area is partitioned from the rest of the attic by a tiny osseous plate extending from the tegmen, called the "cog"[8] (Fig. 4). Posterior to this recess, the epitympanum contains the head of the malleus and both the body and short process of incus. The tip of the incudal short process lies within the so-called incudal fossa.

The lateral epitympanic space is also subdivided into regions, including the lateral epitympanic recess (located superiorly) and the Prussak space (located inferiorly). The Prussak space is an important anatomic landmark as it is often the site of cholesteatoma formation. The space is bound laterally by the pars flaccida of the tympanic membrane and scutum, medially by the malleal neck, superiorly by the lateral malleal ligament, and inferiorly by the lateral process of the malleus.

The aditus ad antrum is an aperture that connects the epitympanum to the mastoid antrum ; its title means "entrance to" the antrum. On axial imaging, the aditus is a relatively narrow pathway

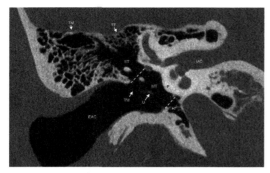

Fig. 3. Boundaries of the tympanic cavity, shown on a coronal CT. The mesotympanum (MT) sits between the tympanic membrane (TM) and promontory (P). The tympanic membrane has a natural concavity into the mesotympanum at its attachment site to the malleus, called the umbo (U). The epitympanum (ET) is above the superior border of the tympanic membrane, while the hypotympanum (HT) is below its inferior border. The roof of the epitympanum is a thin layer of bone called the tegmen tympani (TT); this continues laterally as the tegmen mastoideum (TM) which acts as the roof of the mastoid air cells. Also seen is the EAC and IAC.

set between variably sized mastoid air cells and a rounded eminence formed by the lateral semicircular canal. Together with the larger epitympanum and mastoid antrum that the aditus connects, the structures make a characteristic hourglass shape on axial images.

The hypotympanum, conversely, is located just below the mesotympanum. Along its inferior margin lies the middle ear floor, which is made up of a thin plate of bone called the fundus tympani or jugular plate that lies between the tympani cavity and jugular bulb. The anterior hypotympanum (or protympanum, depending on nomenclature

preference) forms the osseous component of the Eustachian tube, called the tympanic orifice.[9]

The posterior retrotympanic wall is made up of a complex series of protuberances ("crests") and depressions ("sinuses"). The medial retrotympanum, from superior to inferior, includes the posterior sinus (near the oval window), sinus tympani, subtympanic sinus, and hypotympanum. The crests that separate these are the ponticulus (between the posterior sinus and sinus tympani), the subiculum (between the sinus tympani and subtympanic sinus), and the funiculus (between the subtympanic sinus and hypotympanum). The lateral retrotympanum is divided, superiorly to inferiorly, into the facial sinus, lateral tympanic sinus, and hypotympanum, which are separated by the chordiculus and styloid ridge, respectively. However, these anatomic structures tend to be both minute in size and variably present.[10] On CT imaging, radiologists tend to compartmentalize the retrotympanum into the medial sinus tympani (which communicates with the round window niche), the lateral facial recess, and the pyramidal eminence, which separates them.

Ossicles

The ossicular chain consists of three bones that bridge between the tympanic membrane and the oval window.[11] Vibration across these ossicles accounts for more than 90% of sound energy transmission.[12] The malleus, incus, and stapes—from lateral to medial—are connected by minute synovial articulations, named the malleo-incudal and incudo-stapedial joints.[13] These joints, and the subregions of the ossicles, are typically discernible on high-resolution CT imaging.

The malleus is made up of a head and neck, from which three processes project. The

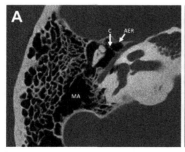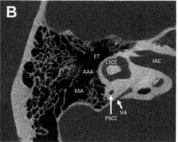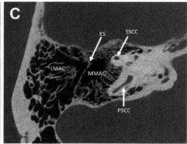

Fig. 4. Epitympanum and mastoid air cells, shown on axial images, from inferior (A) to superior (C). At the level of the short process of the incus, the anterior epitympanum recess (AER) can be seen, separated from the rest of the epitympanum (ET) by a thin ridge of bone called the cog (C). The epitympanum connects to the mastoid antrum (MA) via the aditus ad antrum (AAA), which is bound by the mastoid air cells laterally and the prominence formed by the LSCC medially. Also seen are the PSCC, VA, and IAC (B). Superiorly, Koerner's septum (KS) separates the lateral mastoid air cells (LMAC) and medial mastoid air cells (MMAC). Also seen at this level are the superior semicircular canal (SSCC) and PSCC.

manubrium (also known as the "handle") is the longest and tapers toward its most distal point. Its lateral margin connects to the tympanic membrane, while a slight projection on its medial side serves as the attachment site of the tensor tympani tendon.[7] The lateral and anterior processes are relatively small projections. The lateral process attaches to the tympanic membrane, immediately below the pars flaccida, while the anterior process extends toward the nearby petrotympanic fissure.

The incus is subdivided into three parts. A concavity in its body articulates with the malleus, creating a so-called "ice cream cone sign" appearance on axial CT. Two processes emerge from the body: the short process, which projects posteriorly; and the long process, which projects inferiorly into the mesotympanum. At the far end of the long process is a tiny projection called the lenticular process, which articulates with the stapes.

The stapes is the smallest bone in the human body. Its head, or capitulum, has a concave surface that articulates with the incus at the incudostapedial joint. Connected to the stapedial head is its neck, from which the thin anterior and posterior crura splay within the oval window fossa. Together, these three structures—the head, neck, and crura—form the "superstructure" of the stapes. Its base, or footplate, is connected to the oval window by a rind of connective tissue named the annular ligament (Fig. 5).

Muscles, Tendons, and Ligaments

The two major muscles within the middle ear are the stapedius and tensor tympani. The stapedius muscle, like the ossicle in which it inserts, is the smallest skeletal muscle. It both stabilizes the stapes and serves to dampen excess sound by decreasing ossicular vibration. The muscle emerges from a small foramen at the tip of the pyramidal eminence and inserts into the neck of the stapes.[14] Its belly, located in the temporal bone, sits anterior and medial to the mastoid segment of the facial nerve.[15]

The tensor tympani muscle originates along the superior aspect of the cartilaginous portion of the Eustachian tube. The semicanal in which the muscle sits, together with the Eustachian tube, makes up the two openings into the anterior wall of the tympanic cavity.[16] Both the semicanal and the Eustachian tube run nearly parallel to one another, though the semicanal extends more posteriorly and passes below the genu of the facial nerve canal. From there, it enters the medial aspect of the tympanic cavity just anterior to the oval window. The cochleariform process—a tiny osseous

structure along the anterior tympanic cavity—serves both as a fulcrum for the muscle and a boundary between the muscle and tendon.[17] There, the tensor tympani tendon turns 90° before inserting into the malleal manubrium (Fig. 6). Like the stapedius muscle, the tensor tympani has a protective function against excessive sound.

In addition, four major suspensory ligaments provide support for the ossicles. The incus is held in place by the posterior incudal ligament (divided into both medial and lateral parts), which connects to the short process of the incus from the incudal fossa. The other three ligaments that support the malleus are the anterior, superior, and lateral malleal ligaments. The anterior ligament extends from the malleal head and/or neck to the anterior epitympanic wall; the lateral ligament originates at the malleal neck and inserts into the osseous margin of the tympanic notch; and the superior ligament traverses between the malleal head and the roof of the tympanic cavity (Fig. 7). In addition, medial and lateral incudo-malleal ligaments exist at the first ossicular articulation, though these are often invisible on imaging.[18]

Mastoid

The mastoid part of the temporal bone is highly pneumatized, though the pattern of pneumatization is highly variable between patients.[16] As stated earlier, the mastoid communicates with the epitympanum via the aditus ad antrum. The antrum itself is an airspace, typically 1 to 1.5 cm in size, which is roofed by the tegmen mastoideum. At its margin, the antrum communicates with many of the much smaller-sized mastoid air cells. Also in close proximity to the antrum is the Koerner septum, a thin ridge of bone arising from the petrosquamosal suture, which divides the air cells into lateral and medial compartments.[5]

INNER EAR AND INTERNAL AUDITORY CANAL
Otic Capsule

The term "inner ear" refers to the structures included in the otic capsule (also known as the bony labyrinth) and the membranous labyrinth. The otic capsule is the dense osseous structure that houses the membranous labyrinth. It is divided into three parts (cochlea, vestibular, and semicircular canals) and has four openings (the oval and round windows, and the vestibular and cochlear aqueducts).

The cochlea is spiral-shaped and characteristically makes 2½–2¾ turns from its base to its apex. Each turn is separated by interscalar septae. The modiolus is the central column of bone around which the cochlea spirals. The three

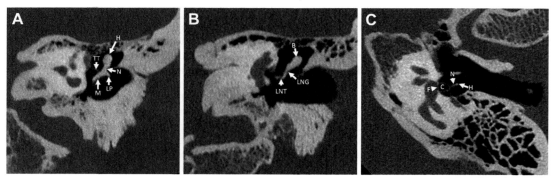

Fig. 5. Ossicular anatomy, shown in images reformatted along the long axes of the malleus (A), incus (B), and stapes (C). The malleus is divided into a bulbous head (H), neck (N), and three processes: the long manubrium (MM), lateral process (LP), and anterior process (not shown). The tensor tympani tendon (TT) is also clearly visible on this image. The subcomponents of the incus include the body (B), long process (LNG), and tiny lenticular process (LNT) which articulates with the stapes; the short process is not shown. The stapes is subdivided into its head (H) and neck (N) which together form the superstructure. The bone then splays into two crura (C placed between them) before terminating at the flat footplate (F) against the oval window.

compartments making up the membranous labyrinth within the cochlea cannot be visualized on CT imaging. However, the delicate osseous spiral lamina, projecting from the modiolus, can be faintly visualized on most images, bisecting through the cochlear turns (Fig. 8).[5] The cochlear aperture is a small foramen at the base of the cochlea, which transmits the cochlear nerve from the adjacent internal auditory canal (IAC).

The vestibule is ovoid in shape. Its internal membranous labyrinth structures are invisible on CT imaging. Anatomically, it is located between the cochlea and the semicircular canals. On its lateral

surface lies the oval window, to which the stapes footplate attaches.

The three semicircular canals—superior (SSCC), lateral (LSCC), and posterior (PSCC) —are attached to the vestibule in anatomic positions that mirror their names. The LSCC typically sits in a plane that is 30° off the true horizontal axis. The superior limb of the PSCC and the posterior limb of the SSCC come together as a common crus near the posteromedial wall of the vestibule. The superior aspect of the SSCC is just inferior to the so-called arcuate eminence—a ridge of bone separating the canal from the overlying middle cranial fossa.

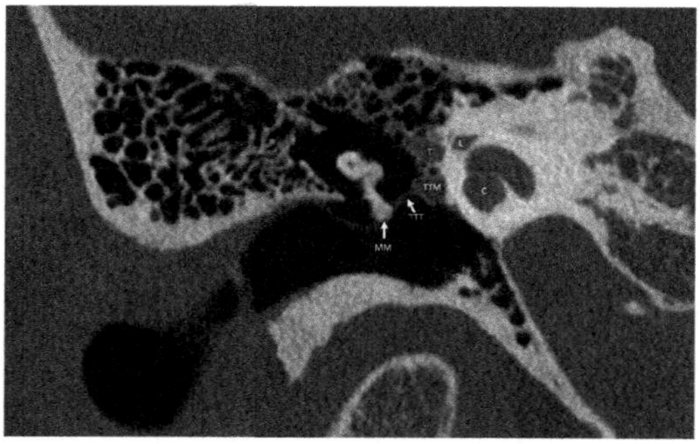

Membranous Labyrinth

Housed within the otic capsule is the membranous labyrinth. It is separated into endolymphatic and perilymphatic spaces, both of which contain fluid by the same name. Within the cochlea, the endolymph-containing scala media is flanked on both sides by the perilymph-containing scala vestibuli and scala tympani. Fluid waves propagate through the oval window into the scala vestibuli and are transmitted to the cochlea apex. There, at the helicotrema, the scala vestibuli meets the scala tympani, which transmits the fluid waves back down the cochlear spirals to the round window. Similar to CT, MR is typically only able to delineate the spiral lamina/basilar membrane complex; the normal scala media is invisible on standard in vivo MR imaging.[19]

In the vestibule, the endolymphatic structures are the saccule and the utricle, connected via the utriculosaccular duct. Both the saccule and the utricle are components of the vestibular system and are responsible for sensing linear

Fig. 6. Tensor tympani, shown on an oblique image reformatted perpendicular to the tendon. At this level, the distal tensor tympani muscle (TTM) is seen along the medial wall of the tympanic cavity. The muscle then hooks around a small osseous process, proceeding as the tensor tympani tendon (TTT) which ultimately attaches to the manubrium of the malleus (MM). In this plane, the tympanic (T) and labyrinthine (L) segments of the facial canal are also seen. Together with the cochlea (C), this anatomic configuration is often referred to as the "snail eyes" view.

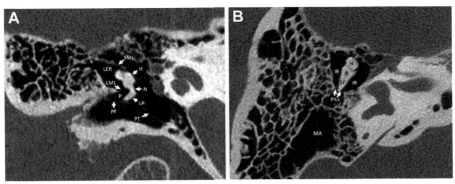

Fig. 7. Suspensory ligaments of the malleus (A) and incus (B). The malleus is supported by the lateral malleal ligament (LML) which attaches to the neck (N) and the superior malleal ligament which attaches to the head (H). In this image, the lateral epitympanum is well defined. Prussak's space (P) is bordered by the lateral process of the malleus (LP), lateral malleal ligament, pars flaccida of the tympanic membrane (PF), and scutum (S). Above Prussak's space is the lateral epitympanic recess (LER). The pars tensa (PT) is also seen. The incus is supported by the medial and lateral posterior incudal ligaments (PILs), which connect to the short process (SP). At this level, the ossicles take on the so-called ice cream cone appearance, in which the body (B) of the incus articulates with the head (H) of the malleus. The short process rests in the similarly shaped incudal recess (IR) of the epitympanum. Also seen is the mastoid antrum (MA).

acceleration. The saccule, located near the cochlea, detects vertical linear acceleration; the utricle, near the semicircular canals, detects horizontal linear acceleration.[20]

The osseous semicircular canals contain three endolymphatic ducts surrounded by perilymphatic fluid. Each duct is dilated at the so-called ampulla, a sac that contains the sensory apparatus. During rotational movement, the relative lag of the endolymph within the ducts deflects the cupula, thereby generating a neurologic response within its embedded hair cells. The cupula, together with the rest of the crista ampullaris that makes up the sensory organ, can sometimes be seen on high resolution MR imaging (Fig. 9).

The endolymphatic and perilymphatic spaces are indistinguishable from one another on standard MR imaging. However, gadolinium preferentially collects within the perilymphatic spaces during both intratympanic gadolinium administration and delayed post-contrast imaging, allowing visualization of the nonenhancing endolymphatic structures.[21–23] Such methods have been employed by some institutions to assess for endolymphatic hydrops in patients suspected of having Meniere's disease. However, these techniques remain outside of the mainstay of imaging in most institutions.

Aqueducts

The vestibular aqueduct (VA) is a J-shaped osseous channel that runs from the vestibule to the posterior cranial fossa near the sigmoid sinus. Within it are the endolymphatic duct and sac, which are thought to play a role in the regulation

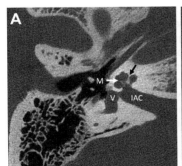
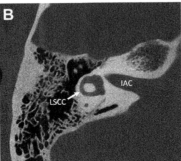
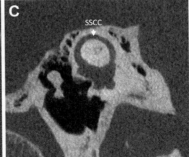

Fig. 8. Various anatomic structures of the otic capsule. Axial (A and B) images show the turns of the cochlea around the modiolus (M). Each turn is separated by an interscalar septum (black arrow). The vestibule (V), LSCC, and IAC are also seen. A Pöschl view (C), often used to assess for semicircular canal dehiscence, clearly delineates the curve of the SSCC.

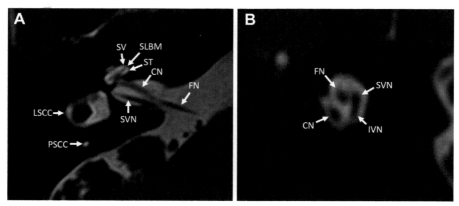

Fig. 9. T2 space MR imaging of the right inner ear and IAC. Axial (A) image demonstrates the cochlear nerve (CN), facial nerve (FN), and superior vestibular nerve as they transverse the IAC. The LSCC and part of the PSCC are also visible. Within the cochlea, the scala vestibuli (SV) is separated from the scala tympani (ST) by the thin spiral lamina/basilar membrane complex (SLBM). An image reformatted perpendicular to the mid-portion of the IAC (B) shows the anterosuperior facial nerve (FN), anteroinferior cochlear nerve (CN), superior vestibular nerve (SVN), and inferior vestibular nerve (IVN). The vestibular nerves are often conjoined at this part of the IAC.

of endolymph fluid.[24] Its origin, in the vestibule, is often invisible on CT imaging. From there, the VA gently widens into the isthmus, which is the curved portion of the aqueduct near the common crus of the semicircular canals. It continues to widen in its straight distal part, ultimately opening at the so-called operculum into the posterior cranial fossa.[25] The VA's size is of particular interest since an enlarged aqueduct is often associated with sensorineural hearing loss. Most commonly, the Cincinnati criteria are used to define normal size: the VA is considered enlarged if it is ≥ 1 mm at the midpoint and/or ≥ 2 mm at the operculum.[26]

The cochlear aqueduct, conversely, contains the perilymphatic duct and thus serves as a potential conduit for perilymphatic fluid, though it is not always patent. It runs obliquely downward from the scala tympani at the base of the cochlea to the jugular foramen. The course of the cochlear aqueduct is divided into four portions: the lateral orifice located near the round window at the scala tympani; the otic capsule segment; the petrous apex segment; and the medial orifice at the jugular foramen. Like the VA, the cochlear aqueduct is funnel-shaped and widens as it gets further from the otic capsule. Its lateral aspects are particularly small, and they are often invisible on imaging (Fig. 10).[27]

Internal Auditory Canal

The IAC is a passageway extending through the petrous segment of the temporal bone. It extends from the porus acusticus—its internal os—to the fundus. The lamina cribosa, located at the fundus,

separates the IAC from the adjacent inner ear vestibule.[28]

The IAC is divided into three canals by the horizontally oriented falciform crest and a vertical bone that divides the upper half of the canal, called Bill's bar. The facial nerve (anterosuperior), cochlear nerve (anteroinferior), and superior and inferior vestibular nerves (posterior) pass through the IAC. In some patients, the nervus intermedius (also known as the nerve of Wrisberg)—a separate root of cranial nerve VII that carries sensory and parasympathetic fibers—is distinctly visible on MR imaging.[29] The labyrinthine artery routinely traverses the IAC. In a minority of patients, a segment of the anterior inferior cerebellar artery loops into the IAC, an anatomic variation of no clinical consequence.[30]

IAC diverticula are a benign normal anatomic variant, occurring in up to 5% of patients.[31] They appear as well-defined lucencies within the anteroinferior IAC. One retrospective series reported an association between IAC diverticula and sensorineural hearing loss, but multiple subsequent studies found no such association.[31–33] IAC diverticula can mimic retrofenestral otosclerosis involving the anteroinferior aspect of the IAC fundus ("cavitary otosclerosis"), prompting close evaluation of the oval window and other more common sites of this disease.

NERVES, FORAMINA, CANALS, AND CLEFTS
Facial Nerve

The facial nerve is segmented into the cisternal, canalicular (also known as meatal), labyrinthine, tympanic, mastoid, and extratemporal portions.[34]

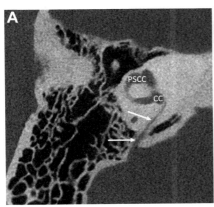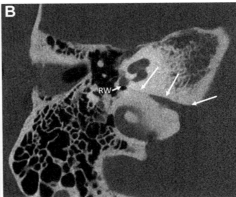

Fig. 10. Long axis views of the vestibular and cochlear aqueducts. The vestibular aqueduct (*A*) extends from the posterior cranial fossa to the vestibule. Along its course, it curves around the common crus (CC) of the semicircular canals. The PSCC is also seen. The cochlear aqueduct (*B*) runs from the jugular foramen to the lateral orifice near the round window (RW). Both structures taper as they near the otic capsule.

The cisternal segment extends from the brainstem, through the cerebellopontine angle, to the porus acousticus of the IAC. The canalicular segment is entirely within the IAC, located in the anterosuperior quadrant. Neither the cisternal nor the canalicular segments give off branches. Once through the internal acoustic meatus—a tiny foramen in the lateral aspect of the IAC—the nerve becomes the labyrinthine segment, traveling within the facial (or Fallopian) canal. The labyrinthine portion of the facial canal, typically about 3 to 5 mm in length, passes by the cochlea and vestibule before bending posteriorly at what is called the "first genu," located at the geniculate ganglion.[35]

Here, at the geniculate ganglion, the facial nerve and nervus intermedius join. Also, three branches arise: the greater superficial petrosal nerve, the lesser petrosal nerve, and the external petrosal nerve. The greater superficial petrosal nerve leaves through a hiatus in the petrous part of the temporal bone, passes through the middle cranial fossa, and joins together with the deep petrosal nerve to form the Vidian nerve within the pterygoid canal. The lesser petrosal nerve—composed of the tympanic branch of Jacobson's nerve, Arnold's nerve (both discussed later), and the nervus intermedius—passes through the hiatus of the lesser petrosal nerve into the middle cranial fossa before exiting the skull, usually through the canaliculus innominatus (a variably present foramen adjacent to the foramen spinosum and foramen ovale).[36] The external petrosal nerve is variably present and supplies sympathetic fibers to the middle meningeal artery.

The tympanic segment, usually 8 to 11 mm in length, travels posteriorly from the geniculate ganglion to the second genu, seen just below the lateral semicircular canal. It lacks any branches. The terminus of the tympanic segment is the second genu, or curve of the Fallopian canal, located posterolateral to the pyramidal process. At the second genu, the orientation of the Fallopian canal becomes vertical. This marks the beginning of the mastoid segment, which travels inferiorly and exits the stylomastoid foramen.

From the mastoid segment of the facial nerve, branches the chorda tympani. In the majority of patients, this branch occurs from the mid-mastoid segment of the facial nerve (**Fig. 11**).[37] From there, the course of the chorda tympani through the temporal bone is divided into three segments. First, within the posterior canaliculus segment, the nerve ascends toward the middle ear. The chorda tympani then traverses the middle ear in its so-called tympanic segment, coursing along the tympanic membrane and between the malleus and incus. This segment is not easily discernible on imaging. The nerve exits the anterior aspect of the middle ear as its anterior canaliculus segment before passing through the petrotympanic fissure. Ultimately, the chorda tympani joins with the lingual nerve, providing an afferent taste sensation from the anterior two-thirds of the tongue.

The mastoid segment of the facial nerve branches out as the nerve to the stapedius, which innervates the stapedius muscle. It also has a branch from the hitchhiking fibers of Arnold's nerve, which provides sensory information from the EAC.

Jacobson's Nerve

Jacobson's nerve is the eponym given to the tympanic branch of the glossopharyngeal nerve. It is

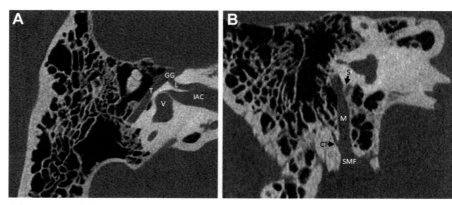

Fig. 11. Facial nerve canal, shown in images reformatted along the course of the proximal (*A*) and distal (*B*) aspects of the canal. Proximally, the labyrinthine segment (L) extends off of the IAC. It curves at the first genu, located at the site of the geniculate ganglion (GG), at which point it becomes the tympanic segment (T). It then curves again at the second genu (not shown) before coursing inferiorly at its mastoid segment (M), ultimately exiting the temporal bone at the stylomastoid foramen (SMF). Tiny channels extending from the mastoid segment hold a branch of the facial nerve innervating the stapedial muscle (S) and the chorda tympani (CT).

the first branch of the glossopharyngeal nerve and arises from the inferior ganglion of cranial nerve IX just below the jugular foramen outlet.[38] The nerve enters the temporal bone via the inferior tympanic canaliculus (also known as Jacobson's canal), located medial to the styloid process and the stylomastoid foramen.[39] Within the inferior tympanic canaliculus, the nerve first follows a vertical course before turning anterolaterally toward the cochlear promontory. The length of the canal is, on average, 9.5 mm.[40] Jacobson's nerve then splays over the promontory as the tympanic plexus, usually located in submucosal grooves on the bone. The parasympathetic fibers of the nerve then exit the middle ear as a contributor to the lesser petrosal nerve. Other branches provide innervation to the Eustachian tube and both oval and round windows.

Clinically, Jacobson's nerve is best known for its association with paragangliomas, which are benign but locally destructive tumors that often occur in the head and neck. Glomus tympanicum tumors—a subset of paragangliomas located along the cochlear promontory—arise from the tympanic plexus of Jacobson's nerve.[41] On imaging, these tumors appear as variably sized soft tissue masses along the promontory, with or without destruction of the adjacent structures. Careful evaluation of such tumors on imaging is needed, as their appearance can mimic that of an aberrant internal carotid artery.[42]

Arnold's Nerve

Arnold's nerve is also known as the auricular branch of the vagus nerve. It arises from the superior ganglion of the vagus nerve, with a minor

contribution from the glossopharyngeal nerve's inferior ganglion. The nerve passes behind the internal jugular vein before entering the mastoid canaliculus, also known as Arnold's canal. This canal travels from the lateral margin of the pars vascularis of the jugular foramen to the mastoid segment of the facial nerve canal.

Historically, Arnold's nerve was best known for the somatovisceral reflexes that occurred following its stimulation. The nerve is sometimes called Alderman's nerve, in reference to the Alderman in the city of London who would dab a napkin dipped in rosewater behind their ears after eating in an effort to aid digestion.[43] Its most recent eponymous name came from Friedrich Arnold, an anatomist who discovered the ear-cough reflex, in which mechanical stimulation of the EAC can activate a cough reflex.[44]

Radiologists should be aware of Arnold's nerve because of its proclivity to form paragangliomas. Paragangliomas are classified by their anatomic location, rather than their nerve root origins. As such, glomus jugulare paragangliomas—those arising within the jugular foramen—can grow from either Arnold's nerve or the proximal aspect of Jacobson's nerve. Because they typically grow superiorly and often invade the tympanic cavity, differentiating between glomus jugulare and glomus tympanicum tumors is often difficult, and such lesions are often referred to as jugulotympanic tumors.[45]

Petromastoid Canal

The petromastoid canal, also known as the subarcuate canaliculus, is a tiny curved osseous channel that extends from the posterior cranial

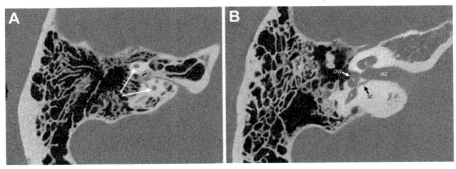

Fig. 12. Petromastoid canal (*A*) and singular canal (*B*), shown in images reformatted along the path of both. The petromastoid, or subarcuate, canal runs from the posterior cranial fossa to the mastoid antrum or adjacent air cells (short red *arrows*). It characteristically passes through the hoop of the superior semicircular canal (long *white arrows*). The singular canal (SC) extends from the posterior IAC to the ampulla of the posterior semicircular canal (P) and transmits a branch of the inferior vestibular nerve. Also seen are the vestibule (V), oval window (OV), and cochlea (C).

fossa to the medial mastoid antrum. It contains the subarcuate artery and vein, providing vascular supply to the otic capsule of the vestibule, semicircular canals, the mastoid antrum, and portions of the facial nerve canal.[46] On imaging, it is closely entwined with the semicircular canals: the canal runs through the "hoop" of the superior semicircular canal and is superior to the lateral semicircular canal.[47] It also has an "inverted V" appearance in coronal oblique images.[46] The petromastoid canal is rarely of clinical importance other than serving as an anatomic landmark. Still, radiologists should be wary of confusing it for a fracture or other pathology.

Singular Canal

The singular canal is a channel that runs from the ampulla of the posterior semicircular canal to the posterior margin of the IAC (Fig. 12).[48] The channel is typically just over 3 mm in length in most patients.[49] It houses the posterior ampullary nerve, also known as the singular nerve, which is a branch of the inferior vestibular nerve. Transmitted through the singular nerve are afferent vestibular signals from the posterior semicircular canal.[50] Like the petromastoid canal, the singular canal is rarely of radiologic interest, though it does serve as a landmark during some procedures.[51]

CLINICS CARE POINTS

- Numerous sutures, fissures, and canals exist within and around the temporal bone, which should not be confused for fractures.

- Thorough knowledge of the anatomy of cranial nerves IX and X may be useful to distinguish between subtypes of paragangliomas. Glomus tympanicum paragangliomas arise from the tympanic plexus of Jacobson's nerve and are typically located along the cochlear promontory. Glomus jugulare paragangliomas arise from either Arnold's nerve or Jacobson's nerve in the jugular foramen. These tumors may be difficult to distinguish, and the term "jugulotympanic" is often used to describe tumors with an indeterminate pattern.

- Both CT and MRI offer specific advantages in temporal bone imaging. CT is typically used to evaluate osseous structures such as the ossicles, middle ear, mastoid air cells, and shape of the otic capsule. MRI is used to evaluate the fluid within the membranous labyrinth, proximal cranial nerves, and various soft tissue pathologies such as tumors.

DISCLOSURE

The authors have nothing to disclose.

CONFLICTS OF INTEREST

None.

REFERENCES

1. Gunlock MG, Gentry LR. Anatomy of the temporal bone. Neuroimaging Clin N Am 1998;8(1):195–209.
2. Kurihara YY, Fujikawa A, Tachizawa N, et al. Temporal Bone Trauma: Typical CT and MRI Appearances and Important Points for Evaluation. RadioGraphics 2020;40(4):1148–62. https://doi.org/10.1148/rg.2020190023.

3. Kwong Y, Yu D, Shah J. Fracture Mimics on Temporal Bone CT: A Guide for the Radiologist. Am J Roentgenol 2012;199(2):428–34. https://doi.org/10.2214/AJR.11.8012.

4. Isaacson B. Anatomy and Surgical Approach of the Ear and Temporal Bone. Head Neck Pathol 2018;12(3):321–7. https://doi.org/10.1007/s12105-018-0926-2.

5. Juliano AF, Ginat DT, Moonis G. Imaging Review of the Temporal Bone: Part I. Anatomy and Inflammatory and Neoplastic Processes. Radiology 2013;269(1):17–33.

6. Nelson G, Ricardo S, Pedro S, et al. Pars tensa and tympanicomalleal joint: proposal for a new anatomic classification. Eur Arch Otorhinolaryngol 2019;276(8):2141–8.

7. Juliano AF. Cross Sectional Imaging of the Ear and Temporal Bone. Head Neck Pathol 2018;12(3):302–20.

8. Petrus LV, Lo WW. The anterior epitympanic recess: CT anatomy and pathology. AJNR Am J Neuroradiol 1997;18(6):1109–14.

9. Pauna HF, Monsanto RC, Schachern P, et al. A 3-D Analysis of the Protympanum in Human Temporal Bones with Chronic Ear Disease. Eur Arch Otorhinolaryngol 2017;274(3):1357–64. https://doi.org/10.1007/s00405-016-4396-4.

10. Burd C, Pai I, Connor S. Imaging anatomy of the retrotympanum: variants and their surgical implications. Br J Radiol 2020;93(1105):20190677. https://doi.org/10.1259/bjr.20190677.

11. Abele TA, Wiggins RH. Imaging of the temporal bone. Radiol Clin North Am 2015;53(1):15–36. https://doi.org/10.1016/j.rcl.2014.09.010.

12. Kamrava B, Roehm PC. Systematic Review of Ossicular Chain Anatomy: Strategic Planning for Development of Novel Middle Ear Prostheses. Otolaryngol–head Neck Surg Off J Am Acad Otolaryngol-head Neck Surg 2017;157(2):190–200. https://doi.org/10.1177/0194599817701717.

13. Luers JC, Hüttenbrink K-B. Surgical anatomy and pathology of the middle ear. J Anat 2016;228(2):338–53. https://doi.org/10.1111/joa.12389.

14. Wojciechowski T, Skadorwa T, Nève de Mévergnies J-G, et al. Microtomographic morphometry of the stapedius muscle and its tendon. Anat Sci Int 2020;95(1):31–7. https://doi.org/10.1007/s12565-019-00490-6.

15. Rubini A, Jufas N, Marchioni D, et al. The endoscopic relationship of the stapedius muscle to the facial nerve: implications for retrotympanic surgery. Otol Neurotol 2020;41(1):e64–9. https://doi.org/10.1097/MAO.0000000000002454.

16. Virapongse C, Rothman S, Kier E, et al. Computed tomographic anatomy of the temporal bone. Am J Roentgenol 1982;139(4):739–49. https://doi.org/10.2214/ajr.139.4.739.

17. Komune N, Matsuo S, Miki K, et al. The endoscopic anatomy of the middle ear approach to the fundus of the internal acoustic canal. J Neurosurg 2016;126(6):1974–83. https://doi.org/10.3171/2016.5.JNS16261.

18. Lemmerling MM, Stambuk HE, Mancuso AA, et al. CT of the normal suspensory ligaments of the ossicles in the middle ear. Am J Neuroradiol 1997;18(3):471–7.

19. Benson JC, Carlson ML, Lane JI. MRI of the Internal Auditory Canal, Labyrinth, and Middle Ear: How We Do It. Radiology 2020;297(2):252–65. https://doi.org/10.1148/radiol.2020201767.

20. Purves D, Augustine GJ, Fitzpatrick D, et al. The otolith organs: the utricle and sacculus. Neurosci 2nd Edition. Published online 2001. Available at: https://www.ncbi.nlm.nih.gov/books/NBK10792/. Accessed May 20, 2021.

21. Baráth K, Schuknecht B, Naldi AM, et al. Detection and grading of endolymphatic hydrops in Ménière disease using MR imaging. AJNR Am J Neuroradiol 2014;35(7):1387–92. https://doi.org/10.3174/ajnr.A3856.

22. Steekelenburg JM van, Weijnen A van, Pont LMH de, et al. Value of Endolymphatic Hydrops and Perilymph Signal Intensity in Suspected Ménière Disease. Am J Neuroradiol 2020. https://doi.org/10.3174/ajnr.A6410. Published online February 6.

23. Attyé A, Eliezer M. Endolymph magnetic resonance imaging: Contribution of saccule and utricle analysis in the management of patients with sensorineural ear disorders. Eur Ann Otorhinolaryngol Head Neck Dis 2020;137(1):47–51. https://doi.org/10.1016/j.anorl.2019.11.001.

24. Nordström CK, Laurell G, Rask-Andersen H. The Human Vestibular Aqueduct: Anatomical Characteristics and Enlargement Criteria. Otol Neurotol 2016;37(10):1637–45. https://doi.org/10.1097/MAO.0000000000001203.

25. Vijayasekaran S, Halsted MJ, Boston M, et al. When Is the Vestibular Aqueduct Enlarged? A Statistical Analysis of the Normative Distribution of Vestibular Aqueduct Size. Am J Neuroradiol 2007;28(6):1133–8. https://doi.org/10.3174/ajnr.A0495.

26. Boston M, Halsted M, Meinzen-Derr J, et al. The large vestibular aqueduct: a new definition based on audiologic and computed tomography correlation. Otolaryngol–head Neck Surg Off J Am Acad Otolaryngol-head Neck Surg 2007;136(6):972–7.

27. Mukherji SK, Baggett HC, Alley J, et al. Enlarged cochlear aqueduct. Am J Neuroradiol 1998;19(2):330–2.

28. Joshi VM, Navlekar SK, Kishore GR, et al. CT and MR Imaging of the Inner Ear and Brain in Children with Congenital Sensorineural Hearing Loss. RadioGraphics 2012;32(3):683–98.

29. Burmeister HP, Baltzer PA, Dietzel M, et al. Identification of the nervus intermedius using 3T MR imaging. AJNR Am J Neuroradiol 2011;32(3):460–4.

30. Valvassori GE, Palacios E. Magnetic resonance imaging of the internal auditory canal. Top Magn Reson Imaging TMRI 2000;11(1):52–65.

31. Mihal DC, Feng Y, Kodet ML, et al. Isolated internal auditory canal diverticula: a normal anatomic variant not associated with sensorineural hearing loss. AJNR Am J Neuroradiol 2018;39(12):2340–4.

32. Pippin KJ, Muelleman TJ, Hill J, et al. Prevalence of internal auditory canal diverticulum and its association with hearing loss and otosclerosis. Am J Neuroradiol 2017;38(11):2167–71.

33. Muelleman TJ, Kavookjian H, Asmar J, et al. Internal auditory canal diverticula in children: a congenital variant. Laryngoscope 2021;131(5):E1683–7. https://doi.org/10.1002/lary.29278.

34. Seneviratne SO, Patel BC. Facial Nerve Anatomy and Clinical Applications. In: StatPearls. StatPearls Publishing; 2021. Available at: http://www.ncbi.nlm. nih.gov/books/NBK554569/. Accessed May 7, 2021.

35. Chhabda S, Leger DS, Lingam RK. Imaging the facial nerve: A contemporary review of anatomy and pathology. Eur J Radiol 2020;126:108920.

36. Kakizawa Y, Abe H, Fukushima Y, et al. The Course of the Lesser Petrosal Nerve on the Middle Cranial Fossa. Oper Neurosurg 2007;61(suppl_3). https://doi.org/10.1227/01.neu.0000289707.49684.a3. ONS-15.

37. Rao A, Tadi P. Anatomy, Head and Neck, Chorda Tympani. In: StatPearls. StatPearls Publishing; 2021. Available at: http://www.ncbi.nlm.nih.gov/books/NBK546586/. Accessed May 7, 2021.

38. Benson JC, Eckel L, Guerin J, et al. Review of Temporal Bone Microanatomy : Aqueducts, Canals, Clefts and Nerves. Clin Neuroradiol 2019. https://doi.org/10.1007/s00062-019-00864-3. Published online December 5.

39. Kanzara T, Hall A, Virk JS, et al. Clinical anatomy of the tympanic nerve: A review. World J Otorhinolaryngol 2014;4(4):17–22. https://doi.org/10.5319/wjo.v4.i4.17.

40. Tekdemir I, Aslan A, Tüccar E, et al. An anatomical study of the tympanic branch of the glossopharyngeal nerve (nerve of Jacobson). Ann Anat Anat Anz Off Organ Anat Ges 1998;180(4):349–52.

41. Sweeney AD, Carlson ML, Wanna GB, et al. Glomus tympanicum tumors. Otolaryngol Clin North Am 2015;48(2):293–304.

42. Nicolay S, De Foer B, Bernaerts A, et al. Aberrant internal carotid artery presenting as a retrotympanic vascular mass. Acta Radiol Short Rep 2014;3(10). https://doi.org/10.1177/2047981614553695.

43. Butt MF, Albusoda A, Farmer AD, et al. The anatomical basis for transcutaneous auricular vagus nerve stimulation. J Anat 2020;236(4):588–611.

44. Ryan NM, Gibson PG, Birring SS. Arnold's nerve cough reflex: evidence for chronic cough as a sensory vagal neuropathy. J Thorac Dis 2014;6(Suppl 7):S748–52.

45. Rao AB, Koeller KK, Adair CF. From the archives of the AFIP. Paragangliomas of the head and neck: radiologic-pathologic correlation. Armed Forces Institute of Pathology. Radiogr Rev Publ Radiol Soc N Am Inc 1999;19(6):1605–32.

46. Akyol Y, Galheigo D, Massimore M, et al. Subarcuate artery and canal: an important anatomic variant. J Comput Assist Tomogr 2011;35(6):688–9.

47. Migirov L, Kronenberg J. Radiology of the petromastoid canal. Otol Neurotol 2006;27(3):410–3.

48. Silverstein H, Norrell H, Smouha E, et al. The singular canal: a valuable landmark in surgery of the internal auditory canal. Otolaryngol–head Neck Surg Off J Am Acad Otolaryngol-head Neck Surg 1988;98(2):138–43.

49. Fatterpekar GM, Mukherji SK, Lin Y, et al. Normal canals at the fundus of the internal auditory canal: CT evaluation. J Comput Assist Tomogr 1999;23(5):776–80.

50. Muren C, Wadin K, Dimopoulos P. Radioanatomy of the singular nerve canal. Eur Radiol 1991;1(1):65–9.

51. Agirdir BV, Sindel M, Arslan G, et al. The canal of the posterior ampullar nerve: an important anatomic landmark in the posterior fossa transmeatal approach. Surg Radiol Anat SRA 2001;23(5):331–4.

Oral Cavity and Salivary Glands Anatomy

Akinrinola Famuyide, MD[a],*, Tarik F. Massoud, MD, PhD[b], Gul Moonis, MD[c]

KEYWORDS

● Anatomy ● Oral ● Cavity ● Salivary ● Glands ● Radiology

KEY POINTS

- Oral cavity anatomy is divided into multiple subsites.
- There are various conditions that affect the oral cavity including congenital, infectious, inflammatory, and neoplastic processes.
- The salivary glands are found throughout and adjacent to the oral cavity.
- Salivary gland pathology can affect or occur within the oral cavity.

INTRODUCTION

The oral cavity is involved in many functions including speech, ingestion, mastication, and propulsion of food into the oropharynx. The oral cavity also serves as a secondary airway additional to the nasal cavity. The oral cavity can be a challenging area to evaluate because of the complex anatomy resulting in particular challenges encountered in imaging this area. The presence of glandular tissue, opposing mucosal surfaces, muscles, soft tissues, and their proximity to osseous structures all contribute to these imaging challenges when viewing normal anatomy or complex pathology.[1]

Oral cavity pathologies are common. Broad categories of conditions affecting the oral cavity include infectious/inflammatory processes, benign and malignant masses, and congenital/developmental lesions. Anatomic variants or pseudolesions mimicking pathologic processes are also encountered in the oral cavity.[2,3]

ANATOMY

The oral cavity is separated into the oral cavity proper and vestibule. The oral cavity is bordered by the lips anteriorly, the mylohyoid muscle inferiorly, the buccomasseteric region bordered by the gingivobuccal sulcus and retromolar trigone laterally, the hard palate superiorly, and circumvallate papillae, tonsillar pillars, and the soft palate posteriorly (Figs. 1 and 2).[4] The circumvallate papillae are immediately adjacent to the sulcus terminalis, which separates the oral cavity from the base of tongue, a structure that is part of the oropharynx (see Fig. 4).

The vestibule is the area between the lateral aspect of the teeth and gums and lateral cheek. The remainder of the oral cavity proper includes the lips, gingivobuccal region, the oral tongue (anterior two-thirds of the tongue), the floor of the mouth, sublingual space, submandibular space, hard palate, and adjacent maxillary and mandibular alveoli (see Figs. 1 and 2; Figs. 3–8).

LIPS

The lips are responsible for phonation, facial expression, sensation, and mastication. The upper lip is known as the labium superius oris and the lower lip is known as the labium inferius oris. The lips contain the vermillion border which serves to separate the skin from the mucosa of the oral

[a] Columbia University Irving Medical Center, 622 West 168th Street, New York, NY 10032, USA; [b] Division of Neuroimaging and Neurointervention, Department of Radiology, Stanford University School of Medicine, Center for Academic Medicine, Radiology, MC: 5659, 453 Quarry Road, Palo Alto, CA 94304, USA; [c] NYU Langone Medical Center, 222 East 41st Street, New York, NY 10017, USA
* Corresponding author.
E-mail address: af3169@cumc.columbia.edu

Neuroimag Clin N Am 32 (2022) 777–790
https://doi.org/10.1016/j.nic.2022.07.021

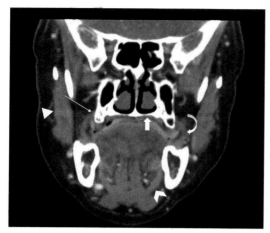

Fig. 1. Boundaries of the oral cavity. Coronal CT demonstrates hard palate (*thick arrow*), upper gingivo-buccal sulcus (*thin arrow*), mylohyoid muscle (*arrow head*), buccinator muscle with buccal mucosa just deep (*curved arrow*), and masseter muscle (*triangle*).

cavity. The upper lip extends from the nasolabial folds to the inferior margin of the nose.[5]

The upper and lower lips meet at the angle of the mouth also known as the commissure. The lower lips extend from the lateral commissures to the chin. The vermillion border of the lip is a modified mucous membrane that is hairless and vascularized. There are no hair follicles, salivary glands, or sebaceous glands. The transition from the dry portion of the lip to the wet mucosa is marked by the presence of submucosal salivary glands.[5]

The lips are supplied primarily by the facial artery branch of the external carotid artery (ECA). The more distal branching superior and inferior labial arteries are located within the submucosal

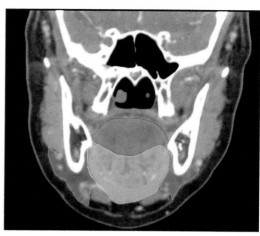

Fig. 3. Boundaries and subsites of the oral cavity. Coronal CT showing the floor of mouth (*yellow*), tongue (*red*), and submandibular space (*green*).

layers of the lips. Venous drainage is through the superior and inferior labial veins. Lymphatic drainage from the lateral aspect of the upper and lower lips is to the ipsilateral submandibular nodes (level Ib).[6] The medial aspect of the lips drains to the submental nodes (level Ia). The branches of cranial nerve (CN) VII (facial nerve) provide motor innervation to the orbicularis oris and muscles responsible for elevating and depressing the mouth. Multiple branches of the trigeminal nerve, CN V, are responsible for sensory innervation of the lips. The maxillary division (V2) supplies the upper lip, and the mandibular division (V3) supplies the lower lip.[2]

The primary muscles of the lips are the muscles of facial expression. This includes the orbicularis oris that acts to close the mouth. It is attached to

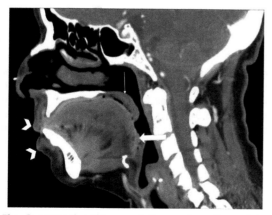

Fig. 2. Normal anatomy of the oral cavity and its boundaries. Sagittal CT showing soft palate (*thin arrow*), lips (*arrow heads*), and base of tongue (*thick arrow*).

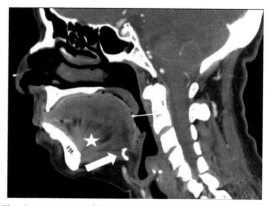

Fig. 4. Anatomy of the oral cavity. Sagittal CT showing the hyoid bone (*thick arrow*), root of tongue (*star*), and approximate location of the sulcus terminalis/circumvallate papilla (*thin arrow*).

with squamous cell carcinoma (SCC) more commonly affecting the lower lip at the vermillion border. Risk factors for SCC include actinic cheilitis, also known as farmer's lips secondary to chronic sun exposure, alcohol, tobacco, fair skin, and immunosuppression.[5]

ORAL TONGUE

The tongue is responsible for deglutition by the formation of a food bolus. In addition, it allows for taste and also the formation of speech. The oral tongue is a subsite of the oral cavity and includes the portion anterior to the sulcus terminalis along with the circumvallate papilla, which is approximately two-thirds posterior from the tip of the tongue. The posterior one-third is developmentally different and has different innervations that form the oropharyngeal aspect of the tongue. The sensory supply of the oral tongue is from the lingual nerve which is a branch of the mandibular division of the trigeminal nerve.[2,8]

The tongue has a dorsal aspect, an apex (which forms the most anterior aspect), an inferior surface that also contains the frenulum, and the root of the tongue, which is attached to the hyoid bone and mandible (see Figs. 4 and 5). The oral tongue is bounded anteriorly and laterally by the alveolar processes of the mandible and maxilla. The internal architecture of the tongue demonstrates a fibrous network known as the lingual septum and hyoglossus membrane.[9] This membrane connects the root of the tongue to the hyoid bone. The lingual septum is a vertical band of fibrous tissue extending in the midline of the long axis of the tongue (see Fig. 6). This restricts any significant vascular anastomosis except for the tongue apex.

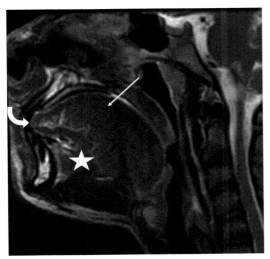

Fig. 5. Anatomy of the oral cavity. Sagittal MR imaging showing the dorsum of the oral tongue (*thin arrow*), root of tongue (*star*), and apex of the tongue (*curved arrow*).

the other muscles of facial expression without an osseous insertion or origin. The modiolus is a fibromuscular structure situated superolateral to the angles of the mouth. The intersection of several facial muscles including the orbicularis oris, levator and depressor anguli oris, risorius, platysma, buccinator, and zygomaticus major converge on the modiolus. It functions to anchor the muscles to act as a functional unit for phonation, mastication, and facial expression.[7]

A variety of disorders can present with lip symptoms, however, in imaging it is often in the context of malignancy or suspected malignancy. The upper lip is usually affected by basal cell carcinoma

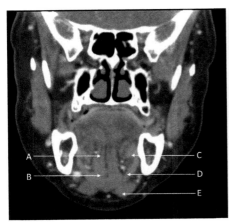
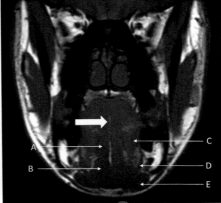

Fig. 6. Tongue and floor of mouth anatomy. Coronal CT (*A*) and coronal T1W MR imaging (*B*) showing muscles of the oral cavity. Genioglossus (A), geniohyoid (B), hyoglossus (C), mylohyoid (D), and anterior belly of the digastric (E). Lingual septum is represented by the thick arrow. T1W, T1-weight.

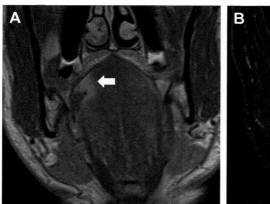
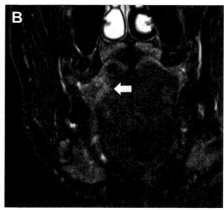

Fig. 7. Squamous cell carcinoma of the oral tongue. Coronal MR imaging T1 post-gadolinium (*A*) and coronal T2 fat-saturated image (*B*) show a right lateral oral tongue lesion (*arrow*) with post-contrast enhancement. The lesion does not cross midline and does not extend into the floor of mouth.

The tongue is primarily composed of skeletal muscle with overlying mucosa. The muscles are divided into the intrinsic and extrinsic tongue muscles. The intrinsic muscles are within the tongue without an osseous origin or insertion. These include the superior and inferior longitudinal, vertical, and transverse bands. The extrinsic muscles have osseous attachments and include the genioglossus, hyoglossus, styloglossus, and palatoglossus. The extrinsic muscles are responsible for stabilizing the tongue, changing its position, and changing its shape.[8]

The genioglossus is the largest of the extrinsic tongue muscles (see Fig. 6). It originates from the genial tubercle and fans out and inserts into the hyoid bone, tongue, and inferior surface of the tongue. The hyoglossus is a thin muscle arising in the hyoid bone, ascending superiorly, and intersecting with the fibers of the styloglossus before attaching to the side of the tongue.

The tongue receives arterial supply from the lingual artery which is an ECA branch. The lingual veins drain into the internal jugular vein. There is additional supply to the root of tongue from the facial artery and ascending pharyngeal branches of the ECA. Innervation of the tongue includes motor, sensory, general sensory, and special sensory for taste. Motor innervation for all intrinsic and extrinsic muscles of the tongue is supplied by the hypoglossal nerve (CN XII), with the exception of the palatoglossus, which is innervated by the vagus nerve (CN X).[10]

Innervation of taste and sensation is different for the anterior two-thirds and posterior one-third of the tongue. The oral tongue is supplied by the chorda tympani branch of the facial nerve (CN VII) for taste and the lingual branch of the mandibular branch (V3) of the trigeminal nerve (CN V) for general sensation. Lymphatic drainage of the apex of the tongue is to the submental lymph nodes (level Ia), with the lateral halves draining to the submandibular lymph nodes (level Ib).

Imaging malignancy of the tongue is used for mapping the extent of tumor, areas of osseous

Fig. 8. Surface anatomy of the oral cavity. Oral cavity anatomy showing the frenulum of the tongue (*thin arrow*), vermillion border of the lips (*thick arrow*), retromolar trigone (*circle*), mucosa overlying the floor of mouth (*triangle*), gingiva (*arrow head*), and buccal mucosa (*angled arrow*).

invasion, and invasion into adjacent structures (see Fig. 7). Lymphadenopathy and distant metastatic disease are also evaluated using imaging. MR imaging is generally the preferred modality owing to dental amalgam and beam hardening artifacts from the teeth obscuring computed tomography (CT) evaluation. However, CT is necessary for evaluation of osseous invasion.[11,12]

The root of the tongue is an important area of the oral cavity particularly in the setting of oral cavity and oropharyngeal cancers. Few lesions arise from the root of the tongue, but invasion from adjacent mucosal surfaces must be adequately evaluated.[13] The root of the tongue includes the lingual septum, bilateral genioglossus, and geniohyoid muscle. The geniohyoid and genioglossus muscles originate at the genial tubercle and insert into the hyoid bone. The genioglossus also inserts into the underside of the tongue. The anterior border of the root of the tongue is the mandible, whereas laterally it is the sublingual spaces, and inferiorly it is the mylohyoid muscle.

FLOOR OF THE MOUTH

The floor of the mouth is a U-shaped space below the tongue. Surgeons will typically consider the floor of the mouth to include the mucosal surface overlying the floor of the mouth and the mylohyoid muscle sling (see Fig. 8). The mylohyoid muscle is a U-shaped muscle that forms the boundary of the floor of the mouth and separates the mouth from the submandibular spaces. Some radiologists consider the sublingual space to be a part of the floor of the mouth along with the mylohyoid muscle, whereas some consider the sublingual space to be a separate compartment. The posterior free edge of the mylohyoid muscle results in communication between the floor of the mouth and the submandibular space. At this location, the upper aspect of the submandibular gland hooks around the posterior edge of the mylohyoid muscle and into the posterior aspect of the floor of the mouth. A defect in the mylohyoid muscle known as boutonniere's deformity is a common normal anatomic variant (Fig. 9). This is a fascial or muscular defect that can allow sublingual gland, fat, minor salivary glands and vascular structures to protrude into the submandibular space, which can result in a pseudomass.[13,14]

The bilateral sublingual spaces are superior and medial to the mylohyoid muscle and lateral to the genioglossus and genioglossus muscles. The sublingual space contains fat, a portion of the hyoglossus muscle that inserts into the lateral tongue, sublingual glands, and minor salivary glands. The neurovascular bundle (NVB) comprising the lingual artery, vein, and nerve, and the hypoglossal nerve traverse the sublingual space. If tumor invades the ipsilateral NVB, partial glossectomy can be performed.[15] However, if tumor extends to the contralateral NVB bundle, it necessitates total glossectomy with sacrifice of both NVBs. The sublingual glands empty through several small ducts into the floor of the mouth known as Rivinus's ducts. The anterior ducts may coalesce to form a common duct known as Bartholin's duct which empties into the submandibular duct (SMD) known as Wharton's duct. Wharton's duct runs anteriorly in the sublingual space. The mucosal impression of the duct is the sublingual papilla and is situated on both sides of the frenulum of the tongue just anterior to the sublingual glands.[14]

The floor of the mouth is typically imaged using CT, which is widely available, quick, and useful at evaluating acute infectious and inflammatory processes, masses, osseous erosions, overlying skin changes, and salivary gland duct calculi. MR imaging provides improved soft tissue resolution and is useful in staging oral cavity malignancies that invade the floor of the mouth, trans-spatial extension, and perineural spread. Ultrasonography can be useful in soft tissue delineation, sialoliths, submandibular gland infectious/inflammatory processes, masses, and cysts. Sialography can be used in selected cases, and there are endoscopic techniques used by surgeons.

There is an array of pathologic processes that affect the floor of the mouth including cystic lesions, infectious processes, inflammatory processes, vascular lesions, and benign and malignant neoplasms (Figs. 10 and 11). In evaluating SCC of the oral cavity and floor of the mouth, assessment of the extrinsic muscles and surrounding osseous structures for invasion is important (Fig. 12).

TEETH

The teeth within the oral cavity are routinely encountered on head and neck imaging, and they are a common site of disease. To appropriately communicate findings, an understanding of normal anatomy, terminology, and morphology is essential. See also article by Hatcher in this issue for greater details.

Teeth can be referred to by name or a universally accepted numbering scheme. Two main classification systems exist: the universal system and the Federation Dentaire International system. The authors only describe the universal system that has been adopted for use in the United States (Fig. 13). Teeth are numbered starting in the right upper quadrant with #1 representing the right third

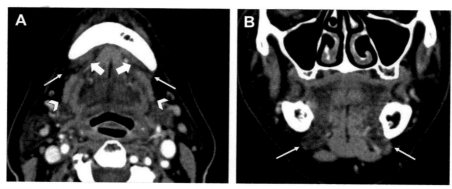

Fig. 9. Boutonniere deformity. Axial post-cotrast CT shows herniation of the sublingual glands (thin arrows) from the sublingual space through a defect in the mylohyoid muscles (thick arrow). known as the mylohyoid boutonniere.

molar. It continues along the maxillary teeth with #8 representing the maxillary central incisor and #16 representing the left maxillary third molar. The number then continues in the left lower quadrant where the left mandibular third molar is assigned #17, the left mandibular central incisor assigned #24, and the right third mandibular molar assigned #32.[16]

Objects within the tooth closer to the crown are termed coronal and when closer to the apex are termed apical, similar to superior and inferior, respectively (Fig. 14A). Medial, lateral, anterior, and posterior tooth surfaces are named in relation

to the alveolar arch (Fig. 15). Mesial and distal are similar to anterior and posterior but refer to how close objects are to the arch midline. Objects closer to the midline are mesial, and those farther are distal. Lingual and facial are similar to medial and lateral, respectively, with the reference point being the alveolar arch. Palatal is a term similar to lingual, and labial and buccal are terms similar to facial. Labial is used for teeth closer to the lips (anterior) and buccal for those closer to the posterior teeth (see Fig. 15).[17]

Teeth are made up of two basic components: a crown and one or more roots (Fig. 14). The crown

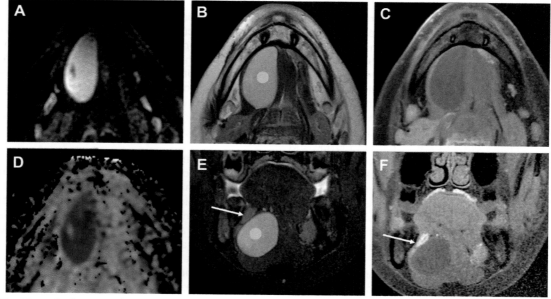

Fig. 10. Right floor of mouth epidermoid cyst. Axial DWI (A), axial T1 pre-contrast (B), axial T1 post-contrast with fat-saturation (C), ADC (D), coronal T2 with fat-saturation (E), and coronal T1 post-contrast with fat-saturation (F) show a cystic right floor of mouth lesions (star) displacing the sublingual gland (*thin arrow*) superolaterally. There is high DWI (A), signal and low ADC, (D), compatible with restricted diffusion. DWI, diffusion weight imaging; ADC, apparent diffusion coefficient.

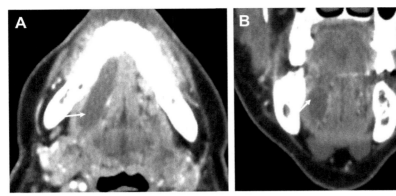

Fig. 11. Right floor of mouth ranula. Axial and coronal CT show a cystic right floor of mouth lesion (*arrow*) centered within the right sublingual space. It replaces the sublingual gland.

is the visible portion when viewing inside the open mouth when there is no periodontal bone loss. The boundary between the crown and tooth is the cementoenamel junction (CEJ) (see Fig. 14B). The portion above the CEJ is covered by enamel and is called the crown. Differences in the morphology of the teeth reflect their different function. The incisional edges of the anterior teeth are for cutting, whereas the posterior teeth with broad surfaces are for chewing. Teeth can either have a single root or have multiple roots. The incisors, canines, and premolars generally have single roots.[16]

The teeth are made up of four dental tissues that include enamel, dentin, and cementum, which are mineralized hard tissue (see Fig. 14). The fourth, that is, the pulp, is a non-mineralized soft tissue. Enamel is the most mineralized substance in the human body and can distinctly be seen on radiographs and CT.[1] Deep to the enamel is dentin that makes up most of the crown and root, which is less calcified. Dentin surrounds the pulp within the tooth. The dentinoenamel junction is where the dentin and enamel meet.[18] Within the root, cementum is the outermost tissue and surrounds the dentin. This is difficult to differentiate from dentin on radiographs and CT owing to similar mineralization. The pulp which has nutritive and sensory function fills the internal cavity of the tooth and is made up of nerves and vessels that enter through the apical foramen of the tooth. It is radiolucent on imaging. The pulp in the crown is called the pulpal chamber and within the root is called the pulpal canal (see Fig. 14).[16]

Periodontal tissues refer to the portions of the maxilla and mandible that surround the roots of the teeth and include the alveolar bone, the

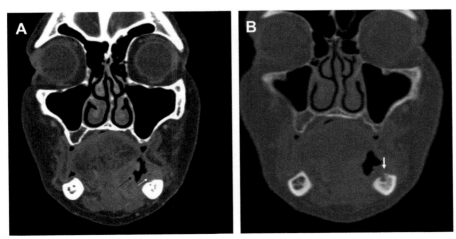

Fig. 12. Left floor of mouth squamous cell carcinoma. Coronal soft tissue (*A*) and bone window (*B*) reformats from a CT scan of the face demonstrate a left floor of mouth mass (*black arrow*) extending to the buccal mucosa across the alveolar ridge gingiva (*white arrow*). Subtle bony erosion is noted on the bone window (*thick white arrow*).

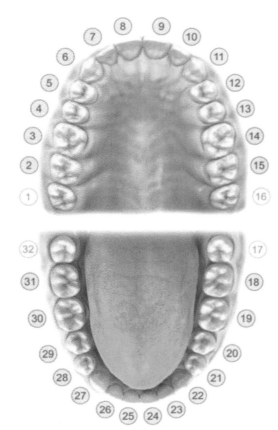

Fig. 13. Upper and lower jaw with numbering of the teeth according to the American dental scheme (Universal Numbering System). Teeth are numbered starting in the right upper quadrant with #1 representing the right third molar. It continues along the maxillary teeth with #8 representing the maxillary central incisor and #16 representing the left maxillary third molar. The number then continues in the left lower quadrant where the left mandibular third molar is assigned #17, the left mandibular central incisor assigned #24 and the right third mandibular molar assigned #32. (*Courtesy of* MedicalGraphics (www.MedicalGraphics.de), Köln, Germany. Copyright Notice Creative commons - Attribution-NoDerivatives 4.0 International (CC BY-ND 4.0) https://creativecommons.org/licenses/by-nd/4.0/.)

periodontal ligament (PDL), and gingiva. The alveolar bone is the thickened portion of bone of the maxilla and mandible that surround and form the tooth socket.[19] The corticated portion surrounding the tooth socket is called the lamina dura. Between the lamina dura and the root is a radiolucent area that contains the PDL (see Fig. 14A). This is made of fibers that attach the root of the teeth to the alveolar socket and are used for proprioception. Widening of the PDL with loss of corticated

bone of the alveolus and lamina dura is a sign of pathology. The gingiva, or gums, is the mucosa that surrounds and protects the teeth. The gingiva can act as a barrier to mechanical trauma and bacterial infection specifically at the gingival sulcus, where the gingiva attaches to the tooth. The gingiva functions in sensation within the mouth, absorption of micronutrients, and has an important role in the innate immune response.[1,18]

GINGIVA, RETROMOLAR TRIGONE, AND GINGIVOBUCCAL SULCUS

The gingiva covers the lingual and buccal aspects of the alveolar process of the mandible and maxilla (Fig. 16). The junction of the gingiva with the buccal mucosa forms the gingivobuccal sulcus and is a common location for SCC.[2,14] There is a triangular shaped area posterior to the last mandibular molar covered by gingival mucosa called the retromolar trigone (Fig. 17). This covers the lower part of the ramus of the mandible and is another common site of SCC. These cancers can arise from the retromolar trigone and extend to or from the oropharynx and tonsils.

The space between the lips and cheeks, lined by buccal mucosa and bounded medially by the teeth and gums, is known as the vestibule. Puffed cheek views on CT distend the vestibule to help differentiate the site of disease pathology between the gingiva and the buccal mucosa. The buccinator muscle is situated in the soft tissue deep to the buccal mucosa (see Fig. 16).[4,20]

The buccinator is one of the muscles of facial expression and innervated by CN VII. It functions to compress the cheeks, which is useful in mastication.[1] It originates on the alveolar process of the maxilla and mandible opposite the sockets of the molar teeth and the anterior border of the pterygomandibular raphe. The buccinator then inserts on the fibers of the orbicularis oris surrounding the mouth.

The pterygomandibular raphe is a fascial band extending from the hamulus of the medial pterygoid to the posterior border of the mylohyoid ridge of the mandible. It serves as a site of attachment for the buccinator and the superior pharyngeal constrictors between the anterior tonsillar pillars and retromolar trigone (see Fig. 17). It is important as a route of transspatial spread of malignancies in the retromolar trigone can extend along the pterygomandibular raphe superiorly to the buccomasseteric region, superiorly to the masticator space, inferiorly to the mylohyoid and floor of mouth, and posteriorly to the prestyloid parapharyngeal space or masticator space.[9,18]

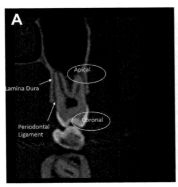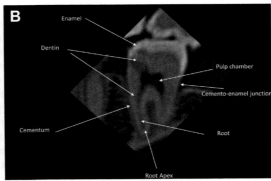

Fig. 14. Tooth anatomy. Coronal CT images. (*A*) Corticated portion surrounding the tooth socket called the lamina dura. Between the lamina dura and the root is a radiolucent area that contains the periodontal ligament which attaches the tooth to the lamina dura. This is made up for fibers that attach the root of the teeth to the alveolar socket and are used for proprioception. (*B*) Enamel; the most mineralized substance in the human body. Deep to the enamel is dentin that makes up most of the crown and root which is less calcified. Dentin surrounds the pulp within the tooth where the dentin and enamel meet the dentinoenamel junction. Within the root, cementum is the outermost tissue and surrounds the dentin. The cementoenamel junction (CEJ) represents the anatomic limit between the crown and root surface and is defined as the area of union of the cementum and enamel at the cervical region of the toot.

HARD PALATE AND MAXILLARY ALVEOLUS

The hard palate and maxillary alveolus will be discussed together because of their close anatomic relationship. Similar pathologies affect these regions, and extension of pathologic processes, particularly malignancies, tends to affect each other (Fig. 18). Together, the hard palate and maxillary alveolus, along with the overlying gingiva form the roof of the oral cavity. The hard palate and maxillary alveolus separate the oral cavity from the nasal cavity and maxillary sinuses, respectively.[21]

The anterior two-thirds of the hard palate are formed by the palatine process of the maxilla with the posterior one-third from by the horizontal plate of each palatine bone. Torus palatinus, a benign osseous overgrowth, can occur at the junction of these four bones. The NVB is situated laterally in the roof of the mouth. The blood supply to the hard palate is from the greater palatine artery, arising from the maxillary branch of the ECA. Sensory innervation is from the greater palatine nerve and nasopalatine branches of the maxillary nerve, which courses within the pterygopalatine (greater

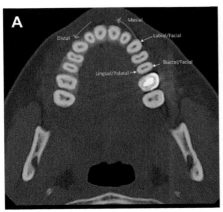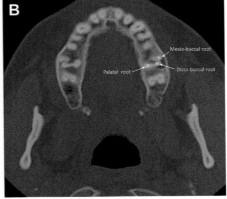

Fig. 15. Tooth relationships. (*A*) Medial, lateral, anterior, and posterior tooth surfaces are named in relation to the alveolar arch. Mesial and distal are similar to anterior and posterior but refer to how close objects are to the arch midline. Objects closer to the midline are mesial, and those farther are distal. Lingual and facial are similar to medial and lateral, respectively, with the reference point being the alveolar arch. (*B*) Palatal is a term similar to lingual, and labial and buccal are terms similar to facial. Labial is used for teeth closer to the lips (anterior) and buccal for those closer to the posterior teeth.

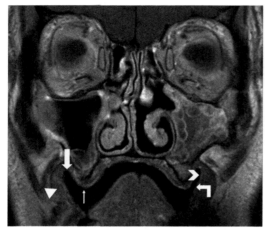

Fig. 16. Oral cavity anatomy. Coronal T1 post-contrast MR imaging showing the gingiva (*thin arrow*), gingivobuccal sulcus (thick arrow), vestibule (angled arrow), buccal mucosa (*arrow head*), and buccinator muscle (*triangle*).

palatine canal) to the greater palatine foramen. It innervates the gums, mucosa, and glands of the hard palate.

SALIVARY GLANDS AND THEIR DUCTS

The salivary glands include the three paired major salivary glands (parotid, submandibular, and sublingual) and an estimated 1000 minor salivary glands scattered throughout the aerodigestive tract. They all serve important functions in normal digestion and oral hygiene. Imaging interpretation of the salivary glands relies heavily on understanding their anatomy and that of the structures that

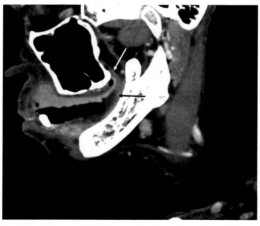

Fig. 17. Retromolar trigone. Post-contrast sagittal oblique image shows the retromolar trigone (*black arrow*) and pterygomandibular raphe (*white arrow*).

reside within or beside them, because salivary gland diseases can easily spread to or from their surroundings.[22] In addition, our ability to identify pathology in a gland requires familiarity with the appearances of normal anatomy of each gland when using different imaging techniques. For a detailed description of anatomy of the three major salivary glands, please see the recent *Neuroimaging Clinics* article by Atkinson and colleagues.[22] Of particular anatomic interest, Valstar and colleagues have recently described the presence of previously unnoticed bilateral macroscopic salivary gland locations in the human nasopharynx, for which they proposed the name tubarial glands. These were suspected after visualization by PET/CT when using prostate-specific membrane antigen ligands.[23]

Here, the authors briefly describe the anatomy of the ductal systems of the major salivary glands—intraglandular and extraglandular structures that receive little attention in the neuroimaging literature. Nonetheless, knowledge of detailed anatomy and morphometrics for these ducts would be useful for therapeutic planning of luminal procedures on the salivary ducts, including sialography, sialoendoscopy, interventional therapies, and lithotripsy.[24]

All major and minor salivary glands arise by ingrowth of oral epithelium into the underlying mesenchyme. The submandibular and parotid glands are the only salivary glands that migrate during embryological development; they therefore acquire long ducts that drain saliva, and accessory glands may be seen along their course. The SMD of Wharton begins by numerous branches that emerge from the deep surface of the gland. It bends sharply around the posterior margin of mylohyoid to form the genu of the SMD, then runs anteriorly and lateral to hyoglossus and genioglossus, and medial to the attachment of mylohyoid to the mandible along the lower edge of the mylohyoid muscle. It then runs forward and slightly upwards along the medial side of the sublingual gland more anteriorly. It is crossed laterally by the lingual nerve at the anterior border of the hyoglossus muscle. It opens by a narrow orifice on the summit of the sublingual papilla.

Two main ductal tributaries within the anterior part of the parotid gland unite to form the parotid duct (PD) of Stenson. It emerges from the anterior border of the upper part of the gland and passes horizontally across the lateral surface of masseter, and then takes a right-angle turn medially at its anterior edge to penetrate the buccal fat, buccopharyngeal fascia, and buccinator. Here, PD then runs obliquely forward for a short distance

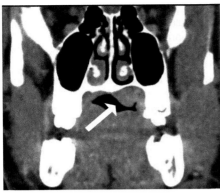
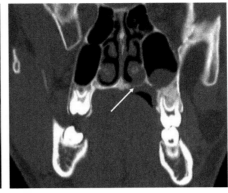

Fig. 18. Clear cell carcinoma of the hard palate. Coronal CT in soft tissue and bone windows showing a left hard palate lesion (*thick arrow*). There is erosion of the hard palate, maxillary sinus, and maxillary bone (*thin arrow*).

between buccinator and the oral mucosa before it penetrates the oral mucosa at a small papilla in the oral vestibule opposite the maxillary second molar. There is a degree of individual variation in the location of the PD orifice in relation to the maxillary molars. An accessory PD may join the PD as the latter passes over the masseter muscle.

Sialography remains the only imaging study for examining the fine anatomy of the salivary ductal system. The technique is described in detail elsewhere and has been reviewed by Horsburgh and Massoud.[24] They analyzed normal digital subtraction sialograms (Figs. 19 and 20) and found the mean PD length was 50 mm, with a mean width of its proximal, mid, and distal segments of 1.8, 1.1, and 1.6 mm, respectively (see Fig. 19). An accessory parotid gland was present in 68% of patients, with a mean angle of confluence of its tributary duct with the PD of 53°. The mean length of the SMD was 58 mm, with a mean width of its proximal, mid, and distal segments of 2.0, 2.7, and 2.1 mm, respectively. The SMD genu had a mean angle of 115°. Thus, on average, the PD is narrower and shorter than the SMD. Therefore, the PD may be more difficult to negotiate with interventional instruments than the SMD.[24]

The sublingual ducts (SLDs) have been described as especially difficult to visualize when dedicated sialography of this gland is attempted owing in great part to the technical challenges in cannulating the small and numerous draining ducts, and the rare need for radiologists to define this particular aspect of anatomy of the sublingual glands.[25] However, a renewed interest in the potential practical use and benefit of SLD sialography may arise from the occasional need to preoperatively map out the precise anatomical relationship between Wharton's and Bartholin's ducts at the oral floor prior to microvascular autologous submandibular gland surgical transfer to replace the lacrimal gland in severe keratoconjunctivitis sicca.[26]

The sublingual glands are the last of the major salivary glands to appear and are the smallest, but, unlike the parotid and submandibular glands, the SLDs do not acquire lengthy ducts as they migrate during development. Bilateral sublingual glands lie under the tongue beneath the mucous membrane of the floor of the mouth. Anatomically, each SLG is subdivided into anterior and posterior parts, and each part has a different drainage system. The smaller or minor ducts of Rivinus, 8 to 20 in number, from the posterior part of each sublingual gland empty at the sublingual fold (plica

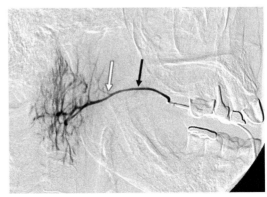

Fig. 19. Digital subtraction sialogram of the parotid duct of Stenson (*black arrow*) and the angle between the accessory parotid duct and main duct (*white arrow*). Patient facing the right. (*From* Horsburgh A, Massoud TF. The salivary ducts of Wharton and Stenson: analysis of normal variant sialographic morphometry and a historical review. Ann Anat. 2013 May;195(3):238-42.)

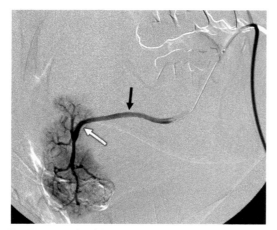

Fig. 20. Digital subtraction sialogram of the submandibular duct of Wharton (*black arrow*) showing its angle (*white arrow*). Patient facing the right. (*From* Horsburgh A, Massoud TF. The salivary ducts of Wharton and Stenson: analysis of normal variant sialographic morphometry and a historical review. Ann Anat. 2013 May;195(3):238-42.)

fimbriata or sublingualis) in the floor of the mouth, formed by the gland and located on either side of the lingual frenulum. The major SLDs were first described by Bartholin—ducts from each anterior SLG may unite to form a larger SLD of Bartholin, which either joins Wharton's duct or drains into the floor of the mouth at the sublingual papilla (caruncle). The exact microanatomic relationship between these ducts at the caruncle has been investigated in detail by Zhang and colleagues[26]

Horsburgh and Massoud presented the first series of patients who had high-resolution digital subtraction sublingual sialograms after unintended cannulation of Bartholin's duct during planned submandibular sialography by cannulating Wharton's duct[25] (Fig. 21). They found that knowledge of the unique histology of the sublingual gland can help explain why the normal imaging anatomy of the sublingual ductal system and secretory units on sialography may cause potential imaging misdiagnosis as severe sublingual sialectasis, with consequent clinical mismanagement. In fact, the salivary glands are compound exocrine tubuloacinar glands composed of aggregated secretory units. These consist of acini that produce secretions and ducts that carry the secretions to the mouth and regulate water and electrolyte contents. There are three types of secretory units: serous, which contain amylase, mucus, and mixed mucus and serous ones, with a greater contribution from either. The sublingual gland is mixed with a predominance of mucous secretions. Mucous acini are larger than serous ones and have an irregular pattern. Intercalated ducts are in direct contact with acini, but in the sublingual glands these are so short to be hardly visible. Therefore, the distinctive microscopic structure of the sublingual glands, with their large mucous-type acini and inconspicuous intralobular ducts, explains the appearances of normal sublingual sialograms as well as contrast retention within the gland following attempted sialogogue provocation. The paucity of branching ducts and apparent immediate contrast medium acinarization of the gland on injection should therefore be considered a normal sialographic finding in the sublingual gland and should not be misdiagnosed as severe sialectasis.

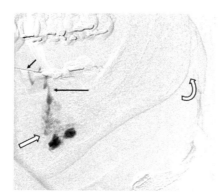
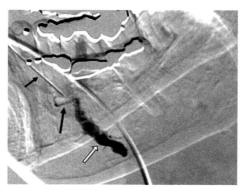

Fig. 21. Lateral projection DSSs of the sublingual glands performed on two separate patients (see Fig. 1A, B) with a straight cannula (*short arrow*) show two examples of inadvertent filling of the duct of Bartholin with contrast medium (*long arrow*) and the sublingual intraglandular ductal system (*hollow straight arrow*). Angle of mandible (*curved arrow*). Patients facing the left. *Reprinted from* Horsburgh A, Massoud TF. Lessons learned from unintended sublingual sialography: imaging anatomy, technical considerations, and diagnostic implications. AJR Am J Roentgenol. 2013 Apr;200(4):879-83. Copyright © 2013 American Roentgen Ray Society.

SUMMARY

The oral cavity is made of many subdivisions and spaces that experience pathology unique to those locations. An understanding of the anatomy and relationships of these compartments is required to form an accurate differential diagnosis of oral cavity pathology. Although unique pathologies are found in the different compartments, there are areas of communication that also extend within the oral cavity or to adjacent spaces of the head and neck. SCC affects multiple subsites (see Fig. 7 and Fig. 12) within the oral cavity, and an understanding of the anatomy allows for accurate radiologic staging. CT and MR imaging play important roles in evaluation of oral cavity pathology and delineation of anatomy. Ultrasonography is an important adjunct and is often the initial imaging technique.

CLINICS CARE POINTS

- Although there are boundaries defined for the different compartments of the oral cavity, these compartments also communicate, and pathology in one area can spread to other areas of the oral cavity and spaces of the head and neck. These are usually malignant neoplasms, aggressive infectious processes, or congenital/developmental lesions.

- Dissemination of oral cavity squamous cell carcinoma can occur by direct extension, via lymphatics, or along neurovascular structures.

- Consider anatomic variants, particularly boutonnière defects of the mylohyoid muscle, as these can mimic disease.

DISCLOSURE

The author A. Famuyide, have no commercial or financial conflicts of interest or funding sources to disclose. G. Moonis, royalties from Walter Kluwers ($100/year).

REFERENCES

1. Som PM, Curtin HD. Head and neck imaging - 2 volume set: expert consult- online and print. Staint Louis, Missouri: Mosby Elsevier; 2011.

2. Law CP, Chandra RV, Hoang JK, et al. Imaging the oral cavity: key concepts for the radiologist. Br J Radiol 2011;84:944–57.

3. Standring S. Gray's anatomy: The anatomical basis of clinical practice. 39th edition. London, England: Churchill Livingstone; 2004.

4. Yousem DM, Chalian AA. Oral cavity and pharynx. Radiol Clin North Am 1998;36:967–81, vii.

5. Piccinin MA, Zito PM. Anatomy, head and neck, lips. In: StatPearls. Treasure Island (FL): StatPearls Publishing; 2021. p. 1–2.

6. Doescher J, Veit JA, Hoffmann TK. The 8th edition of the AJCC cancer staging manual : updates in otorhinolaryngology, head and neck surgery. HNO 2017; 65:956–61.

7. Chapman MC, Soares BP, Li Y, et al. Congenital oral masses: an anatomic approach to diagnosis. Radiographics 2019;39:1143–60.

8. Ong CK, Chong VFH. Imaging of tongue carcinoma. Cancer Imaging 2006;6:186–93.

9. Aiken AH. Pitfalls in the staging of cancer of oral cavity cancer. Neuroimaging Clin N Am 2013;23:27–45.

10. Drake R, Drake RL, Gray H, et al. Gray's anatomy for students. NX Amsterdam, The Netherlands: Elsevier/Churchill Livingstone; 2005.

11. Garcia MRT, Passos UL, Ezzedine TA, et al. Postsurgical imaging of the oral cavity and oropharynx: what radiologists need to know. Radiographics 2015;35:804–18.

12. Trotta BM, Pease CS, Rasamny JJ, et al. Oral cavity and oropharyngeal squamous cell cancer: key imaging findings for staging and treatment planning. Radiographics 2011;31:339–54.

13. Fang WS, Wiggins RH 3rd, Illner A, et al. Primary lesions of the root of the tongue. Radiographics 2011; 31:1907–22.

14. La'porte SJ, Juttla JK, Lingam RK. Imaging the floor of the mouth and the sublingual space. Radiographics 2011;31:1215–30.

15. Sobiesk JL, Munakomi S. Anatomy, head and neck, nasal cavity. In: StatPearls. Treasure Island (FL): StatPearls Publishing; 2021. p. 3.

16. Husain MA. Dental Anatomy and Nomenclature for the Radiologist. Radiol Clin North Am 2018;56:1–11.

17. Scheinfeld MH, Shifteh K, Avery LL, et al. Teeth: what radiologists should know. Radiographics 2012;32:1927–44.

18. Koller A, Sapra A. Anatomy, head and neck, oral gingiva. In: StatPearls. Treasure Island (FL): StatPearls Publishing; 2021. p. 1–2.

19. Loureiro RM, Naves EA, Zanello RF, et al. Dental emergencies: a practical guide. Radiographics 2019;39:1782–95.

20. Tibrewala S, Roplekar S, Varma R. Computed tomography evaluation of oral cavity and oropharyngeal cancers. https://doi.org/10.5005/jp-journals-10003-1111.

21. Simental AA, Myers EN. Cancer of the hard palate and maxillary alveolar ridge: technique and applications. Oper Tech Otolaryngology-Head Neck Surg 2005;16:28–35.

22. Atkinson C, Fuller J III, Huang B. Cross-sectional imaging techniques and normal anatomy of the

salivary glands. Neuroimaging Clin N Am 2018; 28(2):137–58.

23. Valstar MH, de Bakker BS, Steenbakkers RJHM, et al. The tubarial salivary glands: a potential new organ at risk for radiotherapy. Radiother Oncol 2021;154:292–8.

24. Horsburgh A, Massoud TF. The salivary ducts of Wharton and Stenson: analysis of normal variant sialographic morphometry and a historical review. Ann Anat 2013;195(3):238–42.

25. Horsburgh A, Massoud TF. Lessons learned from unintended sublingual sialography: imaging anatomy, technical considerations, and diagnostic implications. AJR Am J Roentgenol 2013;200(4): 879–83.

26. Zhang L, Xu H, Cai Z, et al. Clinical and anatomic study on the ducts of the submandibular and sublingual glands. J Oral Maxillofac Surg 2010;68: 606–10.

Anatomy of the Pharynx and Cervical Esophagus

Ayca Akgoz Karaosmanoglu, MD[a], Burce Ozgen, MD[b],*

KEYWORDS

- Pharynx anatomy • Nasopharynx • Oropharynx • Hypopharynx • Magnetic resonance imaging
- Computed tomography

KEY POINTS

- The pharynx has a complex anatomy, allowing breathing, swallowing, and speech through a common multilayered muscular tube.
- Awareness of the multilayered and integrated anatomy is critical for accurate imaging interpretation.
- Knowledge of the anatomical relationships of different constituents of the pharynx is crucial for understanding the extension pattern of mucosal tumors.

INTRODUCTION

The pharynx, continuous with the cervical esophagus, is a sophisticated structure allowing multiple vital functions through a common pathway, with coordination of numerous muscles. This article reviews the imaging anatomy of the pharynx and cervical esophagus and describes the expected spectrum of imaging findings. Familiarization with the normal appearance of the pharynx and upper esophagus on sectional imaging is critical to recognize the pathological changes in those regions that can be seen in a variety of disease processes. Furthermore, the knowledge of anatomic associations and relationships is crucial in the setting of a neoplastic process to better assess the extension of the disease.

OVERVIEW

The pharynx is a muscular tube extending from the skull base to the level of the cricoid cartilage and plays a crucial role in breathing, swallowing, and speech (Fig. 1).[1] It is continuous inferiorly to the cervical esophagus that serves as part of the functional unit. The pharyngeal airway can be thought of as a pliable tube, surrounded by a multilayered wall that is composed of five layers: mucosa, submucosa, pharyngobasilar fascia, muscles, and buccopharyngeal fascia (BPF) (Fig. 2).[2]

The pharyngeal muscles are organized into two groups based on their orientation (Table 1).[3] The overlapping constrictor muscles, each stacked on top of another from the innermost superior pharyngeal constrictors (SPC) to outer inferior constrictors, function in a complex coordination that allows swallowing while protecting the airway (Fig. 3 A and B).[1,4] The thick pharyngobasilar fascia forms the internal lining of a constrictor muscle sleeve, whereas the thin BPF (middle layer of deep cervical fascia) wraps around the muscle wall.[3]

The pharynx is divided into three separate parts: nasopharynx, oropharynx, and hypopharynx, continuous with the cervical esophagus (see Fig. 1A).

NASOPHARYNX

The nasopharynx is the uppermost part of the pharynx and it has mainly a respiratory function (Table 2).[5] Lying immediately below the central

[a] Department of Radiology, Hacettepe University School of Medicine, Sihhiye 06100, Ankara, Turkey;
[b] Department of Radiology, University of Illinois at Chicago, University of Illinois Hospital, 1740 West Taylor Street, MC 931, Chicago, IL 60612, USA
* Corresponding author.
E-mail address: bozgen2@uic.edu
Twitter: @burceozgen (B.O.)

Neuroimag Clin N Am 32 (2022) 791–807
https://doi.org/10.1016/j.nic.2022.07.022
1052-5149/22/© 2022 Elsevier Inc. All rights reserved.

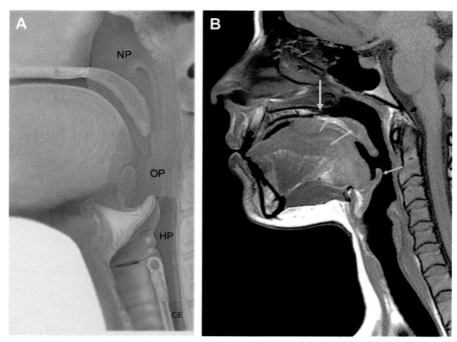

Fig. 1. (A) Sagittal diagram of the pharynx, delineating the pharyngeal subsections (NP, nasopharynx; OP, oropharynx; HP, hypopharynx) and the cervical esophagus (CE). (B) Sagittal T1 W image delineating important anatomical landmarks. Orange arrow: Hard/soft palate junction, short green arrow: aponeurotic segment of SP, green arrow: muscular part of SP, green asterisk: uvula, green shaded area BOT, blue arrow: epiglottis.

skull base, it is bordered supero-posteriorly by the clivus and the anterior aspect of the first two cervical vertebrae (see Fig. 1).[1,6] It extends inferiorly to the level of the hard palate and to the superior surface of the soft palate (SP).[1] It communicates inferiorly with the oropharynx, anteriorly with the nasal cavity through the choanae, and posteriorly with the middle ear cavities.[7]

Posterolateral walls of the nasopharynx are formed and supported by the rigid pharyngobasilar fascia (PBF), which is a tough aponeurosis of the SPC muscle.[1,6] The PBF attaches anteriorly to the medial pterygoid plates, superiorly to the petrous apices, and posteriorly to the pharyngeal tubercle and to the prevertebral muscles (Fig. 4).[8,9] This strong fascia separates the nasopharynx from the adjacent parapharyngeal space and limits tumor spread.[8] Posterior to the medial pterygoid plate, there is a defect in the PBF through which the Eustachian tube and the levator veli palatini (LVP) muscle traverse to enter the nasopharynx.[1,8] This gap in the PBF is known as the sinus of Morgagni.[1,8] The sinus of Morgagni is considered to be a point of weakness for tumor spread, through which nasopharyngeal cancer may spread to the parapharyngeal space.[8,10]

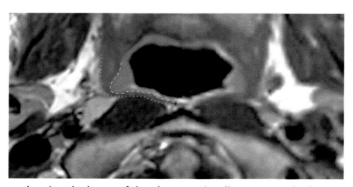

Fig. 2. Axial T2 W image showing the layers of the pharyngeal wall: mucosa and submucosa (pink), pharyngobasilar fascia (yellow line), muscles (red), and buccopharyngeal fascia (blue).

Table 1
Muscles of the pharynx

Muscle	Innervation	Origin	Insertion	Function	Comments
Superior pharyngeal constrictor muscle	CNX through the pharyngeal plexus	Pterygomandibular raphe, pterygoid hamulus, posterior end of mylohyoid line of mandible	Median raphe and pharyngeal tubercle	Constricts the upper portion of the pharynx	Among circular pharyngeal muscles. Innermost location among the pharyngeal constrictors
Middle pharyngeal constrictor muscle	CNX through the pharyngeal plexus	Hyoid bone and stylohyoid ligament	Median raphe	Constricts the middle portion of the pharynx	
Inferior pharyngeal constrictor muscle	CNX through the pharyngeal plexus	Oblique line of the thyroid cartilage and the lateral aspect of the cricoid cartilage	Median raphe and blends inferiorly with circular esophageal muscles	Constricts the lower portion of the pharynx	Two parts: thyropharyngeal part ending in median raphe and cricopharyngeal part blending with circular esophageal muscles
Stylopharyngeus	CN IX	Medial surface of styloid process	Lamina of thyroid cartilage	Elevates the pharynx and expands it laterally	Among inner longitudinal pharyngeal muscles. Passes between the superior and middle pharyngeal constrictor muscle
Salpingopharyngeus	CNX through the pharyngeal plexus	Distal inferior aspect of the cartilaginous ET	Lamina of thyroid cartilage, blends with palatopharyngeus	Opens ET, elevates pharynx	Among inner longitudinal pharyngeal muscles Located posteriorly to torus tubarius
Palatopharyngeus	CNX through the pharyngeal plexus	Upper surface of palatine aponeurosis	Lateral pharyngeal wall, lamina of thyroid cartilage	Depresses soft palate, closes oropharyngeal isthmus	Among inner longitudinal pharyngeal muscles Arch shaped, forms PTP

(continued on next page)

Table 1
(continued)

Muscle	Innervation	Origin	Insertion	Function	Comments
Palatoglossus	CNX through the pharyngeal plexus	Palatine aponeurosis	Lateral BOT	Depresses soft palate, closes oropharyngeal isthmus	Arch shaped, forms ATP
Levator Veli Palatini	CNX through the pharyngeal plexus	Inferior aspect of the petrous bone and medial aspect of the ET	Palatine aponeurosis	Elevates soft palate, opens ET	Located medial to the PBF
Tensor Veli Palatini	CN V mandibular division	Scaphoid fossa, spine of the sphenoid bone and lateral aspect of the ET	Lateral aspect of palatine aponeurosis	Tenses soft palate, opens ET	Located lateral to the PBF
Muscle of uvula	CNX through the pharyngeal plexus	Lower surface of palatine aponeurosis	Tip of uvula and uvular mucosa	Shortens uvula	

Pharyngeal plexus, formed primarily by branches of cranial nerves IX and X, with branches from CN XI and branches from the sympathetic plexus.
Abbreviations: ATP, anterior tonsillar pillar; CN, cranial nerve; ET, eustachian tube; PBF: pharyngobasilar fascia; PTP, posterior tonsillar pillar.

Table 2
Arterial supply, venous, and lymphatic drainage and innervation of the nasopharynx

Arterial supply	Ascending pharyngeal a. Artery of pterygoid canal (vidian a.) Sphenopalatine a.	First-order and second-order (of the maxillary a.) branches of the ECA
Venous Drainage	Pharyngeal venous plexus ⬇ Pterygoid plexus ⬇ Internal jugular vein	The pharyngeal venous plexus has communication with the veins of the orbit via the inferior ophthalmic vein
Lymphatics	Retropharyngeal LNs ⬇ Level II, III and occasionally level V LNs	Extensive lymphatic plexus In adults, nasopharyngeal cancers may metastasize directly to level II and III LNs skipping the retropharyngeal LNs possibly due to obliteration of lymph channels to the retropharyngeal nodes as a result of repeated childhood infections
Innervation	Motor nerve supply—Vagus nerve Sensory innervation—via the glossopharyngeal and the maxillary division of the trigeminal nerve	Exception: tensor veli palatini and stylopharyngeus muscles. Maxillary division of the trigeminal nerve supplies the anterior aspect of the nasopharynx

Abbreviations: a, artery; ECA, external carotid artery; LN, lymph node.

Overlying the PBF and the superior constrictor muscle, the BPF surrounds the nasopharynx, separating it from the deep fascial spaces and acting as an additional barrier limiting the spread of infection and tumor.[1]

Along the lateral walls of the nasopharynx, there are three landmark anatomical structures: the opening of the Eustachian tube, the torus tubarius, and the fossa of Rosenmüller (see Fig. 4).[11] Behind the Eustachian tube orifice, there is a prominent and rounded structure created by the underlying cartilaginous portion of the Eustachian tube, termed the torus tubarius.[7,11] Behind and above the torus tubarius, there is a mucosa-lined recess called the fossa of Rosenmüller (lateral pharyngeal recess), a common site of origin of nasopharyngeal cancers.[1,11] The recess may appear asymmetrical, depending on the amount of lymphoid tissue and the prevertebral muscle thickness.[6]

During swallowing, the salpingopharyngeus, tensor veli palatini (TVP) and LVP muscles pull on the Eustachian tube and ensure its patency while also allowing equalization of pressure between the pharynx and the middle ear.[1]

The adenoids or pharyngeal tonsils are lymphoid tissue lying along the roof and posterior wall of the nasopharynx, a constituent of the Waldeyer's ring (Fig. 5).[8,12] Adenoids are typically enlarged in early childhood but normally regress after puberty.[1,13] However, adenoid enlargement owing to benign lymphoid hyperplasia may persist or recur in some adults.[13] The differentiation of benign lymphoid hyperplasia from nasopharyngeal cancer is best done on contrast-enhanced T1-weighted (T1W) MR images, with symmetric appearance and vertical striping of the adenoid tissue suggestive of benign lymphoid hyperplasia (Fig. 6).[13,14]

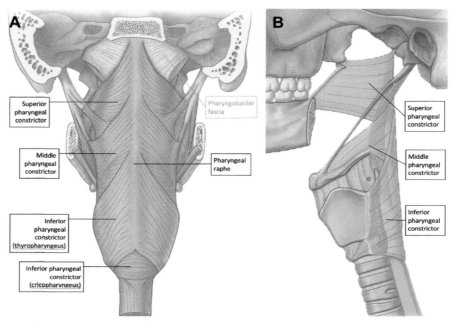

Fig. 3. Pharyngeal constrictors (*A*, *B*). (*Adapted from* Drake RL, Vogl W, Mitchell AWM. Head and Neck. In: Drake RL, Vogl W, Mitchell AWM, Tibbitts R, Richardson P, Horn A, eds. *Gray's basic anatomy.* Second edition. ed. Philadelphia, Pennsylvania: Elsevier; 2018:413-596.)

OROPHARYNX

The oropharynx is the central structure of the upper aerodigestive tract, communicating with the nasopharynx above, the oral cavity anteriorly, and the larynx and hypopharynx inferiorly; serving as a common passageway for food and air (Table 3).[4] It extends craniocaudally from the junction of the soft and hard palate to inferiorly approximately to the level of the hyoid bone and epiglottis.[15] Although the lingual surface of the epiglottis marks the inferior border of the oropharynx, for oncologic purposes, the whole epiglottis is considered as part of the larynx.[16]

Anteriorly, the oropharynx is separated from the oral cavity by an arc-like opening (oropharyngeal isthmus), formed laterally by bilateral mucosal folds (called the anterior tonsillar pillars [ATPs]), and inferiorly by the circumvallate papillae along the posterior aspect of tongue.[17]

In the axial plane, the normal oropharyngeal airway shape is an ellipse with a wide transverse dimension (see Fig. 2).[18] Reduction of the cross-sectional area, especially a decreased transverse dimension plays an important role in the pathophysiology of obstructive sleep apnea (OSA), with a transverse diameter of the airway at the retroglossal level >12 mm especially useful to rule out a severe OSA.[19]

The oropharynx has four subsites that have individual functions and associations that play an important role in disease extension. These subsites include the SP, the base of the tongue

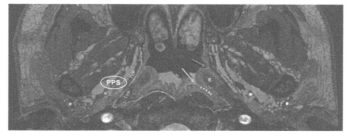

Fig. 4. Axial postcontrast FIESTA image showing the normal anatomy of the nasopharynx. Thin golden line: pharyngobasilar fascia. LVP, levator veli palatini; PPS, parapharyngeal space; tt, torus tubarius; TVP, tensor veli palatini. blue arrow: opening of the Eustachian tube, yellow arrow/line: fossa of Rosenmüller.

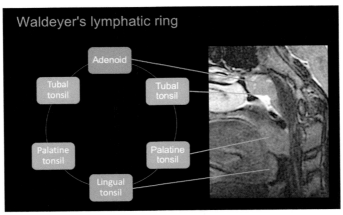

Fig. 5. Location of different constituents of the mucosal-associated lymphoid tissue known as Waldeyer's tonsillar ring; including pharyngeal and tubal tonsils of the nasopharynx, palatine, and lingual tonsils of the oropharynx.

(BOT), the palatine tonsillar fossa, and the posterior pharyngeal wall.

Subsites and Associations

Soft palate

The SP or *velum* is a complex "cape"-like structure, attached to the posterior margin of the hard palate, formed by a midline aponeurosis and interweaving pairs of muscles.[4,20] The uvula sags inferiorly from the dorsal midline edge of the SP and is primarily formed from the insertions of the two muscles of the uvula.[4]

The SP functions as the cock/bar of a three-way stopcock. At rest, during quiet nasal breathing, the SP opposes the tongue, sealing off the oral cavity.[20] During swallowing, complete closure of the nasopharynx is obtained by the superior lifting of the SP to contact the posterior pharyngeal wall and by the contraction of the SPC.[20] The SP has one intrinsic (muscle of the uvula) and several extrinsic muscles (palatoglossus, palatopharyngeus, LVP, and TVP), allowing those functions (see Table 1).[17] LVP is the elevator muscle of the SP, forming 40% of the SP length between the hard palate and base of uvula (Fig. 7).[21] TVL joins its mirror image from the opposite side and with the

LVP, they form a sling that suspends the SP and also tenses the aponeurosis during swallowing.[4,20]

Base of the tongue/lingual tonsil

The tongue base is the posterior third of the tongue, the area posterior to the circumvallate papillae.[15] The tongue base and the free edge of the epiglottis are separated by paired recesses, the valleculae, divided by a median mucosal fold called the glosso-epiglottic fold and bounded laterally by the pharyngoepiglottic folds (Fig. 8).[15,17] Although anatomically the pharyngoepiglottic folds and valleculae are symmetrical, they are more likely to appear asymmetric on imaging.[22]

The BOT contains follicles of lymphatic tissue that form the lingual tonsil, also part of the Waldeyer's ring (Fig. 9).[1] It is variable in size, reported to be 5 mm to 13 mm in the anteroposterior (AP) dimension, and can extend inferiorly and may partially encroach the vallecula; however, extension into the floor or posterior vallecular wall is suspicious for tumoral growth.[1,15,22] The glossotonsillar sulci separate the lingual tonsil from palatine tonsils on each side (Fig. 10).

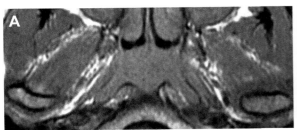
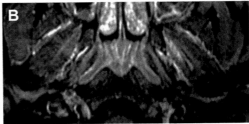

Fig. 6. Axial precontrast (A) and postcontrast fat-suppressed (B) T1-weighted images from the level of the nasopharynx showing adenoidal hypertrophy with striated contrast enhancement (B).

Table 3
Arterial supply, venous, and lymphatic drainage and innervation of the oropharynx

	Soft Palate	Base of Tongue	Palatine Tonsillar Fossa	Posterior Oropharyngeal Wall
Arterial supply	• Lesser palatine a. (br of maxillary a.) • Asc palatine a. (br of the facial a.) • Asc. pharyngeal a (from ECA)	• Lingual a. • Tonsillar br of the facial a. • Asc. pharyngeal a	• Tonsillar br of facial a (main) • Asc. Pharyngeal a • Lingual a • Asc palatine a.	• Asc. Pharyngeal a • Facial artery • Lingual artery • IMA
Venous drainage	Pterygoid venous plexus	Lingual vein → IJV	• Pharyngeal venous plexus • External palatine vein	Pharyngeal venous plexus → IJV
Lymphatics	• Primarily to the retropharyngeal LNs • Secondarily to jugulodigastric LNs	• Primarily to the jugulodigastric LNs • Secondarily the retropharyngeal LNs	• Primarily to the jugulodigastric LNs • Secondarily the retropharyngeal LNs	• Bilat. jugular chain and retropharyngeal LNs
Innervation	Sensory and motor innervation CN V_2 (lesser palatine n.) • special sensory (taste) innervation via the greater petrosal n. (br of facial n)	Sensory and motor innervation of the oropharynx – CN V_2, CN IX &X CN IX (tonsillar br)	• CN IX • CN V_2 (lesser palatine n.)	CN IX

Abbreviations: a, artery; asc, ascending; bilat, bilateral; BOT, base of tongue; br, branch; CN, cranial nerve; ECA, external carotid artery; IJV, Internal jugular vein; IMA, internal maxillary artery; LN, lymph node; n, nerve

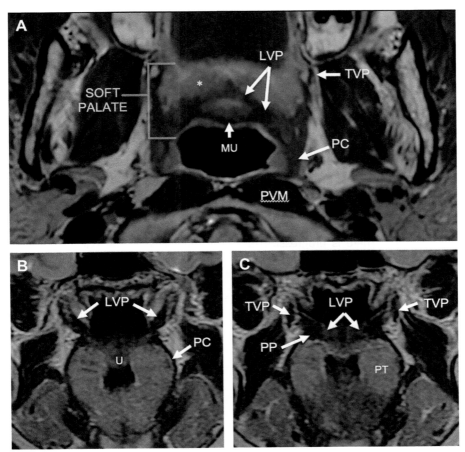

Fig. 7. Axial (*A*) and coronal (*B, C*) T2 W images at the level of the soft palate, illustrating the muscles forming the soft palate: ; LVP, levator veli palatini; MU, muscle of uvula; PC, pharyngeal constrictors; PP, palatopharyngeus; PT, palatine tonsil; TVP, tensor veli palatini; u, uvula; asterisk, palatine glands; PVM, prevertebral muscles.

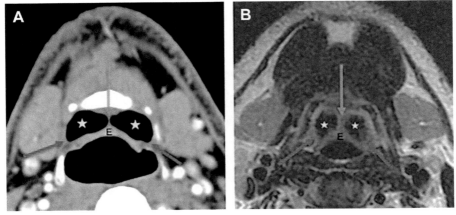

Fig. 8. Axial CT (*A*) and axial T2 W MR *(B)* images showing the valleculae (*stars*) divided by the glossoepiglottic fold (*blue arrow*) and bounded laterally by the pharyngoepiglottic folds (*purple arrows*). E, epiglottis.

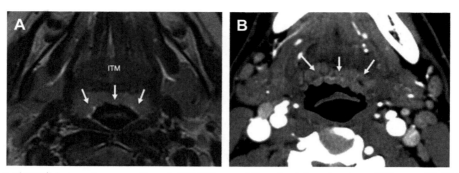

Fig. 9. Lingual tonsil (*arrows*) seen on the axial T2 W image (*A*) and axial postcontrast CT image (*B*). ITM, intrinsic tongue muscles.

Aside from the lymphoid tissue, the BOT is mostly made up of extrinsic and intrinsic tongue muscles (see Fig. 9).[17] There is progressive fat deposition at the tongue base with advancing age and increased body mass index (BMI), an important determinant in OSA. The degree of this fat deposition can be estimated by attenuation measurements on computed tomography (CT) (with 30 HU as the upper limit of normal, corresponding to 32% fat) or by estimating the percentage of fat using Dixon techniques on MR imaging.[18]

The neurovascular bundle (consisting of the hypoglossal nerve, the lingual nerve, and the lingual artery) that supplies the anterior aspect of the tongue, courses in the inferolateral portions of the tongue base, along the styloglossus–hyoglossus complex. With recent advances in transoral robotic surgery for the treatment of oropharyngeal neoplasms and OSA, the detailed anatomical knowledge of the hypoglossal-lingual neurovascular bundle is critical for successful functional outcomes.[23]

Palatine tonsillar fossa

The lateral walls of the oropharynx are demarcated by two pairs mucosal folds called the anterior and posterior tonsillar pillars (PTPs), forming two consecutive arches at the oropharyngeal isthmus (Fig. 11).[1,17] The ATP is the anterior arch formed by mucosa over the palatoglossus muscle and the PTP is the posterior arch formed by mucosa overlying the palatopharyngeus muscle. The tonsillar fossa is located between these arches and contains the palatine tonsil (also called faucial tonsil), another constituent of the Waldeyer's ring. These tonsils can be recognized separately from the ATP and PTP on T2-weighted (T2W) MR images (see Fig. 11B).[17] The tonsils can vary in size with age (usually reaching their maximum size in the adolescence and then gradually regressing)[4] and they can also have an asymmetric appearance with more than 3 mm size difference between the two sides.[17,22,24] The lateral aspect of the palatine tonsils is covered by a hemicapsule, which in turn is surrounded by a loose areolar tissue (forming the peritonsillar space), delineated laterally by the PBF and the SPC muscle (see Fig. 11). In the setting of complicated tonsillar infection, pus can collect in this peritonsillar space and form a peritonsillar abcess.[1] The anatomic relationships of the whole palatine tonsillar fossa region are very crucial for understanding the extension pattern of oropharyngeal tumors as the ATP is the most common site of origin for oropharyngeal squamous cell carcinoma.[25] Tonsillar tumors can spread through

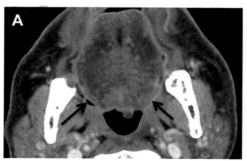
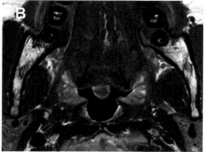

Fig. 10. Axial CT image (*A*) and axial T2W image (*B*) showing the glossotonsillar sulci (*arrows*), between the palatine tonsil and tongue base/lingual tonsil.

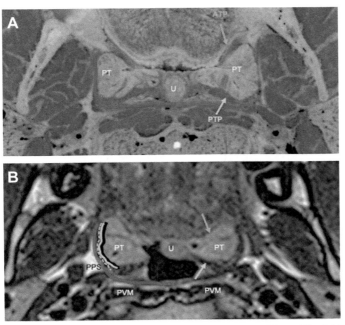

Fig. 11. Axial cross-sectional cryosection from Visible Human Project Data *(A)* and ()axial T2 weighted image *(B)* from the level of the palatine tonsils (PT), bounded anteriorly by the ATP formed by the palatoglossus *(green arrow)* and posteriorly by PTP formed by the palatopharyngeus *(yellow arrow)*. The lateral aspect of the tonsil is delineated by the hemicapsule (in *black*), the peritonsillar space *(white)*, the pharyngobasilar fascia *(dotted yellow line)* and by the pharyngeal constrictor *(red)*, separating it from the parapharyngeal space (PPS). PVM, prevertebral muscles; U, uvula. ([A] *Courtesy of* the U.S. National Library of Medicine, Bethesda, MD.)

the palatoglossus muscle to the SP and to the tongue base, crossing over the glossotonsillar sulcus.[17]

Posterior pharyngeal wall

The posterolateral wall of the pharynx is a continuous structure without any distinctive anatomic markings throughout its course along all subsites of the pharynx.[17] The posterior wall is mainly composed of interweaving SPC and middle pharyngeal constrictor (MPC) muscles, packed between the mucosa and the PBF on the inside and BPF on the outside (Fig. 12). The PBF and musculature often acts as a barrier to contain tumors originating from the underlying mucosa. However, the tumoral infiltration can breach this barrier and involve the retropharyngeal space and then the prevertebral fascia, to reach the cervical spine.

Posterior oropharyngeal wall thickness has been reported to be on average 3.4 ± 0.6 mm.[26] However, age- and sex-related differences exist: with a decreased thickness of the oropharyngeal wall in individuals above 60 years and with increased thickness in men compared with women.[26] Furthermore, the thickness of the oropharyngeal wall is also dependent on the BMI

and obese patients were noted to have significantly increased wall thickness compared with nonobese subjects.[26]

HYPOPHARYNX

The hypopharynx is the most inferior part of the pharynx extending from the level of the hyoid bone to the esophagus (Table 4).[1,27] Its inferior margin is at the level of the lower border of the cricoid cartilage and the 6th cervical vertebra.[3] The hypopharynx is continuous superiorly to the oropharynx and inferiorly to the cervical esophagus without an anatomic barrier, permitting the spread of neoplasms.[27]

Beneath the mucosa and submucosa, the muscular layer of the hypopharynx is composed of inferior pharyngeal constrictor (IPC) muscles posterolaterally, and the posterior cricoarytenoid muscles anteriorly.[28] A fascial layer derived from the BPF surrounds the muscular layer.

At the junction of hypopharynx and the cervical esophagus, the cricopharyngeus muscle forms the lower portion of the IPC muscle.[1,5] The cricopharyngeus muscle attaches to the dorsolateral aspect of the lower part of the cricoid cartilage on each side, forming a horizontal circular

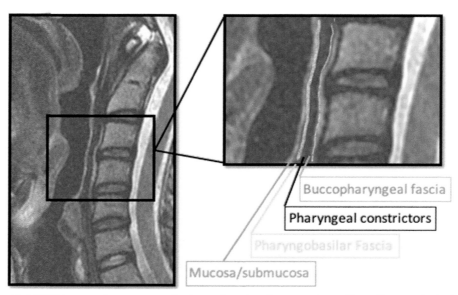

Buccopharyngeal fascia

Pharyngeal constrictors

Pharyngobasilar Fascia

Mucosa/submucosa

Fig. 12. Sagittal T2 W image where consecutive layers forming the posterior wall are illustrated. The buccopharyngeal fascia is separated from the prevertebral fascia by the retropharyngeal space (seen as white strip anterior to vertebra).

muscular band that encircles the lowermost hypopharynx and forming the main component of the upper esophageal sphincter.[1] In the resting state, the cricopharyngeus is normally contracted and closed, to prevent esophagopharyngeal reflux. During swallowing, in response to the volume and pressure of the food bolus, cricopharyngeus relaxes, allowing the luminal content to pass into the esophagus.[1]

Along the posterior wall of the hypopharynx on either side of the raphe, there is a small triangular anatomical area where the upper oblique fibers of the IPC and the cricopharyngeus fibers do not overlap. This area of weakness is called the Killian's dehiscence.[1,29] Herniation of mucosa and submucosa through this area results in a pharyngeal pouch named Zenker's diverticulum.[29]

The three hypopharyngeal subsites are; the paired pyriform sinuses (one on each side), the posterior hypopharyngeal wall, and the postcricoid region.[1,28]

Subsites and Associations

Pyriform sinuses

The pyriform (pear-shaped) sinuses are hypopharyngeal recesses on each side of the larynx.[1,27] They have an inverted pyramid shape with the apex below at the level of the vocal cords and the base at the level of the hyoid bone (Fig. 13).[28] The mucosa of the anterior wall of the pyriform sinus covers the posterior paraglottic space of the larynx.[1] Posteriorly, the pyriform sinus is continuous with the pharyngeal cavity. The

lateral wall of each pyriform sinus is formed by the thyrohyoid membrane (membranous portion) superiorly and the thyroid cartilage (cartilaginous portion) inferiorly.[1,27] Just below the level of the hyoid, the MPC and IPC muscles fail to overlap, leaving the membranous lateral wall as a thin fibrous thyrohyoid membrane that is penetrated by the superior laryngeal neurovascular bundle.[27,29] The medial wall is formed by the lateral surface of the aryepiglottic fold, which is usually considered as a marginal zone as tumors are located at the laryngeal and lateral surface of the aryepiglottic fold behave differently clinically.[1] Tumors involving the laryngeal surface act as a supraglottic tumor whereas, tumors along the lateral wall of the aryepiglottic fold behave more aggressively in a manner similar to hypopharynx tumors.[1]

Pyriform sinus is the most commonly involved subsite of hypopharynx by squamous cell carcinoma.[27,28] Tumors arising on the lateral wall tend to invade the posterior aspect of the thyroid cartilage with extension into the thyroid gland or soft tissues of the neck laterally.[27,28] In contrast, tumors involving the medial wall of the pyriform sinus usually show early laryngeal infiltration with cord fixation.[27,28]

Posterior hypopharyngeal wall

Posterior wall of the hypopharynx is in direct communication with the oropharynx cranially and cervical esophagus caudally.[1] The lateral walls of the pyriform sinuses blend into the posterior

Table 4
Arterial supply, venous, and lymphatic drainage and innervation of the hypopharynx

Arterial supply	Sup. and inf. laryngeal arteries (from sup. and inf. thyroid arteries, respectively)	Sup. laryngeal a and n course through the thyrohyoid membrane to supply the superior aspect of the pyriform sinus Inf. laryngeal a and n travel through a gap inferior to the ipc then course superiorly to supply lower pharynx along with larynx
Venous Drainage	Pharyngeal venous plexus Sup. and inf. thyroid veins ↓ IJV	Hypopharynx also has a rich submucosal venous plexus which then drains to the pharyngeal venous plexus
Lymphatics	*Pyriform sinus*: primarily level II and III LN, secondarily to level V LN *Posterior hypopharyngeal wall*: level II and III LN and retropharyngeal LN *Post-cricoid region*: level III, IV and VI LN	Slightly different lymphatic drainage for subsites of hypopharynx
Innervation	Motor and sensory innervation – pharyngeal nerve plexus	The internal branch of the sup. laryngeal n responsible for referred ear pain in patients with tumor within hypopharynx - courses along the anterior wall of the pyriform sinus. The sensory axons of this nerve carry the stimulus up to the jugular ganglion via CNX *and then the stimulus travels along the Arnold's nerve (the auricular branch of the vagus n).*

Abbreviations: a, artery; IJV, internal jugular vein; Inf, Inferior; IPC, inferior pharyngeal constrictor; LN, lymph nodes; n, nerve; Sup, Superior.

hypopharyngeal wall. Behind the posterior hypopharyngeal wall, there is retropharyngeal space separating it from the cervical vertebrae and prevertebral muscles permitting free movement of the pharynx during swallowing.[28] Posterior hypopharyngeal wall cancers often tend to spread cranio-caudally but can also extend posteriorly, similar to posterior oropharyngeal wall tumors.[27,28]

Post-cricoid region
The post-cricoid area forms the anterior wall of the lower hypopharynx.[1,28] As its name implies, it is the region immediately posterior to the cricoid cartilage. It starts at the level of the cricoarytenoid joints and extends inferiorly to the lower margin of the cricoid cartilage.[1] Owing to its proximity to adjacent structures, tumors involving this site tend to extend to the posterior aspect of the larynx, and also with a high tendency to involve the pyriform sinuses, the trachea, and/or esophagus.[27]

In the resting state, normally the anterior wall (post-cricoid region) and the posterior wall (posterior hypopharyngeal wall) of the hypopharynx

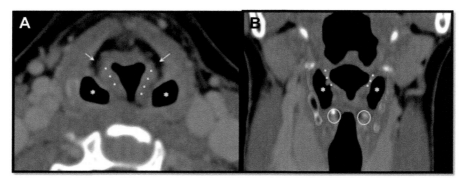

Fig. 13. Pyriform sinuses (*yellow stars*) on axial (*A*) and coronal-reformatted (*B*) contrast-enhanced CT images. Medial walls of the pyriform sinuses are formed by the aryepiglottic folds (*white dots*). Laterally, the pyriform sinuses are bordered by the thyrohyoid membrane (*red curved line* on *B*) and thyroid cartilage (in *blue* on *B*). Inferiorly, the apices of the pyriform sinuses are at the level of the cricoarytenoid joints (*circles*). Paraglottic spaces (*short arrows* in *A*) lie immediately adjacent to the anterior walls of the pyriform sinuses.

cavity are in direct contact with their mucosa in apposition (**Fig. 14**).[28] The AP thickness of the hypopharynx in the post-cricoid region is relatively constant and should be considered abnormal if greater than 10 mm.[30] The anterior wall is slightly thinner than the posterior wall (average 2.5 mm and 3.5 mm, respectively).[30] The transverse diameter of the hypopharynx at the level of the cricoid gradually decreases to approximately 1 cm craniocaudally approaching the esophageal verge.[28] Although the change in size may be indicative of underlying pathology, loss of this normal tapering, especially in combination with obscuration of intramural and/or surrounding fat planes are probably much more reliable imaging findings.[28] The intramural fat planes can be visualized both on CT and MR imaging and normally tend to become less conspicuous from the upper to the lower cricoid cartilage.[30] The transverse diameter of the hypopharynx is wider in men compared with women likely related to the greater size of the thyroid cartilage in men.[30] Other hypopharyngeal anatomic measurements such as volumes of the laryngeal and hypopharyngeal cavities and length of pharynx were also found to be significantly larger in men, even after normalizing for height.[31]

CERVICAL ESOPHAGUS

The cervical esophagus is basically a tubular inferior extension of the pharynx (**Table 5**).[27] The esophagus is arbitrarily subdivided into three segments: cervical, thoracic, and abdominal esophagus.[32] The cervical esophagus is the upper third segment, beginning at the lower border of the cricoid cartilage/upper esophageal sphincter (formed by the cricopharyngeus muscle) and extending to the level of the sternal notch where it becomes the thoracic esophagus.[27,32]

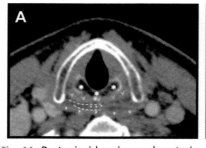
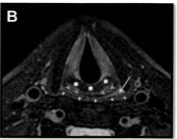
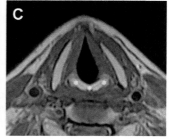

Fig. 14. Post-cricoid region and posterior wall of the hypopharynx delineated on axial contrast-enhanced CT (*A*), fat-saturated T2-W (*B*), and T1-W(*C*) MR images at the level of the cricoid cartilage (*stars* on *A–C*). The opposed mucosal walls of the post-cricoid region and posterior wall can sometimes be appreciated on CT as thin hypodense line (*white dots* on *A*) if intramural fat planes are visible (*dashed yellow lines* on *A*). On T2-weighted images mucosa appears hyperintense (*arrow* in *B*). Anterior wall of the hypopharynx is formed by the posterior cricoarytenoid muscle (*white arrowheads*), whereas the posterior wall of the hypopharynx is formed by the IPC muscle (*yellow arrowheads*). On T1-weighted images, it is hard to appreciate hypopharyngeal walls separately (*C*).

Table 5 Arterial supply, venous and lymphatic drainage and innervation of the cervical esophagus	
Arterial supply	Branches of the inferior thyroid artery
Venous Drainage	Tributaries of the inferior thyroid veins
Lymphatics	Level VI and mediastinal lymph nodes
Innervation	Motor nerve supply-via branches of the recurrent laryngeal nerve Parasympathetic and sympathetic innervation-via the CNX and sympathetic chain, respectively

The esophageal wall is composed of mucosal and submucosal layers, and a muscular layer composed of inner circular and outer longitudinal oriented striated (voluntary) muscle fibers.[5,28] A fascial sheath that is continuous with the BPF surrounds the muscular layer, with no surrounding serosa.[28,32] The absence of a serosal layer may facilitate the spread of disease in the setting of infection or neoplasm.[32]

The inferior border of the cricoid cartilage, pharyngoesophageal junction, and the sixth cervical vertebral body lies on the same plane horizontally.[5] In patients with a high risk of regurgitation, this anatomical relationship can be helpful, permitting usage of a technique called "cricoid pressure," which is compression of the pharyngoesophageal junction in between the cricoid cartilage and the 6th cervical vertebra to prevent passive regurgitation during the induction phase of the anesthesia.[33]

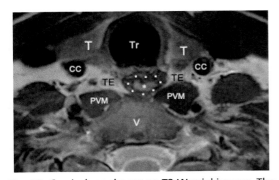

Fig. 15. Cervical esophagus on T2-W axial images. The mucosa appears hyperintense (*yellow star*) and the muscular wall (*white dots*) appears isointense compared with normal muscle. Trachea (Tr), tracheoesophageal groove (TE), prevertebral muscles (PVM), vertebra (V), thyroid gland (T), and common carotid artery (CC).

The cervical esophagus lies posterior to the trachea with a small amount of fatty tissue in-between (Fig. 15).[5,28] Tracheoesophageal groove lies on each side of the cervical esophagus, containing lymph nodes, recurrent laryngeal nerve, and fat tissue.[5]

Posteriorly, the upper esophagus is related to prevertebral fascia, longus colli muscles, and the bodies of C6 and C7 vertebrae.[34]

The lumen of the pharyngoesophageal junction is normally kidney-shaped, a shape preserved even while fully distended, likely owing to the rigidity of the posterior body of the cricoid cartilage forming its anterior wall.[35] Transitioning from the hypopharynx to the esophagus, the AP thickness widens to an average size of 10 mm and the transverse diameter tapers to an average size of 16 mm.[30] Then below, the cervical esophagus continues with little change compared with the pharyngoesophageal junction in terms of AP and transverse diameters.[30] The esophagus may appear contracted or dilated in imaging studies with a variation of the amount of intraluminal air.[28,36] Therefore, while assessing for possible underlying esophageal abnormality, particularly for tumors, esophageal diameter is not as reliable as the esophageal wall thickness, which normally should be less than 5 mm.[28,36] On MR imaging, esophageal mucosa is best seen as a hyperintense structure on T2W images and with diffuse enhancement on contrast-enhanced T1W images.[30] The muscular wall should normally appear isointense to the surrounding musculature on T2W images (see Fig. 15).[28]

SUMMARY

The pharynx and upper esophagus are continuous muscular structures allowing multiple functions. The normal imaging appearance can be challenging owing to the complex muscular framework and surrounding fascial layers forming numerous anatomical landmarks. Knowledge of the expected findings and of the anatomical relations of different pharyngeal subsites are crucial to assess lesions and disease extension in this region.

CLINICS CARE POINTS

- The pharyngobasilar fascia is a natural anatomic barrier preventing the spread of nasopharyngeal tumors from the nasopharynx to the parapharyngeal space.

- The anterior tonsillar pillar is the most common site of origin for oropharyngeal squamous cell carcinoma. This anatomic structure serves as a gateway for extension of these tumors to the soft palate and the base of tongue.
- Tumor laterality is important with regard to the aryepiglottic folds. Laterally located tumors are classified as hypopharyngeal tumors whereas medially located ones are grouped as laryngeal tumors. Among these two, hypopharyngeal tumors tend to be more biologically aggressive.

FUNDING INFORMATION

None (A. Akgoz Karaosmanoglu); None (B. Ozgen).

DISCLOSURE

The authors have nothing to disclose.

REFERENCES

1. Smoker WRK, Som PM. Anatomy and Imaging of the Oral Cavity and Pharynx. In: Som PM, Curtin HD, editors. Head and neck imaging. 5th ed. USA: Elsevier Health Sciences; 2011. p. 1617–42.
2. Norton NS, Netter FH, Machado CAG. Netter's head and neck anatomy for dentistry. Third edition. Philadelphia (PA): Elsevier; 2017.
3. Drake RL, Vogl W, Mitchell AWM. Head and Neck. In: Drake RL, Vogl W, Mitchell AWM, et al, editors. Gray's basic anatomy. Second edition. Philadelphia, Pennsylvania: Elsevier; 2018. p. 413–596.
4. Varghese J, Kirsch C. Magnetic resonance imaging of the oral cavity and oropharynx. Top Magn Reson Imaging 2021;30(2):79–83.
5. Moore KLD, Arthur F. Neck. In: Moore KLD, Arthur F, editors. Clinically oriented anatomy. 5th ed. Baltimore: Lippincott Willams & Wilkins; 2006. p. 1047–122.
6. Chong VF, Khoo JB, Fan YF. Imaging of the nasopharynx and skull base. Neuroimaging Clin N Am 2004;14(4):695–719.
7. Million RRC, Nicholas J. Nasopharynx. In: Million RRC, Nicholas J, editors. Management of head and neck cancer A multidisciplinary approach. Philadelphia: J. B. Lippincott Company; 1984. p. 445–74.
8. Dubrulle F, Souillard R, Hermans R. Extension patterns of nasopharyngeal carcinoma. Eur Radiol 2007;17(10):2622–30.
9. Komune N, Matsuo S, Nakagawa T. The fascial layers attached to the skull base: a cadaveric study. World Neurosurg 2019;126:e500–9.
10. Hyare H, Wisco JJ, Alusi G, et al. The anatomy of nasopharyngeal carcinoma spread through the pharyngobasilar fascia to the trigeminal mandibular nerve on 1.5 T MRI. Surg Radiol Anat 2010;32(10): 937–44.
11. Mukherji SK, Castillo M. Normal cross-sectional anatomy of the nasopharynx, oropharynx, and oral cavity. Neuroimaging Clin N Am 1998;8(1):211–8.
12. Arambula A, Brown JR, Neff L. Anatomy and physiology of the palatine tonsils, adenoids, and lingual tonsils. World J Otorhinolaryngol - Head Neck Surg 2021;7(3):155–60.
13. Bhatia KSS, King AD, Vlantis AC, et al. Nasopharyngeal mucosa and adenoids: appearance at MR imaging. Radiology 2012;263(2):437–43.
14. Wang ML, Wei XE, Yu MM, et al. Value of contrast-enhanced MRI in the differentiation between nasopharyngeal lymphoid hyperplasia and T1 stage nasopharyngeal carcinoma. Radiol Med 2017; 122(10):743–51.
15. Siddiqui A, Connor SEJ. Imaging of the pharynx and larynx. Imaging 2013;22(1). https://doi.org/10.1259/imaging/91047403. 91047403.
16. Hermans R. Neoplasms of oropharynx. In: Hermans R, editor. Head and neck cancer imaging. Berlin Heidelberg: Springer; 2012. p. 147–62.
17. Hermans R, Lenz M. Imaging of the oropharynx and oral cavity. Part I: normal anatomy. Eur Radiol 1996; 6(3):362–8.
18. Whyte A, Gibson D. Imaging of adult obstructive sleep apnoea. Eur J Radiol 2018;102:176–87.
19. Hora F, Napolis LM, Daltro C, et al. Clinical, anthropometric and upper airway anatomic characteristics of obese patients with obstructive sleep apnea syndrome. Respiration 2007;74(5):517–24.
20. Rubesin SE, Jones B, Donner MW. Radiology of the adult soft palate. Dysphagia 1987;2(1):8–17.
21. Perry JL, Sutton BP, Kuehn DP, et al. Using MRI for assessing velopharyngeal structures and function. Cleft Palate Craniofac J 2014;51(4):476–85.
22. Muraki AS, Mancuso AA, Harnsberger HR, et al. CT of the oropharynx, tongue base, and floor of the mouth: normal anatomy and range of variations, and applications in staging carcinoma. Radiology 1983;148(3):725–31.
23. Brennan PA, Standring S, Wiseman SM. Gray's surgical anatomy. Amsterdam: Elsevier; 2020.
24. Mafee MF, Valvassori GE, Becker M. Imaging of the head and neck. 2nd ed. Stuttgart ;: Thieme; 2005.
25. Lin DT, Cohen SM, Coppit GL, et al. Squamous cell carcinoma of the oropharynx and hypopharynx. Otolaryngol Clin North Am 2005;38(1):59–74, viii.
26. Tomblinson CM, Fletcher GP, Hu LS, et al. Determination of posterolateral oropharyngeal wall thickness and the potential implications for transoral surgical margins in tonsil cancer. Head Neck 2021; 43(7):2185–92.
27. Million RRC, Nicholas J. Hypopharynx: Pharyngeal Walls, Pyriform Sinus, and Postcricoid Pharynx. In:

Million RRC, Nicholas J, editors. Management of head and neck cancer A multidisciplinary approach. Philadelphia: J. B. Lippincott Company; 1984. p. 373–92.

28. Schmalfuss IM. Imaging of the hypopharynx and cervical esophagus. Neuroimaging Clin N Am 2004;14(4):647–62.

29. Griffin NL, AG. Oesophagus. In: Griffin NL, AG, editors. Grainger and allison's diagnostic radiology essentials. Churchill Livingstone; 2013. p. 238–53.

30. Schmalfuss IM, Mancuso AA, Tart RP. Postcricoid region and cervical esophagus: normal appearance at CT and MR imaging. Radiology 2000;214(1):237–46.

31. Inamoto Y, Saitoh E, Okada S, et al. Anatomy of the larynx and pharynx: effects of age, gender and height revealed by multidetector computed tomography. J Oral Rehabil 2015;42(9):670–7.

32. Marini T, Desai A, Kaproth-Joslin K, et al. Imaging of the oesophagus: beyond cancer. Insights Imaging 2017;8(3):365–76.

33. Benkhadra M, Lenfant F, Bry J, et al. Cricoid cartilage and esophagus: CT scan study of the dynamic variability of their relative positions. Surg Radiol Anat 2009;31(7):537.

34. Rhyne AL 3rd, Spector LR, Schmidt GL, et al. Anatomic mapping and evaluation of the esophagus in relation to the cervical vertebral body. Eur Spine J 2007;16(8):1267–72.

35. Randall DR, Cates DJ, Strong EB, et al. Three-dimensional analysis of the human pharyngoesophageal sphincter. Laryngoscope 2020;130(12):2773–8.

36. Xia F, Mao J, Ding J, et al. Observation of normal appearance and wall thickness of esophagus on CT images. Eur J Radiol 2009;72(3):406–11.

Anatomy of the Larynx and Cervical Trachea

Kassie L. McCullagh, MD[a],*, Rupali N. Shah, MD[b], Benjamin Y. Huang, MD, MPH[a]

KEYWORDS

• Larynx • Supraglottis • Glottis • Subglottis • Trachea • Anatomy

KEY POINTS

- The major cartilages of the larynx are the thyroid, cricoid, and paired arytenoids. Three additional paired cartilages occasionally seen on imaging are corniculate, cuneiform, and triticeal cartilages.
- The larynx is divided into 3 main regions: the supraglottis, glottis, and subglottis.
- The cervical trachea is a short segment of the trachea, spanning from the inferior edge of the cricoid to the level of the manubrial notch.

Abbreviations	
AC	anterior commissure
AE	aryepiglottic
AJCC	American Joint Committee on Cancer
CAJ	cricoarytenoid joint
CT	computed tomography
FC	false vocal cord
ITA	inferior thyroid artery
MRI	magnetic resonance imaging
NRLN	nonrecurrent laryngeal nerve
PES	preepiglottic space
PGS	paraglottic space
RLN	recurrent laryngeal nerve
STA	superior thyroid artery
TAM	thyroarytenoid muscle
TC	true vocal cord

INTRODUCTION

The larynx is an anatomically complex organ of the upper airway that lies at the crossroads of the upper aerodigestive tract and the tracheobronchial tree. It connects the pharynx with the cervical trachea and serves several key functions related to normal respiration, swallowing, airway protection, and phonation. Cross-sectional imaging plays an important role in the evaluation of the larynx, particularly in the oncologic setting because it allows visualization of submucosal structures and spaces that cannot be readily assessed by direct laryngoscopy. A firm grasp of laryngeal anatomy is therefore critical to providing accurate and useful staging information in patients with cancers

Funding: None.
[a] Division of Neuroradiology, Department of Radiology, University of North Carolina at Chapel Hill, CB #7510, 101 Manning Drive, Chapel Hill, NC 27599, USA; [b] Division of Voice and Swallowing, Department of Otolaryngology-Head & Neck Surgery, University of North Carolina at Chapel Hill, 170 Manning Dr, POB, Ground Floor, G128, Chapel Hill, NC 27599, USA
* Corresponding author.
E-mail address: kassie_mccullagh@med.unc.edu

neuroimaging.theclinics.com

affecting the region; however, owing to its anatomic and functional complexity, the larynx can be a challenging area to master from a diagnostic imaging standpoint.

In this article, we review the anatomy of the larynx, beginning with an overview of the cartilaginous, muscular, and supporting tissues, which make up the organ. This will be followed by a discussion of the clinically defined sites of the larynx that are relevant to cancer staging with an emphasis on critical areas to assess when interpreting an oncologic staging scan. The anatomy of the cervical trachea will also be discussed, and at the conclusion of the article, we briefly review adjunctive imaging techniques that can be useful for more detailed laryngeal assessment in select circumstances.

OVERVIEW OF THE LARYNX

The larynx can be thought of as an undulating air-filled space defined by sets of mucosal folds draped over a cartilaginous and muscular skeleton. Functionally, the larynx acts as an important valve in the upper aerodigestive tract that regulates and directs the transit of air and ingested substances passing from the upper aerodigestive tract into their appropriate lower pathways (ie, the trachea or esophagus). In doing so, the larynx helps to maintain patency of the upper respiratory tract while preventing swallowed substances from being aspirated into the tracheobronchial tree and lungs. The other major function of the larynx is facilitating the act of phonation, in which various tones are produced through vibration of the vocal folds against each other as air is forced between them.[1]

The larynx communicates with the oropharynx above, the hypopharynx behind and around, and the trachea inferiorly. Other notable structures in the vicinity of the larynx include the thyroid gland, which is situated along the anterior and lateral aspects of the lower larynx and trachea and is bound to the larynx by the pretracheal fascia; the carotid spaces, which are situated posterolateral to the larynx; and the infrahyoid strap muscles, which are positioned anterolaterally to the larynx and drape over the thyroid gland more inferiorly.[2]

The larynx is situated in the anterior neck and, in a normal adult, spans from roughly the C3 to C6 levels.[2] In the newborn period, the larynx is located more cranially at the level of the second cervical vertebra, and throughout childhood, it remains more superiorly located relative to its position in adults. During puberty, there is a rapid lowering of the larynx and hyoid bone relative to the tongue base, with the final adult position of the larynx

being as low as the sixth cervical vertebra.[1] In preadolescent children, there is no significant difference in laryngeal size between boys and girls; however in puberty, the male larynx lengthens and grows significantly compared with the female larynx, corresponding to the development of more marked voice changes in men at this stage in life. These age-based and gender-based differences in the size, configuration, and position of the laryngeal structures produce differences in vocal cord length and thickness, which account for the observed differences in vocal pitch between children and adults and between men and women.[2–7]

Bones and Cartilages of the Larynx

The rigid structure of the larynx is provided by the laryngeal cartilages, which are further supported by various anchoring ligaments and muscles that connect the cartilages with one another and to the hyoid bone, skull base, and trachea. There are 4 major laryngeal cartilages—the thyroid, cricoid, paired arytenoids, and the epiglottis—and 3 sets of paired minor cartilages—the cuneiform, corniculate, and triticeal cartilages (**Fig. 1**). The thyroid, cricoid, and arytenoid cartilages are made of hyaline cartilage, which provide a stiffer support system for the mobile components of the larynx, whereas the epiglottis and minor cartilages are composed of elastic fibrocartilage, which allows flexibility needed for airway protection during swallowing.[1,2]

The *hyoid bone* defines the upper extent of the larynx, functioning to suspend and anchor the larynx during movements related to respiration or phonation. It is a shaped like a horseshoe and is made up of a midline body, which is joined on either side to paired greater and lesser horns or cornua (**Fig. 2**). The hyoid bone does not articulate directly with other bones or cartilages but rather has attachments with the styloid processes of the temporal bone above via the stylohyoid ligament and with the thyroid cartilage below via the thyrohyoid membrane and muscle (discussed further later). In addition, it provides attachments for several extrinsic muscles of the floor of mouth, tongue, and anterior neck, as well as the middle pharyngeal constrictor muscle.[8]

The *thyroid cartilage* is the largest of the 4 laryngeal cartilages and is easily identifiable on axial imaging as the inverted "V" or chevron-shaped structure at the anterior most portion of the larynx[9] (**Fig. 3**). It forms protective anterior and lateral walls to the inner laryngeal structures. The thyroid cartilage consists of 2 lateral plates, referred to as the laminae (or alae), each of which gives off 2 sets of horns (or cornua) along their posterior margins

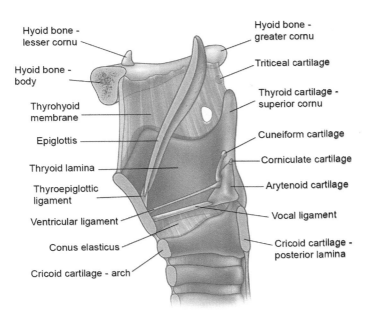

Fig. 1. Midline sagittal cross-sectional illustration of the larynx demonstrating laryngeal cartilages, ligaments, and membranes. (*Courtesy of* Joel Floyd, Jr, MA, CMI, Chapel Hill, NC.)

(Fig. 4). The larger superior horns project upward and posteriorly to anchor the larynx to the hyoid bone through the lateral thyrohyoid ligament. The smaller and shorter inferior horns project downward and medially to articulate with the cricoid cartilage at the cricothyroid joint where rotation of the articular surfaces varies tension and length of the vocal folds.[1,10]

On clinical examination, the thyroid cartilage is palpable as the midline laryngeal prominence where the 2 laminae fuse with one another. Just above the thyroid prominence is a groove where the laminae remain unfused, referred to as the superior thyroid notch. In cadaver studies, the angle formed at the laryngeal prominence, known as the interlaminar angle (ILA), tends to be more acute in men, with reported ILA ranges of between 63° and 90° in men and 80° to 120° in women.[5] As alluded to previously, the thyroid cartilage is also generally

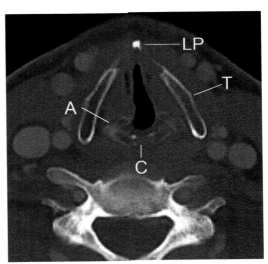

Fig. 3. Cartilages of the larynx on CT. Axial bone window CT at the level the true vocal cords (TC) and laryngeal ventricles demonstrates the cartilages of the larynx. The anteriorly located chevron-shaped cartilage is the thyroid cartilage formed by 2 laminae (T) with the anterior most point representing the laryngeal prominence (LP). The lamina of the cricoid cartilage (C) is partially visible posteriorly. The 2 arytenoid cartilages (A) are visible articulating at the cricoarytenoid joints. (*Courtesy of* University of North Carolina, Chapel Hill, NC.)

Fig. 2. 3D CT reconstruction of the hyoid .bone from a right anterior oblique view. The hyoid bone consists of a midline body joined on either side to paired greater and lesser cornua. (*Courtesy of* University of North Carolina, Chapel Hill, NC.)

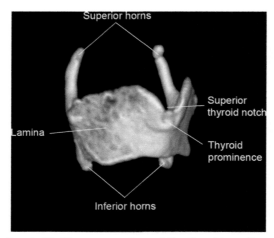

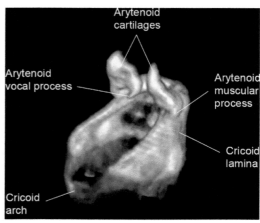

Fig. 4. 3D CT reconstruction of the thyroid cartilage from a right anterior oblique perspective. The thyroid cartilage consists of 2 laminae, which give rise to superior and inferior horns along their posterior margins. Just above where the laminae fuse at the midline, there is a superior midline groove known as the superior thyroid notch. The laryngeal prominence is located just below the notch. (*Courtesy of* University of North Carolina, Chapel Hill, NC.)

Fig. 5. 3D CT reconstruction demonstrating the cricoid and arytenoid cartilages from a left anterior oblique perspective. The cricoid forms a complete ring including a shorter anterior arch and a taller posterior lamina. The pyramid-shaped arytenoids articulate with the lamina at the cricoarytenoid joints. Two processes arise from the base of the arytenoid, including a muscular process extending posterolaterally and a vocal process projecting anteriorly and medially. (*Courtesy of* University of North Carolina, Chapel Hill, NC.)

larger and more anteriorly angulated in men than women.[3-6] In combination, these factors result in the typically more noticeable laryngeal prominence observed in men (the so-called Adam's apple).[1]

The *cricoid cartilage* defines the inferior extent of the larynx and is the only airway cartilage that forms a complete ring. The narrower anterior portion of the cricoid cartilage, known as the arch, measures approximately 0.5 to 1 cm in height, whereas the posterior portion of the ring, referred to as the posterior lamina, is taller, projecting more superiorly, and typically measures approximately 2 to 3 cm in height[1] (**Fig. 5**). The top of the posterior lamina extends to the level of the *true vocal cords* (TC), which is an important landmark in tumor staging. At the superior margins of the lamina are 2 facets that articulate with the arytenoid cartilages to form the cricoarytenoid joints.[10] There are also paired facets along the lateral aspects of the posterior lamina, which articulate with the inferior cornua of the thyroid cartilage to form the previously mentioned cricothyroid joints. The inferior edge of the cricoid demarcates the junction between the subglottic larynx and the trachea.[2]

The paired *arytenoid cartilages*, which are named after a Greek word meaning "ladle" or, more specifically, the "spout" of a ladle or jar,[11] resemble 3-sided pyramids that are located at the superior margins of the posterior lamina of the cricoid (see **Fig. 5**). The triangular base of each arytenoid contains an articular facet that contributes to its respective cricoarytenoid joint. At the cricoarytenoid joint, the primary motions of the arytenoid are translation in an inferolateral or superomedial direction and rocking and twisting motion around the long axis of the facet, which allow the vocal process to rock inferomedially with adduction and superolaterally with abduction.[1] Two processes extend from the base of the arytenoid, including a muscular process extending from the posterior lateral margin of the arytenoid that serves as the attachment site for the cricoarytenoid muscles, and a vocal process projecting anteriorly and medially where the vocal ligament attaches.

Projecting upward from the base of the arytenoid are 3 surfaces forming the respective sides of the pyramid. The posterior facing surface provides attachments for the transverse and oblique interarytenoid muscles; the anterolateral surface gives attachment to the thyroarytenoid muscle and the vestibular ligament; and the medial surface is mucosa covered.[12] The apex of the pyramid formed by each arytenoid cartilage is located at the level of the false vocal cords.[13]

The final major cartilage of the larynx is the *epiglottis*, which is a leaf-shaped structure that narrows inferiorly to a base called the petiole (or stem). It is located at the superior margin of the larynx with the petiole anchored anteriorly to the inner thyroid lamina via the thyroepiglottic ligament (see **Fig. 1**).[2] More superiorly, the epiglottis connects to the back of the body of the hyoid bone by the hyoepiglottic ligament. The mucous membrane covering the anterior aspect of the epiglottis sweeps forward to the tongue base as the median glossoepiglottic fold anteriorly and to the pharyngeal walls laterally as the paired pharyngoepiglottic folds, forming 2 pouch-like areas to either side of the glossoepiglottic fold, which are known as the valleculae.[8] In the center of the posterior wall of the epiglottis there is a normal subtle bump called the tubercle, which can sometimes be observed as a small posterior projection located above the petiole. The hyoid bone is the landmark that divides the epiglottis into 2 portions, a suprahyoid portion, which projects upward into the oropharyngeal airway, and an infrahyoid portion that extends to the inferior tip of the petiole.[14]

Additional small cartilages present in the larynx include the paired *corniculate, cuneiform, and triticeal cartilages* (see **Fig. 1**). These are often not evident on imaging but occasionally they will ossify and be visible as additional small, calcified structures not corresponding to any of the major cartilages. The corniculate cartilages (**Fig. 6**) sit atop the superior processes of the arytenoid cartilages. The cuneiform cartilages are curved cartilages at the margins of the aryepiglottic (AE) folds situated just anterior and lateral to the arytenoid and cuneiform cartilages[8] (see **Fig. 1**). The

triticeal cartilages are located in the free edges of the thyrohyoid membrane above the superior thyroid cornua, within the lateral thyrohyoid ligament (**Fig. 7**).

There is considerable variability in the degree of cartilage ossification, which is frequently discontinuous and asymmetric, occasionally making it difficult to differentiate tumor invasion from normal cortical discontinuity on computed tomography (CT).[14] Ossification of the cartilages typically progresses with age, usually beginning in the second decade of life, and men generally demonstrate greater laryngeal cartilage ossification than women.[15] On CT, nonossified cartilage may only be slightly hyperdense relative to soft tissue (**Fig. 8**).[9] On MR imaging, nonossified cartilage demonstrates intermediate-to-low signal on both T1-weighted and T2-weighted pulse sequences (**Fig. 9**). Ossification of the cartilages is usually best depicted on CT but it can also be appreciated with MR imaging. With progressive ossification, the cortex eventually becomes calcified and demonstrates very-low signal intensity on all MR sequences, whereas the medullary portion transitions to the signal intensity of fat[16–18] (see **Fig. 9**).

Supporting Connective Tissue Structures in the Larynx

In addition to those already mentioned, there are several other ligaments and membranes in the larynx that provide support and connections

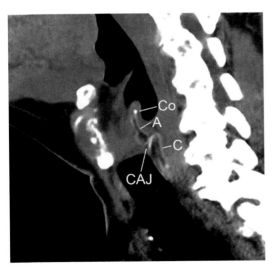

Fig. 6. Sagittal CT showing the ossified corniculate cartilage (Co) at the superior margin of the arytenoid cartilage (A) and the articulation between the arytenoid and cricoid cartilages (C) at the cricoarytenoid joint (CAJ). (*Courtesy of* University of North Carolina, Chapel Hill, NC.)

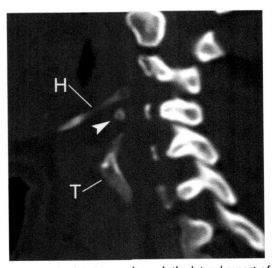

Fig. 7. Sagittal CT image through the lateral aspect of the larynx in a bone window demonstrates an ossified triticeal cartilage (*arrowhead*) positioned between the hyoid bone (H) and the thyroid cartilage (T) within the edge of the thyrohyoid membrane. (*Courtesy of* University of North Carolina, Chapel Hill, NC.)

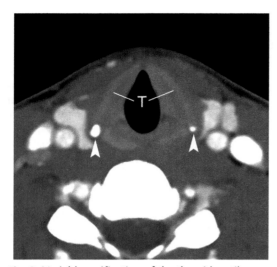

Fig. 8. Variable ossification of the thyroid cartilage on CT in a 17-year-old woman. With the exception of its most posterior margins (*arrowheads*), the thyroid cartilage (T) is mostly unossified and demonstrates densities slightly higher than the adjacent soft tissues (compared with the appearance of the more ossified thyroid cartilage in Fig. 3). (*Courtesy of* University of North Carolina, Chapel Hill, NC.)

The *vocal ligaments* are paired ligaments that attach to the vocal processes of the arytenoids and extend anteriorly and medially to insert on the inner surface of the thyroid lamina, just off midline below the stem of the epiglottis. The small gap between the anterior vocal ligament insertions is referred to as the *anterior commissure* (AC), which is an important landmark in tumor imaging. The AC normally measures no more than 2 mm in thickness, and thickening of the AC can indicate tumor involvement, which may affect surgical treatment options.[19] The AC tendon, also referred to as Broyles ligament, connects the vocal ligaments to the thyroid cartilage and forms part of the AC. The point at which Broyles ligament attaches to the thyroid cartilage lacks perichondrium, leading some authors to think that this site in the cartilage may be particularly susceptible to tumor invasion.[13,20] The space between the posterior insertions of the vocal ligaments on the arytenoids is called the *posterior commissure* (PC) and is wider than the AC at rest and during quiet respiration.

The vocal ligaments actually represent the thickened free margins of an elastic connective tissue structure known as the *conus elasticus* (Fig. 10), which is also variably referred to as the cricothyroid or triangular membrane. The anterior portion of the conus elasticus is made up of the deep fibers of the median (or anterior) cricothyroid ligament, which connects the cricoid arch to the inferior margin of the thyroid cartilage at the midline.[21] Posterior to this, the conus elasticus attaches inferiorly at the superior and medial surfaces of the cricoid cartilage and continues

between the laryngeal cartilages. Several of these membranes also serve a protective function by forming anatomic barriers to disease spread within the larynx and between the larynx and other parts of the neck. Although these connective tissues are not usually resolvable as discrete structures on imaging, their general positions can be inferred based on the locations of the more easily identifiable structures that they attach to and support.

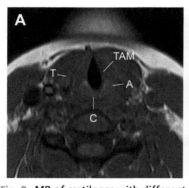
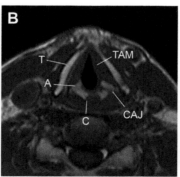
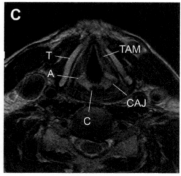

Fig. 9. MR of cartilages with different ossification. (*A*) T1-weighted axial image through the level of the glottis in a 17-year-old woman with mostly unossified laryngeal cartilages. The thyroid (T), cricoid (C), and arytenoid (A) cartilages demonstrate signal intensities very similar to the adjacent strap muscles with only a thin, faintly hypointense rim. In contradistinction, an axial T1-weighted image (*B*) and axial T2-weighted image (*C*) in a 50-year-old man with ossified cartilages demonstrates high signal intensity within thyroid (T), cricoid (C), and arytenoid (A) cartilages owing to the presence of fatty marrow in the medullary spaces, with a more conspicuous low signal intensity rim due to cortical calcification. CAJ, cricoarytenoid joint; TAM, thyroarytenoid muscle. (*Courtesy of* University of North Carolina, Chapel Hill, NC.)

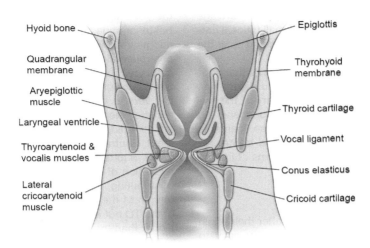

Fig. 10. Coronal cross-sectional illustration of the larynx at the ventricular level showing the relationships of the cartilages, muscles, and ligaments to the mucosal surfaces of the larynx. Note the locations of the quadrangular membrane and conus elasticus, whose free margins form the vestibular and vocal ligaments, respectively. (*Courtesy of* Joel Floyd, Jr, MA, CMI, Chapel Hill, NC.)

superiorly and medially as the lateral cricothyroid ligaments that attach at the AC and vocal processes of the arytenoids, with the superior free margins of the conus elasticus in between forming the vocal ligaments.[1,2,21]

Just above and running parallel to the vocal ligaments are the *ventricular ligaments*. These insert on the anterolateral surface of the arytenoids posteriorly, slightly superior to the level of the vocal processes, and at the inner surface of the thyroid lamina anteriorly, a few millimeters above the vocal ligament insertion. The ventricular ligaments mark the level of the free margin of the *false vocal cords (or vestibular folds)* and represent the lower margins of a second major elastic membrane in the larynx, known as the *quadrangular membrane* (see Fig. 10). The quadrangular membrane is part of the epiglottis support system, attaching to the lateral edges of the epiglottis and extending inferiorly and posteriorly to the arytenoid and corniculate cartilages. The mucosal covered upper margins are the *AE folds*, which separate the laryngeal vestibule anteromedially from the piriform recesses of the hypopharynx posterolaterally. The previously mentioned cuneiform cartilages are contained within the quadrangular membrane, helping to add rigidity to the AE folds.[1] On laryngoscopy, the corniculate and cuneiform cartilages can be identified as elevations of the mucosa (referred to as the corniculate and cuneiform tubercles, respectively) along the posterior aspects of each AE fold, above the arytenoid cartilages[8] (Fig. 11).

The *thyrohyoid membrane* is a fibroelastic sheet connecting the top of thyroid cartilage to the inner

surfaces of the hyoid bone. At the posterior margins of the thyrohyoid membrane lie the paired lateral thyrohyoid ligaments, which extend

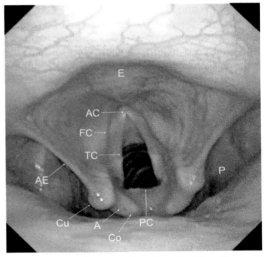

Fig. 11. Image from an in-office flexible fiberoptic laryngoscopy video. Note that the image has been rotated 180° to more closely approximate the typical orientation of the larynx on axial CT imaging. This depicts the major mucosa-lined structures of the larynx including: anterior commissur (AC), false vocal cords (FC), true vocal cords (TC), aryepiglottic folds (AE), arytenoids (A), corniculate tubercles (Co), cuneiform tubercles (Cu), and posterior commissur (PC). The distended piriform sinuses (P) are also well visualized posterolateral to the AE folds. The epiglottis (E) is partially seen as the anterior wall in the image. Portions of the subglottis and upper trachea are also seen deep to the opening between the TC. (Courtesy of R Shah, MD, Chapel Hill, NC.)

between the greater horns of the thyroid cartilage and hyoid bone and contain the small triticeal cartilages. The medial thyrohyoid ligament lies at the midline of the thyrohyoid membrane.

One other important pair of ligaments that support the larynx are the stylohyoid ligaments. Although not technically part of the larynx, the stylohyoid ligaments indirectly help to suspend the larynx through the hyoid bone.[2] These ligaments originate from their respective styloid processes and attach to the ipsilateral lesser horns of the hyoid bone.

Muscles of the Larynx

The laryngeal muscles are named after their origin and insertion sites, making it relatively easy to remember their names, and are traditionally divided into intrinsic and extrinsic groups. The intrinsic muscles facilitate movement of the laryngeal cartilages against one another and directly affect glottic movement, whereas the extrinsic muscles connect the larynx with its anatomic neighbors and act to elevate or depress the larynx.

Intrinsic Muscles

The intrinsic muscles of the larynx are summarized in Table 1 and shown in Fig. 12. Each of the intrinsic laryngeal muscles is confined entirely within the larynx and provides subtle changes in the vocal cord length, tension, and abducted or adducted position, allowing for a wide range of pitches during phonation. These muscles also function to open the vocal cords during inspiration and to close the cords and laryngeal inlet during deglutition and phonation.[8] On imaging, of primary importance are the *thyroarytenoid muscles* (TAMs), which demarcate the level and make up the bulk of the TC.[13]

The TAMs are the dominant component of the vocal folds, running in parallel and just lateral to the vocal ligaments. Each TAM originates on the posterior aspect of the thyroid lamina and median cricothyroid ligament and inserts on the base and anterolateral surface of the ipsilateral arytenoid cartilage. The medial fibers of the TAM are sometimes considered a separate muscle, referred to as the *vocalis muscle*.[8] The vocalis similarly originates at the posterior thyroid lamina and median cricothyroid ligament but inserts on the vocal ligament. Contraction of both the vocalis muscles and TAMs shortens the vocal ligaments (leading to relaxation of the vocal cords) providing bulk and contributing to adduction.[10,22] The superior margin of the TAM demarcates the upper border of the TC but a few fibers of the muscle can insert higher than the AC.

The *lateral cricoarytenoid muscles* originate at the lateral arches of the cricoid and insert on the muscular processes of the arytenoids. They are the primary adductors of the vocal cords, with contraction of these muscles producing rotation of the arytenoids to bring the vocal ligaments together. The *posterior cricoarytenoid muscles* also insert on the muscular processes of the arytenoids but originate on the posterior cricoid lamina. As a result, these muscles work in opposition to the lateral cricoarytenoids to rotate the arytenoid cartilages in the opposite direction thus abducting the vocal ligaments. The posterior cricoarytenoid muscles are the only true abductors of the vocal folds.[8]

The *arytenoid (or interarytenoid) muscle* is unpaired, with 2 components, located on and between the posterior margins of the arytenoid cartilages. The transverse component extends horizontally between the 2 arytenoid cartilages, and the oblique components extend from the muscular process of one arytenoid cartilage to the apex of the other cartilage. Both these components work together to adduct the vocal cords.[8]

Table 1
Intrinsic muscles of the larynx and their innervation

Muscle	Innervation	Function
Cricothyroid	Superior laryngeal	Tenses cords
Posterior cricoarytenoid	Recurrent laryngeal	Abducts vocal cords
Lateral cricoarytenoid	Recurrent laryngeal	Adducts arytenoids and closes glottis
Transverse arytenoid	Recurrent laryngeal	Adducts arytenoids
Oblique arytenoid	Recurrent laryngeal	Closes glottis
Aryepiglottic	Recurrent laryngeal	Closes glottis
Vocalis	Recurrent laryngeal	Relaxes cords
Thyroarytenoid	Recurrent laryngeal	Relaxes cord tension

Adapted from Krohner RG, Ramanathan S. Functional Anatomy of the Airway. In: Hagberg CA, ed. *Benumof's Airway Management: Principles and Practice.* 2nd ed. Mosby Elsevier; 2007:3-21.

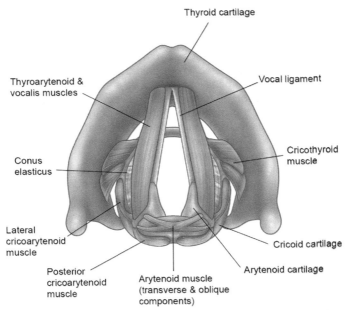

Fig. 12. Superior illustrative view of the larynx without the mucosal covering to show the major intrinsic muscles of the larynx. (*Courtesy of* Joel Floyd, Jr, MA, CMI, Chapel Hill, NC.)

The *cricothyroid muscles* attach to the anterolateral aspects of the cricoid arch and insert on the inferior cornua and laminae of the thyroid cartilage. Contraction of these muscles tips the thyroid cartilage slightly forward and inferiorly, pivoting at the cricothyroid joints. This leads to lengthening of the vocal ligaments and, therefore, increased tension in the vocal cords and pitch. The cricothyroid is the only tensor muscle of the larynx, and some authors consider it to be both an extrinsic and intrinsic muscle because its actions affect both laryngeal movement and glottic tension.[8] It is also the only intrinsic muscle not innervated by the recurrent laryngeal nerve, receiving its innervation from the external branch of the superior laryngeal nerve.

Finally, the *thyroepiglottic and AE muscles* are thin bands of muscle found within the AE folds and along the epiglottis,[13] which work in conjunction with the transverse arytenoid and TAMs to close the epiglottis and laryngeal vestibule during swallowing. The thyroepiglottic muscle actually represents the most lateral portions of the TAM, which attach to the lateral arytenoids, AE fold, and epiglottis, whereas the AE muscle is a continuation of the oblique portion of the arytenoid muscle which courses through the AE fold to attach to the lateral aspect of the epiglottis.[8]

Extrinsic Muscles

The extrinsic muscles of the larynx, also referred to as the strap muscles, act to raise, lower, or stabilize the larynx but have their origins elsewhere in the neck. These muscles are typically divided into an infrahyoid group, which together depress the larynx and displace it downward during inspiration, and a suprahyoid group, which helps suspend the larynx from the skull base and mandible via the hyoid bone and elevates and anteriorly displaces the larynx during swallowing. The infrahyoid group includes the omohyoid, sternothyroid, thyrohyoid, and sternohyoid muscles, which are innervated by the ansa cervicalis. The suprahyoid group includes the digastric, stylohyoid, geniohyoid, mylohyoid, and stylopharyngeus muscles. The middle and inferior pharyngeal constrictor muscles and the cricopharyngeus muscles are also considered extrinsic larynx muscles, which affect the larynx during the act of swallowing.[1]

Mucosa, Submucosal Spaces, and Air-containing Spaces of the Larynx

The laryngeal cartilages, muscles, and ligaments provide a framework for the overlying mucosal surfaces, creating various folds, air-filled spaces, and submucosal spaces. These are important to recognize on imaging because correct anatomic localization provides a better differential of pathologies and allows clearer communication to clinicians regarding sites of tumor involvement. Many of the important mucosal spaces and folds of the larynx have already been mentioned but will be reemphasized here.

The mucosa of the larynx is primarily pseudostratified ciliated columnar epithelium with scattered goblet cells, as seen in the trachea.[23,24] However, regions that often appose other surfaces during phonation and swallowing are covered in nonkeratinized stratified squamous epithelium and include the vocal folds, edges of the AE folds, parts of the epiglottis and parts of the pyriform fossae, although there is variability in the distribution of this squamous epithelium.[23,25] Other important tissues of the mucosa are the small subepithelial mucus secreting glands, which are in higher concentrations along the subglottis, AC, ventricular saccules, false vocal cords, and arytenoid region.[24]

The *laryngeal vestibule* is the superior most air space of the larynx spanning from the superior tip of the epiglottis to the true cord. The lateral margins of the vestibule are formed by the paired AE folds. The inferior aspect of the posterior margin is the interarytenoid fold, which is formed by the mucosal covered interarytenoid muscle.[2,13]

The *laryngeal ventricles* are paired thin air-filled spaces between the true and false vocal cords (see Fig. 10). There is a superior lateral outpouching of each ventricle that protrudes into the paraglottic space (PGS) known as the laryngeal saccule or appendix.[2] The ventricles are best seen on coronal imaging (Fig. 13) and are landmarks for dividing the larynx into supraglottic and glottic regions (as discussed later).

The median slit-like airspace between the TC is referred to as the *rima glottidis*.[2] The more posterior aspect of the rima glottidis is bordered laterally by the mucosally covered medial surfaces of the paired arytenoid cartilages.[12]

Two important submucosal spaces of the larynx are the *preepiglottic space* (PES) and PGS. Above the level of the vocal cords, these spaces are predominantly fat containing and have a rich vascular and lymphatic supply. The PES, as its name suggests, is anterior to the epiglottis and the quadrangular membrane that together comprise its posterior boundary. The anterior boundary is the hyoid bone, thyrohyoid membrane, and the upper thyroid cartilage. The upper boundary is the hyoepiglottic ligament, and the lower boundary is the thyroepiglottic ligament.[26,27] The PES is generally easily visualized on both sagittal (Fig. 14) and axial images. The PGS is located laterally in the larynx, spanning the levels of the true and false cords (FC) and extending slightly below the level of the true cords. The lateral margins are the inner surface of the thyroid, cricothyroid membrane, and, to a lesser extent, the cricoid. It is medially bounded by the quadrangular membrane and conus elasticus.[28]

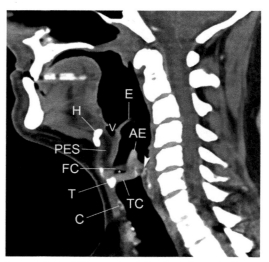

Fig. 14. Paramidline sagittal CT view through the larynx nicely demonstrates the location of the PES in relationship to the surrounding laryngeal structures. The PES is a fat-containing space situated anterior to the epiglottis and the quadrangular membrane and posterior to the hyoid bone, thyrohyoid membrane, and the upper thyroid cartilage. AE, aryepiglottic fold; *arrowhead*, cricoarytenoid joint; *asterisk*, laryngeal ventricle; C, cricoid; E, epiglottis; FC, false vocal cord; H, hyoid; T, thyroid cartilage; TC, true vocal cord; V, vallecula. (*Courtesy of* University of North Carolina, Chapel Hill, NC.)

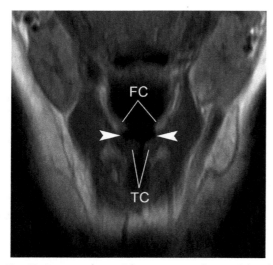

Fig. 13. Laryngeal ventricle on a coronal T1-weighted MR image through the larynx. The laryngeal ventricles (*arrowheads*) are paired thin air-filled spaces located between the FC and TC. The apex of the laryngeal ventricle is the landmark that indicates the transition point from the supraglottis above to the glottis below. (*Courtesy of* University of North Carolina, Chapel Hill, NC.)

A discrete division between the preepiglottic and PGSs is not visible on imaging.[26] The thyroglottic ligament has been described as a division between the spaces but is discontinuous especially at its superior margin.[27] Others have described this ligament as poorly formed and part of the PGS.[28] In either case, the discontinuity of the ligament can allow passage of tumor between the fat of the preepiglottic and PGSs.[26]

Major Larynx Regions Relevant to Cancer Staging

For the purposes of cancer staging, the larynx is traditionally divided into 3 main sites: the supraglottis, the glottis, and the subglottis (Fig. 15), the first 2 of which are further subdivided into additional subsites. Tumor classification (T-category) and treatment planning may differ significantly based on the primary site of disease as well as the extent of spread to other sites within and outside of the larynx, so familiarity with these divisions and their subsites is essential to accurately describe and stage cancers of the larynx. In general, visualization of the mucosal surfaces of the larynx is best achieved by laryngoscopy; however, in cases of confirmed or suspected tumor, imaging plays an important role in evaluating for deep soft

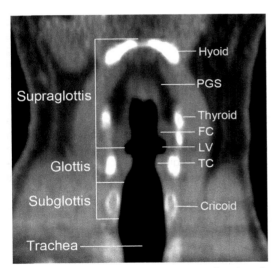

Fig. 15. Reformatted coronal CT image showing the regions of the larynx. The supraglottis is defined superiorly by the epiglottis (not well seen in this plane) and inferiorly by the laryngeal ventricle (LV). The glottis extends from top of the TC, which can be approximated by the apex of the LV to 1 cm inferior to the ventricle. The subglottis extends from the lower margin of the glottis to the inferior margin of the cricoid. Note the fat-containing portion of the PGS at the supraglottic level. FC, false cord. (*Courtesy of* University of North Carolina, Chapel Hill, NC.)

Labels in figure: Hyoid, PGS, Thyroid, FC, LV, TC, Cricoid, Supraglottis, Glottis, Subglottis, Trachea

tissue or cartilaginous involvement and regional nodal spread.

The *supraglottis* (Fig. 16) is defined superiorly by the glossoepiglottic and pharyngoepiglottic folds, although the suprahyoid portion of the epiglottis, which is also a supraglottic structure usually projects above these landmarks, with its free margin extending into the oropharyngeal airway. Inferiorly, the supraglottis is demarcated by and includes the laryngeal ventricle, which separates the supraglottis above from the glottis below. For the purposes of cancer staging, the subsites of the supraglottis are the epiglottis (divided into suprahyoid and infrahyoid components), the laryngeal facing mucosa of the AE folds, the mucosa overlying the arytenoid cartilages, and the false vocal folds.[29] Although not specifically a subsite of the supraglottis, an important midline-imaging landmark in the region is the previously mentioned PES, the fat-containing space situated anterior to the infrahyoid epiglottis.[2,30]

The *glottis* (Fig. 17) is the short segment of the larynx whose subsites include the TC (including its superior and inferior surfaces), the AC, and the PC. The upper limit of the glottis can be identified as the inferior margins of the laryngeal ventricles, which are generally best seen on coronal imaging slices. The histologic landmark that demarcates the lower margin of the glottis is the transition zone from the stratified squamous epithelium covering the TC to the respiratory epithelium of the subglottic airway, which is usually located 5 to 10 mm below the free edge of the TC.[31] However, this zone is not resolvable by imaging, so the inferior limit of the glottis is arbitrarily defined as the plane situated 1 cm inferior to the laryngeal ventricles for imaging purposes.[2,19,29]

Although tumor involvement of the AC and PC alone does not change cancer staging for primary glottic carcinomas, spread to either of these structures can have important treatment implications, particularly when partial laryngectomy is being considered.[30,32] Furthermore, tumors involving the AC are associated with early invasion of the adjacent thyroid cartilage (due to spread along Broyles ligament), subglottic extension, and early extralaryngeal extension; as a result, these tumors tend to be more difficult to treat both surgically or with radiation, are associated with higher recurrence rates, and are frequently understaged initially.[14,20,26,33]

As mentioned earlier, the PGS spans the lateral submucosal portions of the supraglottis and glottis, including the potential space lateral to the laryngeal ventricles. In the supraglottis, the PGS is located lateral to the false cord and is primarily

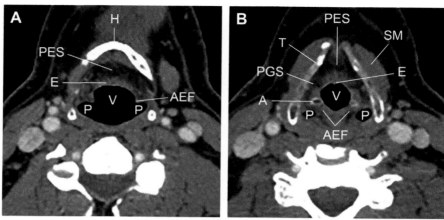

Fig. 16. Axial CT images through the supraglottis. (*A*) Axial slice at the level of the hyoid bone (H) shows the fat-containing PES situated between the hyoid bone and the epiglottis (E). The airspaces visible at this level are the laryngeal vestibule (V) just posterior to the epiglottis and a portion of bilateral piriform sinuses (P), which are separated from the vestibule by the partially imaged aryepiglottic folds (AEF). (*B*) Axial slice slightly inferior to (A) at the level of the false vocal cords. The apices of the arytenoids (A), which mark the false cord level, are visible. The PGSs are the fat-containing space seen bilaterally positioned between the inner surface of the thyroid cartilage (T) and the vestibular airway (V) and communicate anteromedially with the PES. The small pockets of air posteriorly are the inferior aspects or apex of the piriform sinuses (P). SM, infrahyoid strap muscles. (*Courtesy of* University of North Carolina, Chapel Hill, NC.)

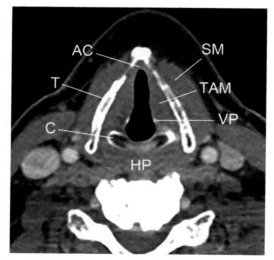

Fig. 17. Axial CT image at the level of the glottis, defined by the TC, which are composed of the vocal ligaments and the TAMs. The AC is located at the insertion site of the vocal ligaments at the inner surface of the thyroid cartilage. The vocal ligaments attach posteriorly to the vocal processes (VP), which are just visible on the slice. The posterior lamina of the cricoid (C) is clearly seen at this level. The airspace between the TC is called the rima glottidis. HP, hypopharynx; SM, infrahyoid strap muscles; T, thyroid cartilage. (*Courtesy of* University of North Carolina, Chapel Hill, NC.)

fat containing, whereas at the level of the glottis, the PGS represents a potential space situated between the TAM and the thyroid cartilage. Unlike in the supraglottis, the PGS at the level of the glottis is not generally resolvable on imaging as a discrete space. Thus, on axial CT and MR images, noting the contents of the space between the laryngeal mucosa and the thyroid cartilage can help determine whether the slice is situated at the supraglottic level, where the PGS will seem primarily fat containing, or the level of the glottis, where there will be almost exclusively soft tissue rather than fat between the airway and the cartilage. From an oncologic imaging standpoint, submucosal invasion of either the PGS or the PES by a laryngeal carcinoma, evident as replacement of the normal fat in these spaces, is critical to recognize because the involvement may not be detectable on laryngoscopic examination but when present, may place the tumor into a higher T-category (at least T3) and prognostic group (at least stage III) than initial clinical staging might suggest.[29] It is also important to remember that the PGS directly abuts the cricoid and thyroid cartilages, so tumors within these spaces can readily erode these cartilages. Furthermore, small defects in the cricothyroid membrane can allow also passage of tumor from the PGS to the overlying extralaryngeal soft tissues.[26]

Finally, the *subglottis* represents the portion of the larynx located immediate inferior to the glottis, extending from the undersurface of the TC to the inferior edge of the cricoid cartilage. The region consists of a single subsite, which is bounded laterally by the cricoid cartilage and the conus elasticus.[2] On axial imaging at the subglottic level, the cricoid can be seen positioned just posterior to the thyroid cartilage with the opening of the ring formed by the anterior arch and lamina visible in plane (Fig. 18). Evaluation of the subglottis on imaging is generally straightforward because the subglottis features only a thin layer of mucosa along the endoluminal surface of the cricoid and tracheal cartilages. Therefore, any soft tissue thickening along the walls of the subglottic airway in this region should be viewed with suspicion on cancer staging scans. Subglottic extension generally precludes most types of partial laryngectomy, leaving only total laryngectomy or near total laryngectomy as the only surgical options.[9]

In addition to closely scrutinizing the structures intrinsic to the larynx on oncologic staging scans, it is also important to look for involvement of neighboring extralaryngeal sites. For tumors of the supraglottis, these include the base of tongue, valleculae, pyriform sinuses, and postcricoid hypopharynx. Other structures that may be involved by advanced primary laryngeal malignancies include surrounding visceral space structures such as the trachea, strap muscles, thyroid gland, and the esophagus, whereas very advanced tumors may involve the carotid and prevertebral spaces or even extend into the mediastinum.

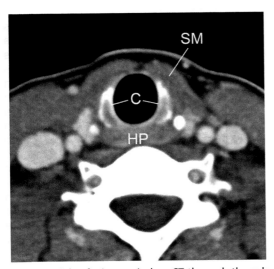

Fig. 18. Axial soft tissue window CT through the subglottis demonstrating the ring of the cricoid cartilage (C). Notice the lack of soft tissue along the wall of the laryngeal airway at this level. HP, hypopharynx; SM, infrahyoid strap muscles. (*Courtesy of* University of North Carolina, Chapel Hill, NC.)

Blood Supply, Innervation, and Lymphatics of the Larynx

Vasculature
The primary blood supply to the larynx is through the *superior thyroid artery* (STA) and *inferior thyroid artery* (ITA; Fig. 19). The STA arises from the external carotid artery and divides into several branches including the superior laryngeal artery and the cricothyroid artery. The internal branch of the superior laryngeal artery pierces through the thyrohyoid membrane along with the superior laryngeal nerve to supply the deeper structures of the larynx.[23] Rarely the superior laryngeal artery may enter the larynx more inferiorly through a foramen in the thyroid cartilage lamina or through the cricothyroid ligament.[34]

The ITA is a branch from the thyrocervical trunk, which arises from the subclavian artery. The ITA branches into the inferior laryngeal artery, which follows the course of the recurrent laryngeal nerve to enter the larynx superior to the cricothyroid joint and below the inferior pharyngeal constrictor muscle.

Venous drainage of the larynx reflects the arterial supply with superior and inferior laryngeal veins. Each superior laryngeal vein drains to the ipsilateral superior thyroid vein, then to the internal jugular vein. The inferior laryngeal vein drains to the middle thyroid vein, then to the internal jugular vein. Some of the veins along the cricothyroid membrane also drain into the thyroid isthmus and then to the inferior thyroid veins, which typically drain to the brachiocephalic veins.[23,35]

Innervation
The larynx is innervated by the vagus nerve via 2 major branches, the *superior laryngeal nerve* and the *recurrent (or inferior) laryngeal nerve* (RLN; see Fig. 19). The dual innervation is explained by the embryologic divisions of the larynx, which are formed by the fourth and sixth branchial arches, respectively. The superior laryngeal nerve supplies the fourth arch derivatives, which include the epiglottis, thyroid and cuneiform cartilages, cricothyroid muscles, and pharyngeal constrictor muscles, whereas the recurrent laryngeal nerve supplies the sixth arch derivatives including the arytenoid, corniculate and cricoid cartilages, and the remaining intrinsic larynx muscles.[36,37]

Sensory innervation above the vocal cords is through the internal laryngeal branch of the superior laryngeal nerve. The internal branch courses with the superior laryngeal artery through the thyrohyoid membrane to reach the mucosa of the epiglottis, AE folds, and larynx. Taste buds located in this region are also innervated by the internal

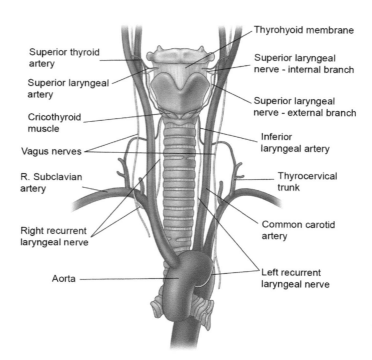

Fig. 19. Coronal illustrative view of the blood supply and innervation to the larynx and trachea. (*Courtesy of* Joel Floyd, Jr, MA, CMI, Chapel Hill, NC.)

laryngeal branch.[38] The superior laryngeal nerve also gives off a smaller external branch that descends along the anterolateral aspect of the larynx to innervate the cricothyroid muscle, which, being a fourth branchial arch derivative, is the only intrinsic larynx muscle not innervated by the RLN.[36]

Motor innervation to all of the other intrinsic muscles of the larynx and sensory innervation below the vocal cords are provided by the RLN. The arytenoid muscles receive bilateral innervation from both RLNs, whereas all of the other laryngeal muscles have unilateral innervation.[13]

It is important to understand the origin and course of the RLN and include its full course from the skull base through the aortic arch in imaging protocols for vocal cord paralysis because an injury or mass effect at any site along this course could produce vocal cord motion abnormalities. The vagus nerve exits the skull through the jugular foramen and runs posterolateral to the carotid artery in the carotid space.[13] The right RLN branches from the vagus nerve just inferior to the right subclavian artery, wraps posteromedially under the origin of the subclavian artery and courses cranially through the right tracheoesophageal groove.[39] Owing to embryologic development, the left RLN has a longer course. It branches from the vagus nerve just inferior to the aortic arch, wraps posteriorly under the arch just lateral to the ligamentum

arteriosum, then courses cranially through the left tracheoesophageal groove to reach the larynx.[39] Each RLN then enters the larynx through a sulcus between the thyroid and cricoid cartilages, just superior to the cricothyroid joint.[13,38]

An important anatomic variant to be aware of is the *nonrecurrent laryngeal nerve* (NRLN), which occurs when the inferior laryngeal nerve enters the larynx directly from the cervical vagus nerve without descending to the thoracic level. This variant almost always appears on the right in association with an aberrant right subclavian artery and has been reported with an incidence of 0.3% to 1.6%.[40] Left-sided occurrence of an NRLN has been described but is extremely rare and seen only in association with situs inversus.[41] Due to its course, an NRLN is highly predisposed to injury during thyroidectomy. Although the nerve cannot be visualized on conventional imaging, its presence can be predicted based on its association with an aberrant right subclavian artery, making it important to identify subclavian artery aberrance preoperatively in patients undergoing thyroid or parathyroid surgery.

Lymphatics
The lymphatic system of the larynx is a complex network with multiple anastomatic communications and directions of flow. However, there are typical patterns of flow that have been documented on

dye injection studies and correlate with common sites of metastatic lymph node spread in cases of laryngeal malignancies.[42–44] The supraglottic and glottic regions drain primarily to the level II and III cervical lymph nodes and the subglottic region drains to levels III and VI.[43,44] In laryngeal cancers, cervical lymph node metastases are typically unilateral on the same side as the tumor, but can be bilateral, or occasionally contralateral.[43]

The lymphatic system of the larynx has 2 networks, one located superficially in the mucosa and one deeper in the submucosal layers with numerous communications between each layer and with the adjacent networks of the hypopharynx and trachea.[44] There is variability in the density of the lymphatic tissue throughout the larynx. It is highest in the supraglottic region, which is extremely rich in lymphatics, with lymphatic density being greatest in the epiglottis, false vocal fold, and AE folds and lowest near the petiole of the epiglottis, thyroepiglottic ligament, and vocal ligament.[44] In fact, some authors note that the free margins of the vocal cords are virtually devoid of lymphatics.[29,45] This may account in part for the higher incidence of occult nodal metastases observed in supraglottic primaries compared with glottic carcinomas. In general, the supraglottic region drains medial to lateral through the thyrohyoid membrane to reach the level II and III cervical lymph nodes.[44]

At the subglottic level, drainage anteriorly is through the cricothyroid ligament and posteriorly through the cricotracheal ligament with subsequent drainage to both level III and VI nodes.[44] In addition, the inferior surface of the vocal cord has been shown to have lymphatic drainage similar to the subglottis.[46] Enlargement of lymph nodes in the level VI station, including the Delphian (or prelaryngeal) lymph node, which is located at the midline anterior to the cricothyroid membrane, can be a sign of metastasis from an AC or subglottic tumor but can also be seen with thyroid gland tumors or from direct extension of tumor to this region.[47]

THE CERVICAL TRACHEA

The trachea serves as the conduit between the larynx and bronchial tree. It typically extends from the C6 level, just below the cricoid cartilage, to the T4–T5 level, bifurcating into the mainstem bronchi at the carina.[48] The extrathoracic or cervical segment of the trachea is a relatively short portion of the trachea, measuring approximately 2 to 4 cm. The average adult trachea is approximately 11 cm in length, with a range of 10 to 13 cm[49,50] (Fig. 20). A segment of the cervical trachea lies superficially in the neck and is only partially covered by the infrahyoid strap muscles. It is palpable between the sternal heads of the sternocleidomastoid muscles and superior to the jugular (suprasternal) notch.[38] As the trachea courses caudally, it tracks posteriorly, and is often displaced just right of midline at the aortic arch.[51] The thyroid gland is just anterior and lateral to the trachea, with the thyroid isthmus typically located at the second or third tracheal ring. The esophagus is closely apposed to the posterior wall of the cervical trachea, usually veering along the left posterior margin of the trachea as it courses inferiorly.[39]

In infancy, the trachea is round in the axial plane. With advanced aging, the trachea may narrow in the transverse diameter and widens in the anteroposterior diameter.[39,52] This change in diameter primarily affects the intrathoracic segment of the trachea.[48]

Composition of the trachea

The trachea is composed of 18 to 22 incomplete cartilage rings that provide structural support to its anterior and lateral walls.[39,49] The trachea generally becomes intrathoracic at the level of the sixth ring.[8] Each tracheal ring is made up of hyaline cartilage and is surrounded by a perichondrium that is composed primarily of collagen with

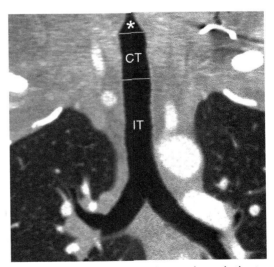

Fig. 20. Obliqued coronal CT image through the trachea. To obtain a single image showing the length of the trachea, an oblique coronal reformatted image was required because the intrathoracic trachea courses slightly posterior as it descends the mediastinum. The coronal view provides an overview of the entire length of the trachea including the cervical (CT) and intrathoracic segments (IT) and can be helpful to assess the length of stenosis or other pathologies (asterisk = subglottis). (Courtesy of University of North Carolina, Chapel Hill, NC.)

a small component of elastin fibers. The cartilage rings are connected to each other by intercartilaginous membranes, also composed of collagen and elastin fibers.[51] The posterior wall of the trachea comprises a fibromuscular membrane. The smooth muscle in this wall is known as the trachealis and runs longitudinally along the length of the trachea.[39] The normal tracheal wall should be thin, measuring 1 to 3 mm, with the mucosa of the trachea being composed of ciliated pseudostratified columnar epithelium with an elastic lamina propria deep to the epithelial layer.[39,50,51] Goblet mucous cells and subepithelial glands are interspersed between and deep to the epithelial layer.[51]

Blood supply, innervation, and lymphatics of the trachea

The arterial supply to the trachea is divided into a cervical (upper) segment and thoracic (lower) segment. The cervical trachea is supplied by the tracheoesophageal branches of the bilateral ITAs, which arise from the thyrocervical trunks of the subclavian arteries. There are several branches of the tracheoesophageal arteries, each supplying short segments of the cervical trachea with anastomoses between each segment. There is some variability to this supply but generally there are 3 major tracheoesophageal branches. Anastomoses with the STA also exist along the anterior tracheal wall, where this artery provides blood supply to the isthmus of the thyroid gland. The thoracic trachea is supplied through multiple bronchial arteries that arise directly from the aorta.[39]

Venous drainage of the trachea is through inferior thyroid veins to the brachiocephalic veins, whereas lymphatic drainage of the proximal two-thirds of the trachea is through the pretracheal and paratracheal lymph nodes of level VI, which subsequently drain to lower jugular nodes of level IV.[51,53]

The trachea is innervated by branches of the vagus nerve. Sensory fibers to the inner tracheal mucosa arise from branches of the bilateral recurrent laryngeal nerves. Parasympathetic innervation to the trachea also arises from the recurrent laryngeal nerves. Sympathetic innervation comes from both cervical ganglia and the second through fourth thoracic ganglia.[51] These autonomic nerves supply the seromucous glands, smooth muscles, and the blood vessels of the trachea.[38]

Imaging techniques for evaluating the larynx and cervical trachea

Larynx

The larynx is frequently evaluated with CT or MR imaging. Contrast-enhanced CT neck is more commonly used owing to wider availability, reproducibility, and decreased risk of motion degradation.[9] At our institution, MR imaging is primarily used to supplement CT when additional assessment is needed.

CT neck imaging with contrast is obtained in the axial plane and coronal and sagittal reconstructed series should also be generated. Because the vocal cords are often not exactly parallel to the plane of the axial images, some advocate for additional reconstructions parallel to plane of the vocal cords, which is generally well approximated by the plane of the C4–C5 or C5–C6 intervertebral disc space (Fig. 21). These reformatted images should typically span from 1 cm above hyoid bone to the inferior margin of the cricoid cartilage.[54]

CT imaging of the neck is primarily obtained during quiet breathing.[54,55] During normal breathing, the vocal cords are abducted and the cords and laryngeal ventricles are not always well demarcated.[9,56] This distinction may be important in assessing transglottic spread of tumors. Therefore, other imaging can be obtained with various breath hold and phonation techniques. The primary additional maneuvers include a modified Valsalva maneuver and phonation with the sound "eee."

Modified Valsalva maneuvers, which include blowing through pursed lips or nose, distend the laryngeal vestibule and piriform sinuses providing better visualization of tumors in the piriform sinus or postcricoid region; however, the true cords and FC are abducted in this maneuver so tumors of the glottic region are not well evaluated with this technique.[26,55,57] Phonation with "eee" produces adduction of the true and FC and distends the laryngeal ventricle. This can aide also in evaluation of transglottic spread of tumors.[57] Use of a high-pitched sound such as "eee" or "hee" requires the vocal cords to be thinner and allows better visualization of abnormalities along the cords. This technique can also be used for the assessment of vocal cord paralysis,[56] although, the best assessment for vocal fold motion remains clinical awake flexible fiberoptic laryngoscopy. In cases of vocal cord paralysis, on standard quiet respiration examinations, the paralyzed cord will be medialized and there will be dilation of the ipsilateral pyriform sinus and laryngeal ventricle, and thickening of the AE fold.[58] This can further be confirmed with a phonation scan, which will demonstrate incomplete adduction of the paralyzed cord and no significant change in the cord position between the quiet respiration and phonation scans.[56] There is some concern that the use of phonation techniques will increase motion artifact but it has been shown that with proper patient

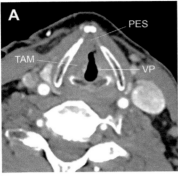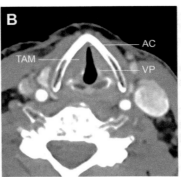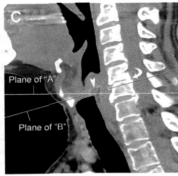

Fig. 21. Value of angled axial images for assessment of the glottis. (*A*) Straight axial CT image through the level of the vocal processes (VP) includes a portion of the PES of the supraglottis anteriorly and the thyroarytenoid muscle (TAM) of the glottis more posteriorly. The anterior extent of the true vocal cord, including the AC, is not seen in plane. (*B*) Angled axial image through the vocal processes (VP) demonstrating the length of the glottis, including the AC, which is normal in this example. (*C*) Parasagittal image through the level of the left cricoarytenoid joint (*arrowheads*) indicating the approximate location and angulation of the previous images. The white line indicates the plane for figure (A), whereas the red line indicates the plane for figure (B). Note how the red line roughly parallels the C5–C6 disc space (*curved arrow*). (*Courtesy of* University of North Carolina, Chapel Hill, NC.)

preparation, motion artifact on phonation examinations can be minimized.[57]

MR imaging is also helpful for the evaluation of the larynx, particularly for the assessment of malignant cartilage invasion. Specifically in cases with AC involvement, MR imaging has been shown to be more accurate than CT in determining cartilage invasion (88.46% for MR imaging vs 57.69% for CT).[59] On CT, cartilage involvement can be demonstrated by cartilage sclerosis, erosion, lysis, or tumor in the extralaryngeal tissues on the other side of the cartilage.[16,17,59] However, because there is variability in ossification of the laryngeal cartilages, these changes can be difficult to distinguish from normal unossified cartilage. Some of this can be overcome with MR imaging but differentiating unossified cartilage from invaded cartilage on MR imaging can also be difficult because one of the best MR imaging markers of cartilage invasion is loss of the normal fatty marrow signal in ossified cartilage.[16–18] Another marker on MR imaging that can be used is the assessment of enhancement. Normally, the cartilage does not enhance, so if contrast enhancement is present, it can indicate invasion. This should also be interpreted with caution, however, because enhancing cartilage can also be seen in peritumoral inflammation without invasion.[16–18] An additional limitation of MR imaging is missing early invasion of just the surface of the cartilage as the rim of ossified cartilage is markedly hypointense on T1-weighted images and may mask early invasion.[18]

Dual-energy CT is a newer technique that can assist in the evaluation of cartilage invasion.[60]

Briefly, 2 different series are provided, the weighted-average (WA) sequence, which seems similar to conventional CT, and an iodine overlay (IO). When there is suspected cartilage invasion on the WA, this area can be confirmed as invasion if there is bright, iodine density in the corresponding area on the IO series. If no corresponding iodine density is seen on the IO, then the region likely represents unossified cartilage. It is important to understand the limitations of dual-energy CT when interpreting a case. One of the major limitations is that bone and calcified cartilage will also seem bright on the IO series; therefore, it should not be confused with enhancing tissue. Evaluation of both the WA and IO series is required to avoid overestimating cartilage invasion.[54]

Ultrasound of the larynx is an alternative option, typically used in the clinical setting and can aid in evaluation of cord mobility; however, it requires the performing physician to have a detailed knowledge of the laryngeal anatomy and understand the limitations of sonography, typically limited by the degree of ossification of the laryngeal cartilages.[61,62]

Trachea

CT is the primary modality for imaging the trachea and advancements in multidetector CT with multiplanar and three-dimensional (3D) reformations allows for a variety of visualization options.[63] Thin section reconstructions using submillimeter slice thicknesses reconstructed in multiple planes should be obtained for the assessment of stenosis of the subglottic trachea, particularly in patients with a history of shortness of breath, stridor, prolonged intubation, or a history of prior tracheostomy. When specifically evaluating the trachea, imaging is mainly obtained with a suspended inspiration; however, the cervical trachea is often seen on neck CTs, which are usually obtained with quiet respiration[9,48] (Fig. 22). Therefore, knowledge of the normal changes in size of the trachea during breathing is needed before assessing for pathologic condition of the trachea.

The diameter of the trachea is dynamic and changes with the phase of respiration. During inspiration, the trachea is rounded or oval shaped, with expiration the posterior wall flattens and can bow forward due to the flexibility of the posterior fibromuscular wall (Fig. 23). Studies have shown the anteroposterior (AP) diameter changes more significantly, up to 35% change, than the transverse diameter, up to 13% change.[48,64] In men, during inhalation, the trachea measures 13 to 25 mm in coronal diameter and 13 to 27 mm in sagittal diameter. In women, during inhalation the trachea measures 10 to 21 mm in coronal diameter and 10 to 23 mm in sagittal diameter. It is important to measure the diameter of the trachea in a true axial plane that is oriented perpendicular to the course of the trachea, which is not always the same as the axial plane of the image. Owing to the advancement of isotropic imaging with the ability to reformat images in any plane, a true axial plane of the trachea is possible and should be used if measurements are needed.[48]

Expiratory imaging can be obtained to assess for tracheomalacia.[65,66] It can also aide in the evaluation of postintubation stenosis because in the chronic state, there may only be minimal wall thickening but on expiratory imaging narrowing of the tracheal lumen can be more pronounced due to cartilage weakening, which is often located 3 to 4 cm below the cricoid cartilage.[63] Expiratory imaging is also often used to evaluate for small airway disease, which will have a mosaic pattern on the expiratory images.[48] Protocols for expiratory imaging can include static end-expiratory CT, or cine imaging during forceful exhalation or coughing.[63]

Three-dimensional images with an external volume rendering can allow easier viewing of subtle narrowing, provide a better view of the length and severity of the stenosis, as well as provide an overview of the full airway with one image.[48,66] This view can also be easier to understand for patients and provide a better anatomic roadmap for preprocedural planning.[65] Off axis coronal 2D projections are also helpful in evaluating the trachea in a single image (see Fig. 20).[66] Virtual bronchoscopy is an internal 3D rendering of the airway to mimic the views as seen in conventional bronchoscopy. This can be used for stenoses that will not allow passage of the bronchoscope, preplanning for transbronchial biopsies, foreign body aspiration evaluation, and tracheomalacia.[48]

Finally, the trachea can be evaluated on MR imaging but respiratory motion artifact makes it more difficult to obtain diagnostic quality imaging. MR imaging can be helpful in cases of mediastinal masses to assess for tracheal compression or invasion or in cases of vascular rings or anomalies. Because these pathologic conditions affect the intrathoracic trachea, further discussion is beyond the scope of this article. To avoid excessive exposure to ionizing radiation, MR imaging should be considered in pediatric patients that may require frequent imaging.[66]

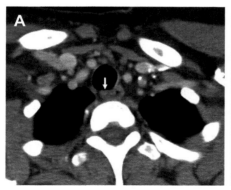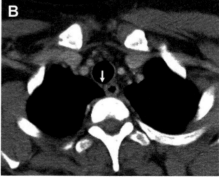

Fig. 22. Normal CT images demonstrating the variation in the shape of the trachea using different breathing techniques. Figure A obtained from a neck CT during quiet respiration showing flattening of the posterior wall of the trachea (*arrow*). Figure B obtained immediately after Figure A from a chest CT from the same patient during end-inspiratory breath hold showing the posterior wall is now convex (*arrow*) and gives the trachea a rounded appearance. (*Courtesy of* University of North Carolina, Chapel Hill, NC.)

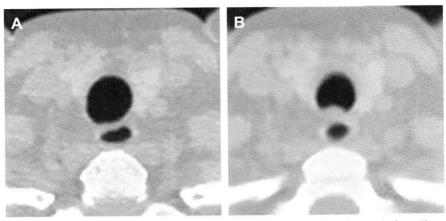

Fig. 23. Axial chest CT images through the cervical segment of the trachea in a lung window. Figure A was obtained during end-inspiratory breath hold and figure B was obtained during end-expiratory breath hold. This shows the normal change of the posterior fibromuscular wall and normal overall reduction in the tracheal diameter in the expiratory phase. At end-expiration the normal inward bowing of the posterior fibromuscular wall (*B*) could be mistaken for pathologic condition if not aware of this normal dynamic change. On these images, the esophagus is also visualized as the air-filled structure located just posterior to the trachea; more commonly the esophagus is collapsed. (*Courtesy of* University of North Carolina, Chapel Hill, NC.)

CLINICS CARE POINTS

- Involvement of the preepiglottic and paraglottic spaces may not be clinically suspected in patients with laryngeal cancers but when present could potentially increase the tumor category (to at least T3) and AJCC prognostic stage (at least stage III).

- Tumors involving the anterior commissure (AC) are associated with early invasion of the adjacent thyroid cartilage, subglottic extension, and early extralaryngeal extension, so this region should be closely scrutinized in patients with laryngeal cancers. The normal AC should measure no more than 2 mm in thickness.

- Subglottic tumor extension precludes most types of partial laryngectomy, leaving only total laryngectomy or near total laryngectomy as the only surgical option.

- Imaging protocols for vocal cord paralysis should cover the entire course of the cervical vagus and recurrent laryngeal nerves from the skull base through the aortic arch because lesions at any site along this course may cause vocal cord weakness.

- In patients potentially undergoing thyroidectomy, it is important to recognize the presence of an aberrant subclavian artery because this anatomic variant is associated with a nonrecurrent course of the inferior laryngeal nerve, which places the nerve at increased risk for injury during surgery.

DISCLOSURE

The authors have nothing to disclose.

REFERENCES

1.. Wadie M, Adam SI, Sasaki CT. Development, Anatomy, and Physiology of the Larynx. In: Shaker R, Belafsky PC, Postma GN, et al, editors. Principles of deglutition: a multidisciplinary text for swallowing and its disorders. New York, NY: Springer; 2013. p. 175–97.

2. Lev MH, Curtin HD. Larynx. Neuroimaging Clin N Am 1998;8(1):235–56.

3. Ajmani ML. A metrical study of the laryngeal skeleton in adult Nigerians. J Anat 1990;171:187–91.

4. Eckel HE, Sittel C, Zorowka P, et al. Dimensions of the laryngeal framework in adults. Surg Radiol Anat 1994;16(1):31–6.

5. Glikson E, Sagiv D, Eyal A, et al. The anatomical evolution of the thyroid cartilage from childhood to adulthood: a computed tomography evaluation. Laryngoscope 2017;127(10):E354–8.

6. Loth A, Corny J, Santini L, et al. Analysis of hyoid-larynx complex using 3D geometric morphometrics. Dysphagia 2015;30(3):357–64.

7. Markova D, Richer L, Pangelinan M, et al. Age- and sex-related variations in vocal-tract morphology and voice acoustics during adolescence. Horm Behav 2016;81:84–96.

8. Krohner RG, Ramanathan S. Functional Anatomy of the Airway. In: Hagberg CA, editor. Benumof's airway management: Principles and Practice. 2nd edition. Philadelphia, PA: Mosby Elsevier; 2007. p. 3–21.

9. Huang BY, Solle M, Weissler MC. Larynx: anatomic imaging for diagnosis and management. Otolaryngol Clin North Am 2012;45(6):1325–61.

10. Sataloff RT, Chowdhury F, Portnoy JE, et al. Anatomy and physiology of the voice: a brief overview. In: Sataloff RT, editor. Surgical techniques in otolaryngology head and neck surgery: laryngeal surgery. 1st edition. New Delhi, India: JP Medical Ltd; 2013. p. 8–15. chap 3.

11. Lydiatt DD, Bucher GS. The historical Latin and etymology of selected anatomical terms of the larynx. Clin Anat 2010;23(2):131–44.

12. Andaloro C, Sharma P, La Mantia I. Anatomy, head and neck, larynx arytenoid cartilage. StatPearls 2021. StatPearls Publishing.

13. Curtin HD. Anatomy, imaging, and pathology of the larynx. In: Som PM, Curtin HD, editors. Head and neck imaging. 5th edition. St. Louis, MO: Mosby Inc. Elsevier Inc.; 2011. p. 1905–2040. chap 31.

14. Baugnon KL, Beitler JJ. Pitfalls in the staging of cancer of the laryngeal squamous cell carcinoma. Neuroimaging Clin N Am 2013;23(1):81–105.

15. Garvin HM. Ossification of laryngeal structures as indicators of age. J Forensic Sci 2008;53(5):1023–7.

16. Becker M, Burkhardt K, Dulguerov P, et al. Imaging of the larynx and hypopharynx. Eur J Radiol 2008; 66(3):460–79.

17. Becker M, Zbaren P, Laeng H, et al. Neoplastic invasion of the laryngeal cartilage: comparison of MR imaging and CT with histopathologic correlation. Radiology 1995;194(3):661–9.

18. Fatterpekar GM, Mukherji SK, Rajgopalan P, et al. Normal age-related signal change in the laryngeal cartilages. Neuroradiology 2004;46(8):678–81.

19. Kallmes DF, Phillips CD. The normal anterior commissure of the glottis. AJR Am J Roentgenol 1997;168(5):1317–9.

20. Chone CT, Yonehara E, Martins JE, et al. Importance of anterior commissure in recurrence of early glottic cancer after laser endoscopic resection. Arch Otolaryngol Head Neck Surg 2007;133(9): 882–7.

21. Reidenbach MM. Normal topography of the conus elasticus. Anatomical bases for the spread of laryngeal cancer. Surg Radiol Anat 1995;17(2):107–11, 4-111.

22. Netter FH. Actions of intrinsic muscles of larynx. Atlas of human anatomy. 7th edition. Philadelphia, PA: Saunders Elsevier; 2019. chap 93.

23. Armstrong WB, Netterville JL. Anatomy of the larynx, trachea, and bronchi. Otolaryngol Clin North Am 1995;28(4):685–99.

24. Bak-Pedersen K, Nielson KO. Mucus-producing elements in the normal adult human larynx. Acta Otolaryngol 1982;93(Suppl 386):170–2.

25. Stell PM, Watt J, Stell IM. Squamous metaplasia of the human larynx: the influence of sex and area of residence in the non-smoking population. Clin Otolaryngol Allied Sci 1982;7(5):335–9.

26. Connor S. Laryngeal cancer: how does the radiologist help? Cancer Imaging 2007;7:93–103.

27. Sato K, Kurita S, Hirano M. Location of the preepiglottic space and its relationship to the paraglottic space. Ann Otol Rhinol Laryngol 1993;102(12): 930–4.

28. Tucker GF Jr, Smith HR Jr. A histological demonstration of the development of laryngeal connective tissue compartments. Trans Am Acad Ophthalmol Otolaryngol 1962;66:308–18.

29. Patel SG, Lydiatt WM, Glastonbury CM, et al. Larynx. In: Armin MB, Edge SB, Greene FL, et al, editors. AJCC cancer staging manual. 8th ed. New York, NY: Springer; 2017. p. 149–61.

30. Blitz AM, Aygun N. Radiologic evaluation of larynx cancer. Otolaryngol Clin North Am 2008;41(4): 697–713, vi.

31. Thurnher D, Moukarbel RV, Novak CB, et al. The glottis and subglottis: an otolaryngologist's perspective. Thorac Surg Clin 2007;17(4):549–60.

32. Ferreiro-Arguelles C, Jimenez-Juan L, Martinez-Salazar JM, et al. CT findings after laryngectomy. Radiographics 2008;28(3):869–82 [quiz: 914].

33. Rodel RM, Steiner W, Muller RM, et al. Endoscopic laser surgery of early glottic cancer: involvement of the anterior commissure. Head Neck 2009;31(5): 583–92.

34. Krmpotic-Nemanic J, Draf W, Helms J. Surgical anatomy of head and neck. 1st edition. Berlin, Heidelberg, Germany: Springer-Verlag; 1988.

35. Netter FH. Thyroid gland: anterior view. Atlas of human anatomy. Philadelphia, PA: Saunders Elsevier; 2019. p. 87.

36. Adams A, Mankad K, Offiah C, et al. Branchial cleft anomalies: a pictorial review of embryological development and spectrum of imaging findings. Insights Imaging 2016;7(1):69–76.

37. Belafsky PC, Lintzenich CR. Development, anatomy, and physiology of the pharynx. In: Shaker R, Belafsky PC, Postma GN, et al, editors. Principles of deglutition: a multidisciplinary text for swallowing and its disorders. New York, NY: Springer; 2013. p. 165–73.

38. Hiatt JL, Gartner LP. Palate, Pharynx, and Larynx. In: McGraw L, editor. Textbook of head and neck anatomy. Philadelphia, PA: Lippincott Williams & Wilkins; 2002. p. 229–45. chap 16.

39. Furlow PW, Mathisen DJ. Surgical anatomy of the trachea. Ann Cardiothorac Surg 2018;7(2):255–60.

40. Toniato A, Mazzarotto R, Piotto A, et al. Identification of the nonrecurrent laryngeal nerve during thyroid surgery: 20-year experience. World J Surg 2004; 28(7):659–61.

41. Henry JF, Audiffret J, Denizot A, et al. The nonrecurrent inferior laryngeal nerve: review of 33 cases,

including two on the left side. Surgery 1988;104(6): 977–84.

42. Pressman J, Dowdy A, Libby R, et al. Further studies upon the submucosal compartments and lymphatics of the larynx by the injection of dyes and radioisotopes. Ann Otol Rhinol Laryngol 1956;65(4): 963–80.

43. Tomik J, Skladzien J, Modrzejewski M. Evaluation of cervical lymph node metastasis of 1400 patients with cancer of the larynx. Auris Nasus Larynx 2001;28(3):233–40.

44. Werner JA, Dunne AA, Myers JN. Functional anatomy of the lymphatic drainage system of the upper aerodigestive tract and its role in metastasis of squamous cell carcinoma. Head Neck 2003;25(4): 322–32.

45. Sanabria A, Shah JP, Medina JE, et al. Incidence of occult lymph node metastasis in primary larynx squamous cell carcinoma, by subsite, T classification and neck level: a systematic review. Cancers (Basel) 2020;12(4). https://doi.org/10.3390/cancers12041059.

46. Liu YH, Xu SC, Tu LL, et al. A rich lymphatic network exists in the inferior surface of the vocal cord. Surg Radiol Anat 2006;28(2):125–8.

47. Forghani R, Yu E, Levental M, et al. Imaging evaluation of lymphadenopathy and patterns of lymph node spread in head and neck cancer. Expert Rev Anticancer Ther 2015;15(2):207–24.

48. Laroia AT, Thompson BH, Laroia ST, et al. Modern imaging of the tracheo-bronchial tree. World J Radiol 2010;2(7):237–48.

49. Epstein SK. Anatomy and physiology of tracheostomy. Respir Care 2005;50(4):476–82.

50. Webb EM, Elicker BM, Webb WR. Using CT to diagnose nonneoplastic tracheal abnormalities: appearance of the tracheal wall. AJR Am J Roentgenol 2000;174(5):1315–21.

51. Sasson JP, Madan N, Gilman MD, et al. Anatomy, imaging, and pathology of the trachea. In: Som PM, Curtin HD, editors. Head and neck imaging. St. Louis, MO: Mosby Inc. Elsevier Inc.; 2011. p. 2041–84. chap 32.

52. Trigaux JP, Hermes G, Dubois P, et al. CT of sabersheath trachea. Correlation with clinical, chest radiographic and functional findings. Acta Radiol 1994; 35(3):247–50.

53. Netter FH. Lymph vessels and nodes of lung. Atlas of human anatomy. Saunders Elsevier; 2019. p. 212.

54. Kuno H, Onaya H, Fujii S, et al. Primary staging of laryngeal and hypopharyngeal cancer: CT, MR imaging and dual-energy CT. Eur J Radiol 2014; 83(1):e23–35.

55. Lell MM, Greess H, Hothorn T, et al. Multiplanar functional imaging of the larynx and hypopharynx with multislice spiral CT. Eur Radiol 2004;14(12): 2198–205.

56. Kim BS, Ahn KJ, Park YH, et al. Usefulness of laryngeal phonation CT in the diagnosis of vocal cord paralysis. AJR Am J Roentgenol 2008;190(5):1376–9.

57. Wear VV, Allred JW, Mi D, et al. Evaluating "eee" phonation in multidetector CT of the neck. AJNR Am J Neuroradiol 2009;30(6):1102–6.

58. Chin SC, Edelstein S, Chen CY, et al. Using CT to localize side and level of vocal cord paralysis. AJR Am J Roentgenol 2003;180(4):1165–70.

59. Wu JH, Zhao J, Li ZH, et al. Comparison of CT and MRI in diagnosis of laryngeal carcinoma with anterior vocal commissure involvement. Sci Rep 2016; 6:30353.

60. Kuno H, Onaya H, Iwata R, et al. Evaluation of cartilage invasion by laryngeal and hypopharyngeal squamous cell carcinoma with dual-energy CT. Radiology 2012;265(2):488–96.

61. Loveday EJ. Ultrasound of the larynx. Imaging 2003; 15(3):109–14.

62. Singh M, Chin KJ, Chan VW, et al. Use of sonography for airway assessment: an observational study. J Ultrasound Med 2010;29(1):79–85.

63. Heidinger BH, Occhipinti M, Eisenberg RL, et al. Imaging of Large Airways Disorders. AJR Am J Roentgenol 2015;205(1):41–56.

64. Ederle JR, Heussel CP, Hast J, et al. Evaluation of changes in central airway dimensions, lung area and mean lung density at paired inspiratory/expiratory high-resolution computed tomography. Eur Radiol 2003;13(11):2454–61.

65. Lee KS, Boiselle PM. Update on multidetector computed tomography imaging of the airways. J Thorac Imaging 2010;25(2):112–24.

66. JO Shepard, Flores EJ, Abbott GF. Imaging of the trachea. Ann Cardiothorac Surg 2018;7(2):197–209.

Anatomy of Neck Muscles, Spaces, and Lymph Nodes

Carrie D. Norris, MD, Yoshimi Anzai, MD, MPH*

KEYWORDS

- Head and neck • Spaces • Muscles • Anatomy • Lymph nodes • Lymphatic drainage • Fascia

KEY POINTS

- Understanding the anatomy and innervation of head and neck muscles helps radiologists recognize potential pathology resulting in neuropathy associated with muscle atrophy or contralateral hypertrophy.
- An essential step to interpreting cross-sectional imaging studies of the head and neck is identifying the space within which a lesion is located. Understanding head and neck spaces and their boundaries and contents is critical to addressing potential etiologies.
- Lymph node metastasis is one of the most significant prognostic factors for head and neck cancer. Therefore, it is critical to learn head and neck lymph node anatomy and the drainage pathways. This allows us to scrutinize high-risk lymph node-bearing regions given a primary tumor location and the location of abnormal lymph nodes, and which primary head and neck site is highly likely to harbor primary cancer.

MUSCLES OF THE HEAD AND NECK

Muscle of Head and Neck Movement and Support

Sternocleidomastoid

- Attachments: The sternal head originates from the superior surface of the anterior manubrium (Fig. 1). The clavicular head originates from the superior surface of the medial third of the clavicle. Both heads insert on the lateral surface of the temporal bone mastoid process and lateral half of the occipital bone superior nuchal line.
- Innervation: Spinal accessory nerve (cranial nerve [CN] XI), branches of the cervical plexus (C2–C3)
- Action
  - Unilateral contraction: Ipsilateral neck flexion, contralateral neck rotation
  - Bilateral contraction: Elevates the head, flexes the lower cervical column.

Trapezius

- Attachments: Originates from the skull, nuchal ligament, and the spinous processes of C7–T12 and inserts on the clavicle, acromion, and the scapular spine.
- Innervation: Spinal accessory nerve (CN XI)
- Action: The upper fibers of the trapezius elevate the scapula and rotate it during abduction of the arm. The middle fibers retract the scapula and the lower fibers pull the scapula inferiorly.

Levator scapulae

- Attachments: Originates from the transverse processes of the C1–C4 vertebrae and inserts on the medial border of the scapula.

The authors have nothing to disclose.
No external funding was received related to this article.
University of Utah, Department of Radiology and Imaging Sciences, 30 North 1900 East #1A071, Salt Lake City, Utah 84132, USA
* Corresponding author.
E-mail address: yoshimi.anzai@hsc.utah.edu

neuroimaging.theclinics.com

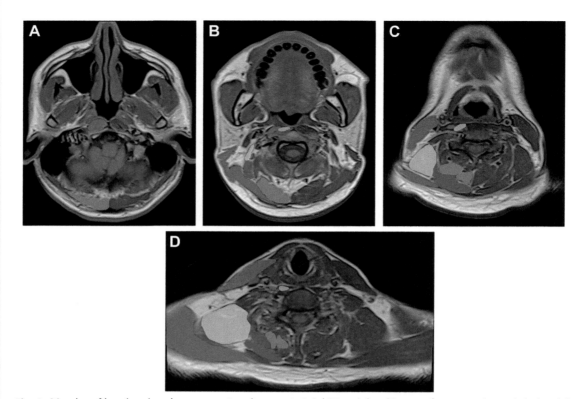

Fig. 1. Muscles of head and neck movement and support. Axial T1-weighted images from superior to inferior: (A) longus capitis (pink), semispinalis capitis (orange), (B) longus capitis (pink), semispinalis capitis (orange), longus colli (gray), splenius capitis (red), trapezius (blue), levator scapulae (yellow), sternocleidomastoid (green), (C) longus capitis (pink), semispinalis capitis (orange), longus colli (gray), splenius capitis (red), trapezius (blue), levator scapulae (yellow), sternocleidomastoid (green), semispinalis cervicis (aqua), (D) longus capitis (pink), semispinalis capitis (orange), longus colli (gray), splenius capitis (red), trapezius (blue), levator scapulae (yellow), sternocleidomastoid (green), semispinalis cervicis (aqua), splenius cervicis (purple).

- Innervation: Dorsal scapular nerve
- Action: Elevates the scapula.

Splenius capitis

- Attachments: Originates from the lower aspect of the nuchal ligament and the spinous processes of C7–T3/4 vertebrae and inserts on the temporal bone mastoid process and the occipital bone.
- Innervation: Posterior rami of spinal nerves C3 and C4
- Action: Ipsilateral head rotation

Splenius cervicis

- Attachments: Originates from the spinous processes of T3–T6 vertebrae and inserts on the transverse processes of C1-3/4.
- Innervation: Posterior rami of the lower cervical spinal nerves
- Action: Ipsilateral head rotation

Semispinalis capitis

- Attachments: Originates from the articular processes of vertebrae C4–C7 and transverse processes of vertebrae T1–T6 and inserts between the superior and inferior nuchal lines of the occipital bone.
- Innervation: Descending branches of the greater occipital nerve (C2) and spinal nerve C3
- Action:
  - Bilateral contraction: Extension of head, cervical and thoracic spine
  - Unilateral contraction: Lateral flexion of head, cervical and thoracic spine (ipsilateral), rotation of head, cervical and thoracic spine (contralateral)

Semispinalis cervicis

- Attachments: Originates from the transverse processes of vertebrae T1–T6, and inserts on the spinous processes of vertebrae C2–C5.

- Innervation: Medial branches of spinal nerve posterior rami
- Action:
  ○ Bilateral contraction: Extension of head, cervical and thoracic spine
  ○ Unilateral contraction: Lateral flexion of head, cervical and thoracic spine (ipsilateral), rotation of head, cervical and thoracic spine (contralateral)

Longus capitis

- Attachments: Originates from the anterior tubercles of the C3–C6 transverse processes and inserts on the base of the occipital bone.
- Innervation: Anterior rami of spinal nerves C1–C3
- Action:
  ○ Bilateral contraction: Head flexion
  ○ Unilateral contraction: Head rotation (ipsilateral)

Longus colli

- Attachments: Originates from the anterior tubercles of the C3–C6 transverse processes (superior part, anterior surface of the C5–T3 vertebral bodies (intermediate part) and anterior surface of the T1–T3 vertebral bodies (inferior part). Inserts on the anterior tubercle of C1 (superior part), anterior surface of the C2–C4 vertebral bodies (intermediate part), and the anterior tubercles of the C5–C6 vertebral bodies.
- Innervation: Anterior rami of spinal nerves C2–C6
- Action:
  ○ Bilateral contraction: Neck flexion
  ○ Unilateral contraction: Lateral neck flexion (ipsilateral), neck rotation (contralateral)[1–3]

Suprahyoid

Stylohyoid

- Attachments: Arises from the styloid process of the temporal bone and inserts on the lateral aspect of the hyoid bone.
- Innervation: Stylohyoid branch of the facial nerve (CN VII)
- Action: Initiates swallowing by pulling the hyoid bone posteriorly and superiorly.

Digastric

- Attachments:
  ○ The anterior belly arises from the digastric fossa of the mandible.

  ○ The posterior belly arises from the mastoid process of the temporal bone.
  ○ The two bellies are connected by an intermediate tendon, which is attached to the hyoid bone via a fibrous sling.
- Innervation:
  ○ The anterior belly is innervated by the inferior alveolar nerve, via a branch of the mandibular nerve (CN V3).
  ○ The posterior belly is innervated by the digastric branch of the facial nerve (CN VII).
- Action: Depresses the mandible and elevates the hyoid bone.

Mylohyoid

- Attachments: Originates from the mylohyoid line of mandible and inserts on the mylohyoid raphe and body of hyoid.
- Innervation: Nerve to mylohyoid, via a branch of the inferior alveolar nerve (CN V3).
- Action: Forms floor of oral cavity, elevates hyoid bone and floor of mouth, and depresses mandible.

Geniohyoid

- Attachments: Originates from the inferior mental spine (inferior genial tubercle) and inserts on the body of the hyoid.
- Innervation: Anterior ramus of spinal nerve C1, via hypoglossal nerve (CN XII)
- Function: Elevates and draws hyoid bone anteriorly, shortens the floor of the mouth, and widens pharynx.[1–3]

Infrahyoid

Omohyoid

- Attachments:
  ○ The inferior belly of the omohyoid arises from the scapula. It is attached to the superior belly by an intermediate tendon, which is anchored to the clavicle by the deep cervical fascia. The superior belly ascends to insert on the hyoid bone.
- Innervation: Anterior rami of C1–C3, carried by a branch of the ansa cervicalis
- Action: Depresses the hyoid bone.

Sternohyoid

- Attachments: Originates from the sternum and sternoclavicular joint and inserts on the hyoid bone.
- Innervation: Anterior rami of C1–C3, carried by a branch of the ansa cervicalis
- Action: Depresses the hyoid bone.

Sternothyroid

- Attachments: Arises from the manubrium of the sternum and inserts on the thyroid cartilage.
- Innervation: Anterior rami of C1–C3, carried by a branch of the ansa cervicalis
- Action: Depresses the thyroid cartilage.

Thyrohyoid

- Attachments: Arises from the thyroid cartilage of the larynx and ascends to insert on the hyoid bone.
- Innervation: Anterior ramus of spinal nerve C1 (via hypoglossal nerve, CN XII)
- Action: Depresses the hyoid bone.[1–3]

Suboccipital

Rectus capitis posterior major

- Attachments: Originates from the spinous process of C2 and inserts on the lateral part on the occipital bone inferior nuchal line (Fig. 2).
- Innervation: Suboccipital nerve (posterior ramus of C1)
- Action: Extension and rotation of the head.

Rectus capitis posterior minor

- Attachments: Originates from the posterior tubercle of C1 and inserts on the medial part on the occipital bone inferior nuchal line.

- Innervation: Suboccipital nerve (posterior ramus of C1)
- Action: Extension of the head.

Obliquus capitis inferior

- Attachments: Originates from the spinous process of C2 and inserts on the transverse processes of C1.
- Innervation: Suboccipital nerve (posterior ramus of C1)
- Action: Extension and rotation of the head.

Obliquus capitis superior

- Attachments: Originates from the transverse process of C1 and inserts on the occipital bone between the superior and inferior nuchal lines.
- Innervation: Suboccipital nerve (posterior ramus of C1)
- Action: Extension of the head.[1–3]

Scalenes

Anterior scalene

- Attachments: Originates from the anterior tubercles of the transverse processes of C3–C6 and inserts on the scalene tubercle, on the inner border of the first rib (Fig. 3).
- Innervation: Anterior rami of C5–C6
- Action: Elevation of the first rib, lateral neck flexion (ipsilateral), anterior neck flexion (bilateral)

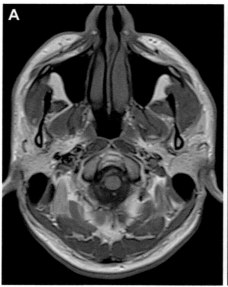 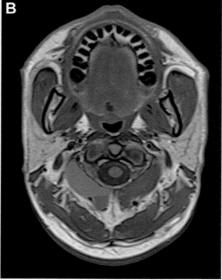

Fig. 2. Suboccipital group. Axial T1-weighted images from superior to inferior: (A) obliquus capitis superior (orange), rectus capitis posterior major (red), rectus capitis posterior minor (blue) and (B) rectus capitis posterior major (red), obliquus capitis inferior (green).

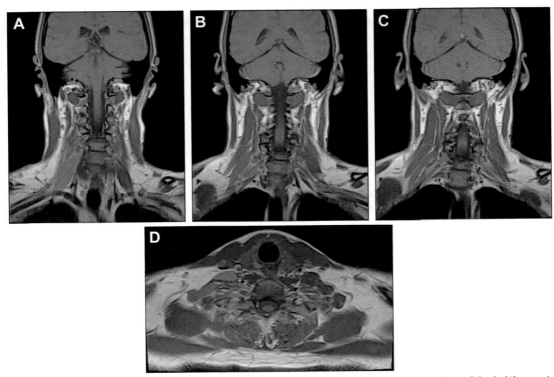

Fig. 3. Scalenes. Coronal T1-weighted images from anterior to posterior: (*A*) anterior scalene (blue), (*B*) anterior scalene (blue), middle scalene (red), posterior scalene (purple), (*C*) middle scalene (red), posterior scalene (purple), and axial T1-weighted image (*D*) anterior scalene (blue), middle scalene (red), posterior scalene (purple).

Middle scalene

- Attachments: Originates from the posterior tubercles of the transverse processes of C2–C7 and inserts on the scalene tubercle of the first rib.
- Innervation: Anterior rami of C3–C8
- Function: Elevation of the first rib, lateral neck flexion (ipsilateral)

Posterior scalene

- Attachments: Originates from the posterior tubercles of the transverse processes of C5–C7 and inserts on the second rib.
- Innervation: Anterior rami of C6–C8
- Function: Elevation of the second rib, lateral neck flexion (ipsilateral)[1–3]

Muscles of Mastication

Masseter

- Attachments: Originates from the inferior margin of the anterior zygomatic arch and inserts onto the outer surface of the mandibular ramus and mandibular coronoid process (Fig. 4).

- Innervation: Mandibular division of the trigeminal nerve (CN V3)
- Action: Elevate the mandible, approximate the teeth, retract, and protrude mandible.

Temporalis

- Attachments: Originates from the inferior temporal line of the lateral skull (temporal fossa) and passes underneath the zygomatic arch to insert on the mandibular coronoid process.
- Innervation: Deep temporal nerve, via the mandibular division of the trigeminal nerve (CN V3)
- Action: Elevate the mandible, side-to-side mandibular motion.

Medial pterygoid

- Attachments: Originates from the pterygoid process (maxillary tuberosity and lateral pterygoid plate) and inserts on the medial ramus of the mandible posterior and inferior to the mylohyoid groove.
- Innervation: Mandibular division of the trigeminal nerve (CN V3)

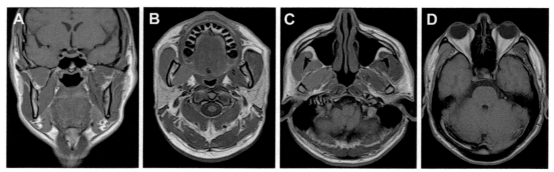

Fig. 4. Muscles of mastication. Coronal T1-weighted image: (*A*) medial pterygoid (blue), lateral pterygoid (red), masseter (purple) and axial T1-weighted images from inferior to superior: (*B*) medial pterygoid (blue), masseter (purple), (*C*) temporalis (green), medial pterygoid (blue), lateral pterygoid (red), masseter (purple), (*D*) temporalis (green).

- Action: Elevation and protrusion of the mandible, side-to-side mandibular motion

Lateral pterygoid

- Attachments: Originates from the infratemporal crest of the greater wing of the sphenoid bone and lateral surface of the lateral pterygoid plate. Inserts on mandibular condylar process and articular capsule of the temporomandibular joint.
- Innervation: Mandibular division of the trigeminal nerve (CN V3)
- Action: Depression and protrusion of the mandible, side-to-side mandibular motion[1–3]

Muscles of the Oral Cavity

Musculus uvulae

- Attachments: Originates from the posterior margin of the hard palate and the posterior

nasal spine of the palatine bone and inserts on the palatine aponeurosis (Fig. 5).
- Innervation: Pharyngeal plexus of the vagus nerve (CN X)
- Action: Shortens the uvula.

Tensor veli palatini

- Attachments: Originates from the scaphoid fossa of pterygoid process, spine of the sphenoid bone, and membranous wall of the auditory tube and inserts on the palatine aponeurosis.
- Innervation: Nerve to medial pterygoid, a branch of the mandibular nerve (CN V3)
- Action: Elevation of the hyoid-laryngeal complex during swallowing, opening of the Eustachian tube

Levator veli palatini

- Attachments: Originates from the petrous temporal bone and inferior cartilaginous

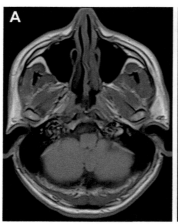
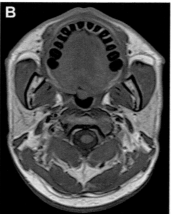
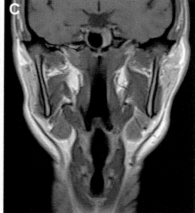

Fig. 5. Muscles of the oral cavity. Axial T1-weighted images from superior to inferior: (*A*) levator veli palatini (orange), tensor veli palatini (green), (*B*) musculus uvulae (purple), palatoglossus (red), palatopharyngeus (blue) and coronal T1-weighted image: (*C*) levator veli palatini (orange), tensor veli palatini (green).

auditory tube and inserts on the palatine aponeurosis.

- Innervation: Pharyngeal plexus of the vagus nerve (CN X)
- Action: Elevation of the soft palate during swallowing

Palatopharyngeus

- Attachments: Originates from the posterior margin of the hard palate and palatine aponeurosis and inserts on the posterior border of the thyroid cartilage.
- Innervation: Pharyngeal plexus of the vagus nerve (CN X)
- Action: Elevates and shortens the pharynx during swallowing.

Palatoglossus

- Attachments: Originates from the palatine aponeurosis of soft palate, inserts on the lateral margins of tongue, and blends with intrinsic muscles of tongue.
- Innervation: Branches of pharyngeal plexus via the vagus nerve (CN X)
- Action: Elevates the root of tongue and constricts isthmus of fauces.[1]

Intrinsic Tongue Muscles

Superior longitudinal

- Attachments: Originates from the submucosa of the posterior tongue and lingual septum and inserts at the apex and anterolateral tongue margins (Fig. 6).
- Innervation: Hypoglossal nerve (CN XII)

- Action: Retracts and broadens tongue and elevates apex of tongue.

Inferior longitudinal

- Attachments: Originates from the root of the tongue and body of the hyoid bone and inserts at the apex of the tongue.
- Innervation: Hypoglossal nerve (CN XII)
- Action: Retracts and broadens tongue and lowers apex of tongue.

Transverse

- Attachments: Originates from the lingual septum and inserts at the apex and lateral tongue margins.
- Innervation: Hypoglossal nerve (CN XII)
- Action: Narrows and elongates tongue.

Vertical

- Attachments: Originates from the root of the tongue and genioglossus muscle and inserts at the lingual aponeurosis.
- Innervation: Hypoglossal nerve (CN XII)
- Action: Broadens and elongates tongue.[1]

Extrinsic Tongue Muscles

Genioglossus

- Attachments: Originates from the superior mental spine of the mandible and inserts along the entire length of dorsum of tongue, lingual aponeurosis, and body of the hyoid bone.
- Innervation: Hypoglossal nerve (CN XII)

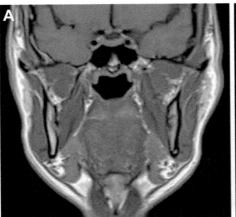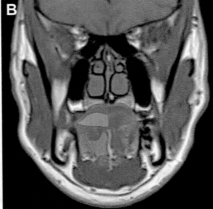

Fig. 6. Intrinsic and extrinsic tongue muscles. Coronal T1-weighted images from posterior to anterior: (A) palatoglossus (red), styloglossus (blue), hyoglossus (green), (B) styloglossus (blue), hyoglossus (green), genioglossus (orange), inferior longitudinal (purple) vertical/transverse (aqua), superior longitudinal (pink) intrinsic tongue muscles.

- Action: Depresses and protrudes tongue (bilateral contraction) and deviates tongue contralaterally (unilateral contraction).

Hyoglossus

- Attachments: Originates from the body and greater horn of the hyoid and inserts on the inferior/ventral parts of the lateral tongue.
- Innervation: Hypoglossal nerve (CN XII)
- Action: Depresses and retracts tongue.

Styloglossus

- Attachments: Originates from the anterolateral aspect of styloid process (of temporal bone), stylomandibular ligament, blends with inferior longitudinal muscle (longitudinal part); blends with hyoglossus muscle (oblique part).
- Innervation: Hypoglossal nerve (CN XII)
- Action: Elevates and retracts lateral aspects of the tongue.

Palatoglossus

- Attachments: Originates from the palatine aponeurosis of soft palate, inserts on the lateral margins of tongue, and blends with intrinsic muscles of tongue.
- Innervation: Branches of pharyngeal plexus via the vagus nerve (CN X)
- Action: Elevates root of tongue and constricts isthmus of fauces.[1]

Pharynx

There are two main groups of pharyngeal muscles (Fig. 7): longitudinal and circular.

There are three circular pharyngeal constrictor muscles: the superior, middle, and inferior pharyngeal constrictors. They are stacked and form an incomplete muscular circle as they attach anteriorly to structures in the neck.

The circular muscles contract sequentially from superior to inferior to constrict the lumen and propel the bolus of food inferiorly into the esophagus.

Superior pharyngeal constrictor

- The uppermost pharyngeal constrictor, located in the oropharynx.
- Attachments: Originates from the pterygomandibular ligament, alveolar process of mandible and medial pterygoid plate and pterygoid hamulus of the sphenoid bone. Inserts posteriorly into to the pharyngeal tubercle of the occiput and the median pharyngeal raphe.

Middle pharyngeal constrictor

- Located in the laryngopharynx.
- Attachments: Originates from the stylohyoid ligament and the horns of the hyoid bone and inserts posteriorly into the pharyngeal raphe.

Inferior pharyngeal constrictor

- Located in the laryngopharynx. It has two components:

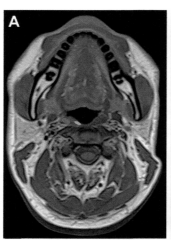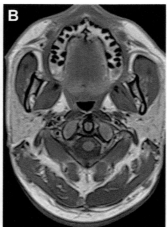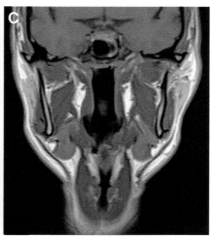

Fig. 7. Pharyngeal muscles. Axial T1-weighted images from inferior to superior: (A) middle constrictor (yellow), stylopharyngeus (green), palatopharyngeus (purple), (B) palatopharyngeus (purple), superior constrictor (red), salpingopharyngeus (blue), stylopharyngeus (green), and coronal T1-weighted image: (C) palatopharyngeus (purple), superior constrictor (red), salpingopharyngeus (blue).

○ Superior component (thyropharyngeus) has oblique fibers that attach to the thyroid cartilage.

○ Inferior component (cricopharyngeus) has horizontal fibers that attach to the cricoid cartilage.

All pharyngeal constrictors are innervated by the vagus nerve (CN X).

The longitudinal muscles are the stylopharyngeus, palatopharyngeus, and salpingopharyngeus. They act to shorten and widen the pharynx and elevate the larynx during swallowing.

Stylopharyngeus

- Attachments: Arises from the styloid process of the temporal bone and inserts into the pharynx.
- Innervation: Glossopharyngeal nerve (CN IX)

Palatopharyngeus

- Attachments: Arises from hard palate of the oral cavity and inserts into the pharynx.
- Innervation: Vagus nerve (CN X)

Salpingopharyngeus

- Attachments: Arises from the Eustachian tube and inserts into the pharynx.
- Innervation: Vagus nerve (CN X)
- Action: In addition to contributing to swallowing, it also opens the Eustachian tube to equalize the pressure in the middle ear.[1–3]

Larynx

The larynx is an organ located in the anterior neck with several important functions, including phonation, the cough reflex, and protection of the lower respiratory tract (Fig. 8).

The muscles of the larynx can be divided into two groups: the external muscles and the internal muscles. The external muscles act to elevate or depress the larynx during swallowing. The internal muscles move the individual components of the larynx, with primary roles in breathing and phonation.[4,5]

Cricothyroid

- Attachments: Originates from the anterolateral aspect of the cricoid cartilage and attaches to the inferior margin and inferior horn of the thyroid cartilage.
- Innervation: External laryngeal nerve, via a branch of the superior laryngeal nerve (CN X)
- Action: Stretches and tenses the vocal ligament.

Thyroarytenoid

- Attachments: Originates from the inferoposterior aspect of the angle of the thyroid cartilage and attaches to the anterolateral part of the arytenoid cartilage.
- Innervation: Inferior laryngeal nerve, via a branch of the recurrent laryngeal nerve (CN X)
- Action: Relaxes the vocal ligament.

Posterior cricoarytenoid

Attachments: Originates from the posterior surface of the cricoid cartilage and attaches to the muscular process of the arytenoid cartilage.

- Innervation: Inferior laryngeal nerve, via a branch of the recurrent laryngeal nerve (CN X)
- Action: Abducts the vocal folds.

Lateral cricoarytenoid

- Attachments: Originates from the arch of the cricoid cartilage and attaches to the muscular process of the arytenoid cartilage.
- Innervation: Inferior laryngeal nerve, via a branch of the recurrent laryngeal nerve (CN X)
- Action: Adducts the vocal folds.

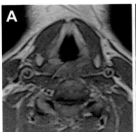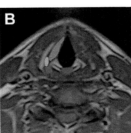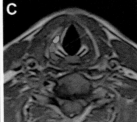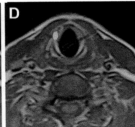

Fig. 8. Laryngeal muscles. Axial T1-weighted images from superior to inferior: (A) transverse/oblique arytenoids (blue), thyroarytenoid (orange), (B) posterior cricoarytenoid (red), lateral cricoarytenoid (yellow), interarytenoid (purple), (C) posterior cricoarytenoid (red), lateral cricoarytenoid (yellow), cricothyroid (green), interarytenoid (purple), (D) lateral cricoarytenoid (yellow), cricothyroid (green).

Transverse/oblique arytenoids

- Attachments: Extends from one arytenoid cartilage to the contralateral arytenoid.
- Innervation: Inferior laryngeal nerve, via a branch of the recurrent laryngeal nerve (CN X)
- Action: Adducts the arytenoid cartilages.[1–3]

Muscles of Facial Expression

Orbital group

Orbicularis oculi The orbicularis oculi muscle surrounds the eye socket and extends into the eyelid. It has three distinct parts—orbital orbicularis, palpebral orbicularis, and lacrimal orbicularis (palpebral, lacrimal, and orbital).

- Attachments: Originates from the medial orbital margin, the medial palpebral ligament, and the lacrimal bone. It then inserts into the skin around the margin of the orbit and the superior and inferior tarsal plates.
- Innervation: Temporal and zygomatic branches of the facial nerve (CN VII)
- Action:
  - Palpebral part—gently closes the eyelids (voluntary and involuntary)
  - Lacrimal part—involved in the drainage of tears
  - Orbital part—tightly closes the eyelids (voluntary)

Corrugator supercilii

- Attachments: Originates from the superciliary arch and inserts onto the skin of the eyebrow.
- Innervation: Temporal branch of the facial nerve (CN VII)
- Action: Draws the eyebrows together, creating vertical wrinkles on the bridge of the nose, assists in shielding the eyes from bright light.

Occipitofrontalis Composed of an occipital belly (occipitalis) and a frontal belly (frontalis). The frontal belly is the major contributor to facial expression.

- Attachments: The occipital belly originates from the occipital bone, as well as the mastoid process of the temporal bone, and inserts into the epicranial aponeurosis. The frontal belly originates from the epicranial aponeurosis and inserts into the fascia of the facial muscles surrounding the eyes and the skin above the eyes.
- Action: Raises the eyebrows and wrinkles the forehead
- Innervation: Temporal branch of the facial nerve (CN VII) innervates frontalis. Posterior auricular branch of the facial nerve (CN VII) innervates occipitalis.

Nasal group

Nasalis The nasalis is the largest of the nasal muscles. It is split into two parts: transverse and alar.

- Attachments: Both portions of the muscle originate from the maxilla. The transverse part inserts on an aponeurosis across the dorsum of the nose. The alar portion of the muscle inserts on the alar cartilage of the nasal skeleton.
- Innervation: Buccal branch of the facial nerve (CN VII)
- Action: The transverse part compresses the nares, and the alar part opens the nares.

Procerus

- Attachments: Originates from the nasal bone, inserting into the lower medial forehead.
- Innervation: Temporal and lower zygomatic branches of the facial nerve (CN VII)
- Action: Contraction of this muscle pulls the eyebrows downward to produce transverse wrinkles over the nose.

Depressor septi nasi

- Attachments: Runs from the maxilla (above the medial incisor tooth) to the nasal septum.
- Innervation: Buccal branch of the facial nerve (CN VII)
- Action: Pulls the nose inferiorly, opening the nares.

Oral group These are the most important group of the facial expressors: responsible for movements of the mouth and lips.

Orbicularis oris

- Attachments: Arises from the maxilla and from the other muscles of the cheek. It inserts into the skin and mucous membranes of the lips.
- Innervation: Buccal branch of the facial nerve (CN VII)
- Action: Purses the lips.

Buccinator

- Attachments: Originates from the alveolar processes of the maxilla and mandible and the pterygomandibular raphe. The fibers run in an inferomedial direction, blending with the orbicularis oris and the skin of the lips.
- Innervation: Buccal branch of the facial nerve (CN VII)
- Action: Pulls the cheek inwards against the teeth, aiding mastication.

Other oral muscles There are other muscles that act on the lips and mouth. Anatomically, they can be divided into upper and lower groups:

The lower group contains the depressor anguli oris, depressor labii inferioris, and the mentalis.

The upper group contains the risorius, zygomaticus major, zygomaticus minor, levator labii superioris, levator labii superioris alaeque nasi, and levator anguli oris.[1,4,5]

Accessory Muscles of the Head and Neck

Levator claviculae

A normal variant that has been hypothesized to be a potential cause of thoracic outlet syndrome.

- Attachments: Originates from the transverse processes of the cervical vertebrae (C1–C6 and variations have been described). Inserts on the middle and/or lateral third of the clavicle.
- Innervation: Variable, but usually branches of the cervical plexus (C2–C4)
- Action: Not definitive, but thought to involve elevation of the clavicle and lateral flexion of the neck.[6]

Spaces of the neck Three layers of deep cervical fascia form the boundaries of the deep spaces in the neck.

The superficial layer: investing fascia of the sternocleidomastoid and trapezius muscles, fascia of the muscles of mastication, fascia between the hyoid and mandible that forms the floor of the submandibular space, and at least some of the fascia covering the parotid gland.

The middle layer: strap muscle fascia and visceral fascia that encloses the thyroid gland and aerodigestive tract (pharynx, larynx, trachea, esophagus).

The deep layer: perivertebral fascia of the prevertebral and paraspinal muscles and the alar fascia.

All three layers contribute to the carotid sheath.[7]

SUPRAHYOID

Parotid Space

The most lateral of the deep spaces of the head and neck, the parotid space is predominantly composed of the parotid gland.

- Borders:
  - Anterior: Masticator space
  - Lateral: Platysma muscle, subcutaneous tissue, and skin (the parotid space is deep to platysma)
  - Medial: Parapharyngeal space
  - Superior: External auditory canal
  - Inferior: Inferior margin of the mandibular margin (including the parotid tail)
  - Posteromedial: Mastoid process of the temporal bone
- Contents:
  - Parotid gland
  - Intraparotid lymph nodes
  - Intraparotid facial nerve
  - External carotid artery
  - Retromandibular vein (posterior facial vein)
- Relationships:
  - The posterior belly of the digastric muscle forms a variable portion of the posteromedial border of the parotid space, and at times, this muscular band helps to differentiate a deep-lobe parotid space lesion to one arising in the carotid space.
  - The facial nerve traverses through the parotid space and separates the superficial and deep lobes of the parotid gland.[7,8]

Submandibular Space

A U-shaped space superficial to the mylohyoid muscle includes the submental space. Some investigators treat the submandibular space as two paired triangular compartments surrounding the submandibular gland and consider the submental space (medial to the paired anterior digastric muscles) as separate.

- Borders:
  - Anterolateral: Medial surface of the mandible
  - Superior: Mylohyoid muscle
  - Posteroinferior: Hyoid bone
  - Inferolateral: Platysma muscle, subcutaneous tissue, and skin (the submandibular space is deep to platysma)
  - Medial: Anterior digastric muscle
- Contents:
  - Superficial (main) portion of the submandibular gland
  - Submandibular lymph nodes (level IB)
  - Branches of the facial artery and vein
  - Branches of the lingual artery
  - Fat
  - Inferior loop of the hypoglossal nerve
  - Nerve to mylohyoid muscle
- Relationships:
  - Unbounded by fascia posteriorly, where it is continuous with the sublingual space and inferior parapharyngeal space at the posterior margin of mylohyoid muscle
  - Communicates with the contralateral submandibular space below the mylohyoid sling.[7,8]

Sublingual Space

A paired, inverted V-shaped space that makes up part of the floor of the mouth.

- Borders:
  - Anterolateral: Medial surface of the mandible

- Superior: Mucosa of the floor of the mouth and tongue
- Inferior: Mylohyoid muscle
- Posterior: Geniohyoid and genioglossus muscles
- Medial: Intrinsic tongue muscles and genioglossus muscle
- Contents:
  - Sublingual gland and duct
  - Lingual artery and nerve
  - Glossopharyngeal (CN IX) and hypoglossal (CN XII) nerves
  - Deep portion of the submandibular gland and duct (Wharton's duct)
- Relationships:
  - Unbounded by fascia posteriorly, where it is continuous with the submandibular space
  - Communicates with the contralateral sublingual space via an isthmus below the frenulum.[7,8]

Masticator Space

Sometimes split into several compartments (ie, sub-masseteric, pteromandibular, temporal and infra-temporal or infrazygomatic and suprazygomatic), the masticator space is primarily composed of muscles.

- Borders:
  - Anterolateral: Buccal space
  - Posterolateral: Parotid space
  - Inferomedial: Submandibular space
  - Medial: Parapharyngeal space
- Contents:
  - Muscles of mastication
  - Inferior alveolar artery and vein
  - Inferior alveolar nerve
  - Pterygoid venous plexus
  - Mandibular division of the trigeminal nerve (CN V3)
- Relationships:
  - Malignancy can spread from the lower face perineurally via the mandibular division of the trigeminal nerve (V3) through foramen ovale and into the middle cranial fossa.
  - Odontogenic and other infections can spread to the middle cranial fossa via foramen ovale.[7,8]

Parapharyngeal Space

Parapharyngeal space is surrounded medially by the pharyngeal mucosal space, anteriorly masticator space, laterally by the parotid space, and posteriorly by the carotid space.

A deep compartment of the head and neck consists largely of fat. Displacement of the space serves as a ueful trait when attempting to delinerate the space of origin when encountering pathology.

- Borders:
  - Anterior: Pterygomandibular raphe and superficial layer of the deep cervical fascia covering the medial pterygoid muscle
  - Posterior: An extension of tensor veli palatini muscle fascia termed the tensor-vascular-styloid fascia or an extension of the fascia of the stylopharyngeus, styloglossus, and levator veli palatini muscles
  - Superior: Skull base
  - Inferior: Greater cornu of the hyoid bone, although some state the space functionally ends higher, with the styloglossus muscle at the level of the angle of the mandible
  - Lateral: Superficial layer of the deep cervical fascia extending between styloid process and mandibular ramus, covering the parotid and lateral pterygoid muscle
  - Medial: Middle layer of the deep cervical fascia covering the superior pharyngeal constrictor and levator and tensor veli palatini muscles
- Contents:
  - Fat
  - Internal maxillary artery (variable)
  - Ascending pharyngeal artery (variable)
  - Pterygoid venous plexus
  - Nerve to the tensor veli palatine, a branch of the trigeminal nerve (CN V3)
  - Minor salivary glands/rests
- Relationships:
  - Posteromedial to the masticator space (medial pterygoid muscle)
  - Anteromedial to the parotid space
  - Posterolateral to the pharyngeal mucosal space
  - Anterolateral to the prevertebral space, retropharyngeal space, and danger space
  - Anterior to the carotid space[7,8]

Buccal Space

A potential space, paired on each side of the oral cavity, continuous with the subcutaneous space, which covers the entire body, head to toe.

- Borders:
  - Anterior: Angle of the mouth
  - Posterior: Masseter muscle
  - Superior: Zygomatic process of the maxilla and the zygomaticus muscles

- Inferior: Depressor anguli oris muscle and the attachment of the deep fascia to the mandible
- Lateral: Platysma muscle, subcutaneous tissue, and skin (the buccal space is deep to platysma)
- Medial: Buccinator muscle (the buccal space is superficial to the buccinator)
- Contents:
  - Buccal fat pad
  - Parotid duct (Stensen's duct)
  - Anterior facial artery and vein
  - Transverse facial artery and vein
  - Minor salivary glands
  - Buccal lymph nodes
  - Buccal branch of facial nerve
- Relationships:
  - Communicates with the parapharyngeal and masticator spaces posteriorly.
  - Communicates with the submandibular space inferiorly.[7,8]

Suprahyoid and Infrahyoid

Pharyngeal mucosal space

A deep compartment of the head and neck, located between the fascia of the pharyngeal constrictor muscles (visceral fascia) and the mucosal surface of the nasopharynx, oropharynx, and hypopharynx (Figs. 9 and 10).

- Borders:

- Posterior: Middle layer of the deep cervical fascia
- Superior: Skull base
- Inferior: Cricoid cartilage
- Lateral: Middle layer of the deep cervical fascia
- Contents:
  - Pharyngeal mucosa
  - Lymphoid tissue of Waldeyer's ring (tonsils and adenoids)
  - Minor salivary glands
  - Muscles (superior, middle, and inferior constrictor muscles, levator veli palatini muscle, and salpingopharyngeus muscle)[7,8]

Carotid Space

Defined by the carotid sheath, a connective tissue boundary in the neck, that is made by the superficial, middle, and deep layers of the deep cervical fascia. The carotid space extends from the jugular foramen at the skull base to the aortic arch at the thoracic inlet and is divided craniocaudally into the suprahyoid and infrahyoid regions.

Suprahyoid Carotid Space (Fig. 11)

- Borders:
  - Anterolateral: Parapharyngeal space, stylopharyngeus and digastric muscles (posterior belly)
  - Lateral: Parotid space
  - Posterior: Perivertebral space
  - Superior: Skull base at the jugular foramen

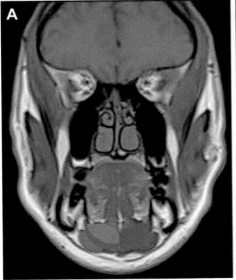
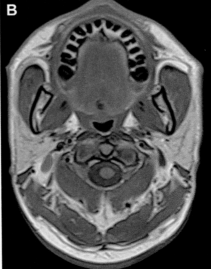

Fig. 9. Muscles of the suprahyoid neck. (A) Coronal T1-weighted image: mylohyoid (red), anterior belly of digastric (blue), geniohyoid (green) and (B) axial T1-weighted image: posterior belly of digastric (blue), stylohyoid (orange).

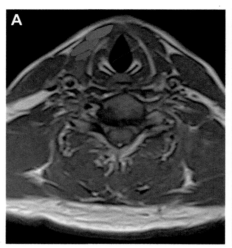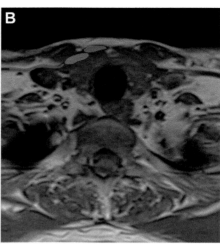

Fig. 10. Muscles of the infrahyoid neck. Axial T1-weighted images from superior to inferior: (A) anterior belly of omohyoid (red), sternohyoid (blue), thyrohyoid (purple) and (B) sternohyoid (blue), sternothyroid (green), posterior belly of omohyoid (red).

- ○ Medial: Retropharyngeal space
- Contents:
  - ○ Internal carotid artery
  - ○ Internal jugular vein
  - ○ Ansa cervicalis
  - ○ Glossopharyngeal nerve (CN IX)
  - ○ Spinal accessory nerve (CN XI)
  - ○ Hypoglossal nerve (CN XII)
  - ○ Sympathetic plexus
  - ○ Deep cervical lymph nodes (levels II and III)

Infrahyoid carotid space

- Borders:
  - ○ Anterolateral: Sternocleidomastoid muscle (inferiorly)
  - ○ Lateral:
  - ○ Posterior: Perivertebral space
  - ○ Superior: Skull base at the jugular foramen
  - ○ Inferior: Aortic arch
  - ○ Medial: Retropharyngeal space
- Contents:
  - ○ Common carotid artery
  - ○ Internal jugular vein
  - ○ Vagus nerve (CN X)
  - ○ Sympathetic nerves
  - ○ Deep cervical lymph nodes (level IV)
- Relationships:
  - ○ The suprahyoid carotid space is sometimes referred to as the poststyloid parapharyngeal space, owing to its location posterior to the styloid process.
  - ○ Within the carotid sheath, the glossopharyngeal nerve (CN IX) is the only nerve anterior to the vessels. From medial to lateral, the nerves that course posterior to the vessels within the

carotid sheath are the hypoglossal nerve (CNXII), sympathetic trunk, vagus nerve (CN X), and spinal accessory nerve (CNXI).[7,8]

Perivertebral Space

The perivertebral space is subdivided into two compartments, the prevertebral (anterior) and paraspinal (posterior) portions, by a deep slip of the deep cervical fascia which inserts onto the transverse processes.

Prevertebral compartment

- Borders:
  - ○ Anterior: Retropharyngeal and "danger" spaces
  - ○ Posterior: Deep fascia on transverse processes
  - ○ Superior: Skull base
  - ○ Inferior: Superior mediastinum
  - ○ Lateral: Posterior cervical space
- Contents:
  - ○ Vertebral bodies and intervertebral disc spaces
  - ○ Prevertebral muscles
  - ○ Scalene muscles
  - ○ Vertebral artery and vein/venous plexus
  - ○ Phrenic nerve
  - ○ Roots of the brachial plexus

Paraspinal compartment

- Borders:
  - ○ Anterior: Deep fascia on transverse processes
  - ○ Posterolateral: Posterior cervical space
  - ○ Superior: Skull base

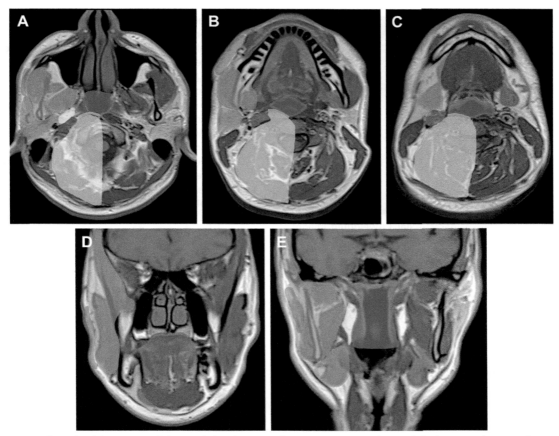

Fig. 11. Suprahyoid spaces. Axial T1-weighted images from superior to inferior: (*A*) pharyngeal mucosal space (pink), masticator space (orange), perivertebral space (gray), carotid space (red), parotid space (blue), parapharyngeal space (yellow), buccal space (purple), retropharyngeal space (aqua), (*B*) pharyngeal mucosal space (pink), masticator space (orange), perivertebral space (gray), carotid space (red), parotid space (blue), buccal space (purple), retropharyngeal space (aqua), submandibular space (green), sublingual space (brown), (*C*) pharyngeal mucosal space (pink), perivertebral space (gray), carotid space (red), retropharyngeal space (aqua), submandibular space (green), and coronal T1-weighted images from anterior to posterior: (*D*) masticator space (orange), buccal space (purple), submandibular space (green), sublingual space (brown), (*E*) pharyngeal mucosal space (pink), masticator space (orange), parotid space (blue), submandibular space (green).

- ○ Inferior: Superior mediastinum
- Contents:
  - ○ Posterior vertebral elements (neural arch)
  - ○ Paraspinal muscles[7,8]

Retropharyngeal space

- Borders:
  - ○ Anterior: Pharyngeal mucosal space
  - ○ Posterior: "Danger" space, prevertebral space
  - ○ Superior: Skull base
  - ○ Inferior: Superior mediastinum (the termination of the true retropharyngeal space (RPS) along the upper thoracic spine [T1–T6] is variable based on where the alar fascia joins and fuses with the visceral fascia)
  - ○ Lateral: Carotid space

- Contents:
  - ○ Areolar fat
  - ○ Retropharyngeal lymph nodes
  - ○ Small vessels
- Relationships:
  - ○ The alar fascia separates the retropharyngeal space (anterior), from the "danger" space (posterior). Infection from the oral cavity can spread down either side of the fascia into the mediastinum.[7,8]

Infrahyoid

Visceral space

- Borders:
  - ○ Anterior: Anterior strap muscles (Fig. 12)
  - ○ Posterior: Middle layer of the deep cervical fascia

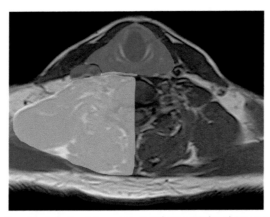

Fig. 12. Infrahyoid spaces. Axial T1-weighted image: visceral space (pink), perivertebral space (gray), carotid space (red), retropharyngeal space (aqua).

- o Superior: Hyoid bone
- o Inferior: Superior margin of the aortic arch/T4
- o Lateral: Carotid space
- Contents:
- o Thyroid gland
- o Parathyroid glands
- o Trachea
- o Esophagus
- o Larynx
- o Hypopharynx
- o Recurrent laryngeal nerve
- o Paraesophageal/paratracheal lymph nodes (level IV)[8]

Lymph nodes in the head and neck

Traditionally, lymph nodes have been divided into superficial and deep groups, relating to the superficial structures from which they drain, and the pattern of drainage. For the purposes imaging description, however, lymph nodes will be grouped into nodal stations and other non-nodal station nodes, a more useful anatomic classification for the head and neck radiologist.

Generally, a short axis diameter of less than 1 cm (or <1.5 cm for the jugulodigastric node) is considered non-pathologic, however, morphology, internal characteristics (preservation of fatty hilum or area of hypodensity), and capsular irregularities may be more important indicators of pathology.[9]

CERVICAL NODAL STATIONS

Level I: Submental (Ia) and submandibular (Ib) (Fig. 13).

- Borders (Ia):
- o Anterior: Platysma muscle
- o Posterior: Mylohyoid muscle
- o Superior: Mandibular symphysis
- o Inferior: Inferior border of the hyoid bone
- o Lateral: Anterior bellies of the digastric muscles
- Borders (Ib):
- o Anterior: Platysma muscle
- o Posterior: Posterior border of the submandibular gland
- o Superior: Mylohyoid muscle and mandible
- o Inferior: Inferior border of the hyoid bone
- o Medial: Anterior bellies of the digastric muscles
- Drainage (Ia):
- o Skin of the mental region, or chin, the mid-lower lip, the anterior portion of the oral tongue, and the floor of the mouth
- Drainage (Ib):
- o Efferent lymphatics from level Ia, the lower nasal cavity, the hard and soft palates, maxillary and mandibular alveolar ridges, skin and mucosa of the cheek, both upper and lower lips, the floor of the mouth, and the anterior oral tongue[9–11]

Level II: Upper jugular.

- Borders (IIa):
- o Anterior: Posterior border of the submandibular gland
- o Posterior: Posterior edge of the jugular vein (inseparable/no fat plane)
- o Superior: Insertion of the posterior belly of the digastric muscle into the mastoid process
- o Inferior: Inferior border of the hyoid bone
- o Medial: internal carotid artery and scalene muscles
- o Lateral: Medial margin of the sternocleidomastoid muscle
- Borders (IIb):
- o Anterior: Posterior border of the jugular vein (separated by fat plane)
- o Posterior: Posterior edge of the sternocleidomastoid muscle
- o Superior: Insertion of the posterior belly of the digastric muscle into the mastoid process
- o Inferior: Inferior border of the hyoid bone
- o Medial: Internal carotid artery and scalene muscles
- o Lateral: Medial margin of the sternocleidomastoid muscle
- Drainage:
- o Efferent lymphatics of the face, parotid gland, level Ia, level Ib, and retropharyngeal nodes. It receives direct drainage from the nasal cavity, the entire pharyngeal axis,

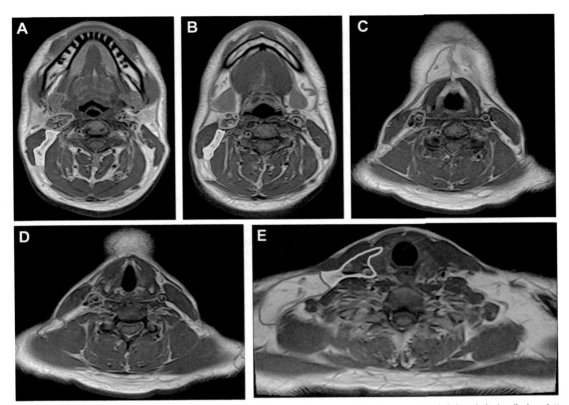

Fig. 13. Cervical nodal stations. Axial T1-weighted images from superior to inferior: (*A*) level Ib (red), level IIa (green), level IIb (yellow), level Va (orange), (*B*) level Ib (red), level IIa (green), level IIb (yellow), level Va (orange), (*C*) level Ia (blue), level VI (purple), level III (pink), level Va (orange), (*D*) level VI (purple), level III (pink), level Vb (brown), (*E*) level VI (purple), level IV (aqua), level Vb (brown).

larynx, external auditory canal, middle ear, and the sublingual and submandibular glands.[9–11]

Level III: Middle jugular

- Borders
  - Anterior: Anterior margin of the sternocleidomastoid muscle or posterior third of the thyrohyoid muscle
  - Posterior: Posterior margin of the sternocleidomastoid muscle
  - Superior: Inferior border of the hyoid bone
  - Inferior: Inferior border of the cricoid cartilage
  - Medial: Internal carotid artery and scalene muscles
  - Lateral: Medial margin of the sternocleidomastoid muscle
- Drainage:
  - Efferent lymphatics from levels II and V and partially from the retropharyngeal, pretracheal, and recurrent laryngeal nodes. It receives direct drainage from the base of the tongue, tonsils, larynx, hypopharynx, and thyroid gland[9–11]

Level IV: Lower jugular

- Borders
  - Anterior: Anterior margin of the sternocleidomastoid muscle
  - Posterolateral: Oblique line connecting the posterior border of the sternocleidomastoid muscle and the posterolateral border of the anterior scalene muscle
  - Superior: Inferior border of the cricoid cartilage
  - Inferior: Clavicle
  - Medial: Medial border of the common carotid artery
  - Lateral: Medial margin of the sternocleidomastoid muscle
- Drainage:
  - Efferent lymphatics from levels III and V and partially from the retropharyngeal, pretracheal, and recurrent laryngeal nodes. It receives direct drainage from the larynx, hypopharynx, esophagus, and thyroid gland.[9–11]

Level V: Posterior triangle

- Borders (Va):
  - Anterior: Posterior margin of the sternocleidomastoid muscle
  - Posteromedial: Levator scapulae
  - Superior: Skull base
  - Inferior: Inferior border of the cricoid cartilage
  - Lateral: Platysma muscle
- Borders (Vb):
  - Anteromedial: Posterior margin of the sternocleidomastoid muscle
  - Posteromedial: Levator scapulae and scalene muscles
  - Superior: Inferior border of the cricoid cartilage
  - Inferior: Clavicle
  - Lateral: Platysma muscle
- Drainage:
  - Efferent lymphatics from the occipital, retro-auricular, occipital, and parietal scalp nodes. It receives direct drainage from the skin of the lateral and posterior neck and shoulder, the nasopharynx, oropharynx, and thyroid gland.[9-11]

Level VI: Anterior compartment

- Borders
  - Anterior: Platysma muscle
  - Posterolateral: Prevertebral space
  - Posteromedial: Trachea
  - Superior: Inferior border of the hyoid bone
  - Inferior: Superior border of manubrium
- Drainage:
  - Skin of the lower face and anterior neck, efferent lymphatics from the anterior floor of the mouth, tip of the oral tongue, lower lip, thyroid gland, larynx, hypopharynx, and cervical esophagus[9-11]

Other Lymph Nodes

Premaxillary/infraorbital and buccinator

- Drainage: Mucous membranes of the nose and cheek, eyelids, and conjunctiva

Suboccipital

- Drainage: Occipital scalp

Parotid

- Contained by the parotid space, also includes peri-parotid nodes
- Drainage: Efferent lymphatics from the frontal and temporal skin/scalp, eyelids, conjunctivae, auricles, external acoustic meatus, tympanum, nasal cavities, the root of the nose, nasopharynx, and the eustachian tube

Retropharyngeal

- Contained by the retropharyngeal space
- Drainage: Efferent lymphatics from the nasopharynx, eustachian tube, and soft palate

Supracalvicular

- Drainage: Efferent lymphatics from the abdomen and chest[10]

CLINICS CARE POINTS

- Head and neck radiologists must understand complex and delicate anatomy to localize pathology and offer a reasonably short list of differential diagnoses. The complex anatomy of the head and neck is defined by many small muscles and fascia, which also serve as the landmark for dividing cervical lymph nodes into various zones/levels.
- For example, the posterior belly of the digastric muscle separates the carotid space from the parotid space; the mylohyoid muscle demarcates the floor of the mouth, which separates sublingual space from submandibular space. Anterior digastric muscle divides submental space from submandibular space.
- Understanding muscle innervation allows us to search for potential cranial nerve(s) that contribute to specific denervation changes. For example, in a case of vocal cord paralysis, radiologists need to search the entire cranial nerve pathway from the origin nucleus to the end organ and its course.

REFERENCES

1. Betts JG, Young KA, Wise HA, et al. Axial Muscles of the Head, Neck, and Back. In: Anatomy and physiology. Houston: OpenStax; 2013.
2. Saladin KS, Gan CA, Cushman HN. Muscles of the Head and Neck. In: Anatomy & physiology: The unity of form and function, 9th edition. McGrew Hill, New York. ISBM13: 978-1260256000, January 8, 2020. Available at: https://openstax.org/books/anatomy-and-physiology-2e/pages/11-3-axial-muscles-of-the-head-neck-and-back.
3. Westbrook KE, Nessel TA, Hohman MH, et al, Anatomy, head and neck, facial muscles.. In: StatPearls [Internet], 2021, StatPearls Publishing; Treasure Island (FL), Available at: https://www.ncbi.nlm.nih.gov/books/NBK493209/. Accessed December 2, 2021.

4.. Harnsberger HR, Glastonbury CM, Michel MA, et al. Diagnostic imaging: head and neck. Philadelphia: Lippincott Williams & Wilkins; 2010. 1931884781.

5. Harnsberger HR. Handbook of head and neck imaging. 2nd edition. St.Louis, MO: Mosby; 1995. p. 3–28.

6. Ferreli F, Mercante G, Spriano G. Levator claviculae muscle: anatomic variation found during neck dissection. Laryngoscope 2019;129(3):634–6.

7. Mukherji SK, Castillo M. A simplified approach to the spaces of the suprahyoid neck. Radiol Clin North Am 1998;36(5):761–80.

8. Aiken AH and Shatzkes DR. Approach to masses in head and neck spaces, In: Hodler J, Kubik-Huch RA, von Schulthess GK. Diseases of the brain, head and neck, spine 2020–2023: diagnostic imaging [internet], 2020, Springer; Cham (CH), Chapter 16. Available at: https://www.ncbi.nlm.nih.gov/books/NBK554341/. Accessed December 2, 2021.

9. Chong V. Cervical lymphadenopathy: what radiologists need to know. Cancer Imaging 2004;4(2):116–20.

10. Koroulakis A, Jamal Z and Agarwal M. Anatomy, head and neck, lymph nodes. In: StatPearls [Internet], 2021, StatPearls Publishing; Treasure Island (FL), Updated 2020 Dec 16 Available at: https://www.ncbi.nlm.nih.gov/books/NBK513317/. Accessed December 2, 2021.

11. Ishikawa M, Anzai Y. MR imaging of lymph nodes in the head and neck. Neuroimaging Clin N Am 2004; 14(4):679–94.

Root of the Neck and Extracranial Vessel Anatomy

Osama Raslan, MD[a], Tarik F. Massoud, MD, PhD[b],
Lotfi Hacein-Bey, MD, FASFNR[a],*

KEYWORDS

• Root of the neck • Arteries • Veins • Nerves • Lymphatics

KEY POINTS

- The root of the neck is an important anatomic area that harbors critical organs.
- Anatomy includes major vessels, nerves, spinal cord, muscles and lymphatics, the cervicothoracic junction, and the thyroid gland.
- Major functions (neurologic, respiratory, digestive, endocrine, immunologic) depend on the integrity of the root of the neck.

INTRODUCTION

The root of the neck is the crossroad between the thorax, the axilla, and the neck. It is bounded anteriorly by the manubrium sterni and the clavicles, laterally by the first ribs, and posteriorly by the body of the first thoracic vertebra (T1) (Fig. 1). The aim of this article is to discuss the radiological anatomy of this vital anatomic structure, highlighting the important muscles, vessels, nerves, and other associated structures.

MUSCLES

Scalenus Anterior

The scalenus anterior (ScA) arises from the anterior tubercles of the transverse processes of cervical vertebrae C3–C6 and inserts via a narrow flat tendon into the scalene tubercle and a ridge in front of the subclavian groove, both on the first rib (Fig. 2).[1] Together with the scalenus medius and posterior scalene muscles, the scalenus anterior muscle forms an important radiological landmark, the "interscalene triangle" with the subclavian artery and brachial plexus passing

through the triangle, and the subclavian vein passing anterior to the triangle, that is, the scalenus anterior muscle (Fig. 2; Fig. 3).[1]

Longus Colli Muscle

The longus colli muscle runs on the anterior surface of the vertebral column from C1 to T3 within the prevertebral space, posterior to the prevertebral layer of the deep cervical fascia and the retropharyngeal space.[2] It consists of the superior oblique, vertical, and inferior oblique portions, all which arise from the anterior tubercles of C3–C5, ventral bodies of C5–T3, and ventral bodies of the first 2 or 3 thoracic vertebra, respectively, and insert on the anterior arch of C1, ventral bodies of C2–C4 and anterior tubercles of the transvers process of C5–C6, respectively.[3–5]

The longus colli meets the scalenus anterior muscle to form the pyramidal colli scalene triangle, with its apex marking the C6 carotid tubercle, an important anatomic landmark for identifying the carotid artery, and its base is bounded inferiorly by the subclavian artery, with vertebral artery,

[a] Neuroradiology, Radiology Department, University of California Davis Medical School of Medicine, 4860 Y Street, Sacramento, CA 95817, USA; [b] Division of Neuroimaging and Neurointervention, Department of Radiology, Stanford University School of Medicine, Center for Academic Medicine, Radiology, MC: 5659, 453 Quarry Road, Palo Alto, CA 94304, USA
* Corresponding author.
E-mail address: lhaceinbey@yahoo.com

Neuroimag Clin N Am 32 (2022) 851–873
https://doi.org/10.1016/j.nic.2022.07.023

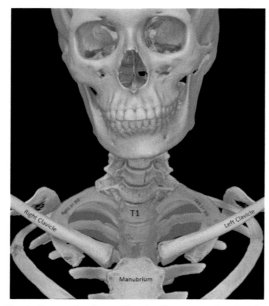

Fig. 1. Coronal volume illumination reconstructed image from CT of the neck showing the boundaries of the root of the neck between the manubrium sterni and clavicles anteriorly, first ribs laterally, and the first thoracic vertebra posteriorly (T1).

cervical sympathetic trunk and the stellate ganglion all lying within this pyramidal space (see Fig. 2; Fig. 4).

VASCULAR STRUCTURES
Subclavian Artery

The subclavian arteries are the main arterial supply to the root of neck. They also supply the occipital lobes, cerebellum, brain stem, upper extremities, and anterior and superior chest wall.[6,7]

Classic anatomy
The right subclavian artery arises as the most lateral terminal branch of the brachiocephalic trunk, while the left subclavian artery arises directly from the aortic arch. The arteries run laterally and superiorly in the superior thoracic outlet, deep to the clavicle and superior to the first rib, passing within the interscalene triangle, between the insertions of the scalenus anterior and medius muscles. The subclavian arteries exit the root of the neck at the lateral border of the first rib continuing as the axillary arteries (Fig. 5).

Variants

Left arch with aberrant right subclavian artery
This is the most common SCA anomaly with a reported incidence of 0.5% to 2.5%[8] where the aberrant right SCA arises as the most distal branch

of the left-sided aortic arch (Fig. 6). The artery will course to the right and in most cases will pass posterior to the esophagus (Fig. 6E, F). Infrequently, however, it may course between the trachea and esophagus or even anterior to the trachea.[9] It is typically seen incidentally on cross-sectional imaging or on an esophagogram as a characteristic persistent oblique indentation and narrowing of the dorsal esophagus frequently known as the "bayonet deformity" (see Fig. 6E, F). During femoral approach angiogram, the guidewire will frequently access the ARSA first as it is the first and lowest aortic branch, appearing as a brachiocephalic artery devoid of a common carotid branch. Also, frequently the right vertebral artery will arise from the proximal right common carotid artery instead of the right SCA (Fig. 6D).[10] Most cases are asymptomatic, however, rarely a patient might present with symptoms of esophageal compression termed "dysphagia lusoria" or tracheal compression.[11] Knowledge of this anomaly is also important in thyroid/parathyroid surgeries to avoid injury of the right recurrent laryngeal nerve, which is commonly nonrecurrent in these cases, and to avoid life threatening bleeding from accidental injury to the ARSA during esophagectomy.[12,13]

Left aortic arch with diverticulum of Kommerell
The diverticulum of Kommerell is a bulbous dilatation of the proximal aberrant right subclavian artery (Fig. 7). It may be asymptomatic, or present with tracheoesophageal compressive symptoms. Tracheal compressive symptoms are more prevalent in children, and esophageal symptoms are more common in adults. Rarely, a diverticulum of Kommerell may dissect or rupture.[14]

Right aortic arch with aberrant left subclavian artery with or without retroesophageal diverticulum
This is one of the most common supraaortic branching patterns of a right-sided aortic arch whereby the left common carotid artery arises first, followed by the right common carotid, right subclavian, and then the ALSA, which could arise with or without a diverticulum also called the Diverticulum of Kommerell. The ALSA is most commonly retroesophageal; however, in 15% of the cases it runs between the trachea and esophagus and in 5% it runs anterior to the trachea. Detecting a right-sided aorta with the corresponding tracheal indentation on a chest X-ray may be the first clue to the presence of ALSA (Fig. 8A). Cross-sectional imaging readily demonstrates an ALSA, its course, the presence of a diverticulum of Kommerell, as well as the mass effect on the esophagus or trachea (Fig. 8B,

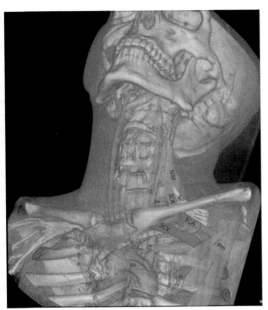

Fig. 2. CT volume rendered (VR) reconstruction of CT Neck demonstrating the main structures of the root of the neck. The interscalene triangle is formed between the scalenus anterior (ScA) and medius (ScM) muscles and the clavicle and contains the subclavian artery (SCA) and the brachial plexus (BP) with the subclavian vein running anterior to the ScA, outside the triangle. The colliscalene triangle lies between the ScA and the longus colli muscle (LC) muscles and SCA inferiorly with the vertebral artery (VA) vertebral artery, cervical sympathetic trunk, and the stellate ganglion all lying within this pyramidal space. Abbreviations: AA, Aortic arch; BP, brachial plexus; CCA, Common carotid artery; LC, Longus coli muscle; Pm, pictorials minor muscle; SCA, subclavian artery; ScA, Scalenus anterior muscle; ScM, Scalenus medius muscle; SVC, Subclavian vein; VA, vertebral artery. Note: the BP, ScA, ScM, LC, Pm, and SVC were diagrammatically added to the VR reformatted image for illustrative purposes.

C).[15,16] An oblique filling defect at the proximal esophagus coursing from right inferior to left superior is a characteristic finding of ALSA on a barium esophagram (Fig. 8D, E).

Right arch with the isolation of the left subclavian artery

This is the least common type of right-sided aortic arch occurring in approximately 0.8% of right-sided aortic arch variants for which the left SCA is not connected to the arch or to the common carotid artery, but rather, is tethered to the left pulmonary artery via a patent or occluded ductus arteriosus. The isolated left SCA is supplied by retrograde filling from the left vertebral artery, that is, creating congenital left subclavian steal phenomena.[17]

BRANCHES OF THE SUBCLAVIAN ARTERY

The subclavian artery branches are fraught with variations and scrutiny of the branches from different views is necessary to confirm the branching pattern. Generally, the subclavian artery is divided by the scalenus anterior muscle into 3 parts, with the first part from its origins to the medial border of the scalenus anterior muscle, the second part deep to the scalenus anterior muscle, and the third part from the lateral border of the scalenus anterior muscle to the lateral border of the 1st rib (Fig. 9).

The SCA branches can be remembered by the popular mnemonic "*VIT C and D*" (Figs. 10 and 11),[18] as follows:

Branches of the first part:
- Vertebral artery (VA): The VAs supply the cerebellum, brainstem, occipital lobes, and the spinal cord. The course of the VAs is divided into 4 parts. The first part (V1) or the preforaminal part extends from its origin from the subclavian artery up to its entrance into the C6 transverse foremen. This part normally arises as the 1st superior posterior branch of the left subclavian artery[19] and courses cranially and posteriorly through the base of the colliscalene triangle (see Figs. 2 and 4; Fig. 12) posterior to the common carotid artery, vertebral vein, as well as the thoracic duct on the left and the lymphatic duct on the right. The artery runs anterior to the ventral rami of C7 and C8 spinal nerves, C7 transverse process, and inferior cervical ganglion, and posterior and lateral to the middle cervical ganglion and inferior thyroid artery. This V1 segment gives off segmental cervical muscular and spinal branches. V2 is the foraminal segment from the transverse foramen of C6 to the transverse foramen of C2. V3 is the atlantic, extradural, or extraspinal segment, starting from C2, whereby the artery loops and turns lateral to ascend into the transverse foramen, then continues through C1 to pierce the dura. V4 is the intradural or intracranial segment.
  - Variants of V1 segment:
    - Variable origin: Single left, single right, and bilateral aberrant origins of the VAs have been described in detail by Yuan and colleagues[20] Left VA origin from the aortic arch is a common variant (incidence ~5%) (Fig. 13A, B). Other described vertebral artery origins include arising as the second (instead of the first) branch of the subclavian artery, arising

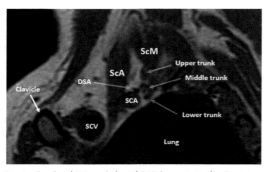

Fig. 3. Sagittal T1-weighted MR image at the interscalene triangle. The subclavian artery (SCA) contained in the interscalene triangle is used as a landmark to identify the triangle which lies between the scalenus anterior (ScA) and medius/posterior (ScM) muscles. The upper (C5–C6) (*arrow*) and middle (C7) (*arrow*) trunks of the brachial plexus pass superior to the SCA, in the superior part of the triangle, while the lower trunk (C8–T1) (*arrow*) passes posterior to the SCA in the lower part of the triangle. Note the subclavian vein (SCV) lies outside of the interscalene triangle in the prescalene space, separated from the SCA by the anterior scalene muscle. Also, note the dorsal scapular artery (DSA) (*arrow*) between the middle and lower trunks.

with a common origin with the thyrocervical trunk, and rarely arising from the common (see **Fig. 6**D), internal, or external carotid arteries.

- Variable orientation of the ostium: The VA is oriented cranially in ~47%, posteriorly in ~45%, caudally in ~5%, and anteriorly in ~3%.[21]
- Asymmetric VAs: Left dominant VAs are more common than right dominant, followed by codominant VAs.[22,23]
- Complete or partial duplication of the VA (**Fig. 13**C, D).

- Internal mammary artery (IMA) (internal thoracic artery): The IMA arises from the 1st part of the SCA and passes caudally, posterior to the subclavian vein and the first rib, and slightly lateral to the sternum, to supply the anterior chest and abdominal walls from the clavicle to the umbilicus, including the mammary tissue, the phrenic nerves, thymus, mediastinum, and pericardium. Knowledge of this branch and its variants is pivotal as the IMA is frequently harvested for coronary artery bypass grafting.[24]
  - Variants of IMA (20%):
    - The IMA can arise from the second (~7%) or third (~1%) parts of the SCA.[25]

- The IMA and thyrocervical trunk sharing a common origin from the SCA.
- The IMA arising from other SCA branches, for example, transverse cervical arteries, and subscapular arteries.[26]

- Thyrocervical trunk (TCT): The TCT most commonly arises as the second superiorly directed branch of the SCA at the inner border of the scalenus anterior muscle, just distal to the VA origin. It is very short and almost immediately divides into 4 branches:
- Inferior thyroid artery (ITA): It is the primary visceral artery of the neck, typically arising from the TCT, ascending just anterior to the medial border of the scalenus anterior muscle, and then arching medially at the C7 vertebral level to supply the inferior thyroid gland. It gives off several branches along its course to supply the adjacent muscles, esophagus, trachea, larynx, and thyroid and parathyroid glands. To avoid recurrent laryngeal nerve (RLN) iatrogenic injury during thyroidectomy, the ITA is used as an important landmark in identifying the RLN, which most commonly runs posterior to the ITA, less commonly anterior to the ITA, and least commonly between the ITA branches.[27,28]
  - Variants of ITA:
    - In their meta-analysis, Toni and colleagues, found that the ITA originated from the TCT, SCA, VA, and CCA in 90%, 10%, 0.6%, and 0.2% of cases, respectively[29]
    - When the ITA is absent or hypoplastic, it can be replaced by the *thyroidea ima artery* with variable origin from the BCT (most commonly), right CCA, aortic arch, IMA, CCA, or SCA.[30,31]
- Suprascapular artery (SSA): The SSA passes inferolaterally, anterior to the scalenus anterior muscle and phrenic nerve, and then the third part of the SCA and the brachial plexus, supplying the subclavius muscle and the inferior belly of the omohyoid muscle, then passing posteriorly above (~80%) or below (~20%) the superior transverse scapular ligament whereby it is occasionally accompanied by the suprascapular nerve, to end by contributing to the scapular anastomosis.[28] Its proximity to the suprascapular nerve has been implicated in suprascapular entrapment neuropathy.[32]
  - Variants of SSA:
    - Tountas and Bergman described the SSA arising from different parts of the SCA or the axillary artery with a median incidence of 10%.[33] Singh and

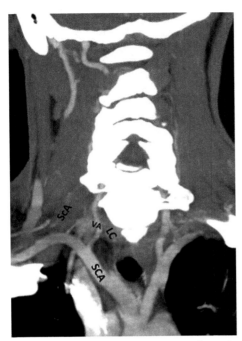

Fig. 4. Contrast-enhanced oblique coronal MIP CT images showing the pyramidal colliscalene triangle formed by the scalenus anterior muscle laterally (ScA), longus colli muscle medially (LC), and the subclavian artery (SCA) at the base, with the vertebral artery (VA) traversing the base of the pyramidal space. The cervical sympathetic trunk and the stellate ganglion also lie in this triangle.

colleagues, described the SSA arising from the first part of the AXA artery.[34] Overall, the SSA most commonly arises from the subclavian artery, but it may also arise from the internal thoracic artery (1%–5.1%), from the costocervical

trunk (1%), or from the dorsal scapular artery.[35,36]

- Ascending cervical artery (AsCA): The AsCA ascends on the prevertebral fascia medial to the phrenic nerve giving off multiple muscular and spinal branches. The ascending cervical artery also anastomoses with the vertebral, occipital, and ascending pharyngeal arteries, providing perfusion to the vertebral bodies, spinal cord, and meninges.[37] Munger and colleagues described the first case of catheterization of an anastomosis between an ascending cervical artery and the proximally occluded ipsilateral cervical vertebral artery to perform coil embolization of a ruptured basilar apex aneurysm.[38]

- Transverse cervical artery (TCA): after arising from the TCT, the TCA branches early into superficial and deep branches both of which run laterally and superficially across the scalenus anterior muscle and phrenic nerve, crossing, or passing through the brachial plexus trunk supplying their vasa nervorum. It branches into the superficial cervical artery, which runs adjacent to the spinal accessory nerve (CN XI). It also frequently branches into the dorsal scapular artery. The TCA may also arise directly from the 2nd or 3rd parts of the SCA.[39]

Branches of the 2nd part:

- Costocervical trunk: This arises from the posterior surface of the 2nd part of the SCA and passes cranially and posteriorly above the copula of the pleura dividing into its 2 terminal branches at the neck of the first rib.[40]
  ○ Supreme (superior) intercostal artery: This passes posteroinferiorly along the medial aspect of the thorax between the

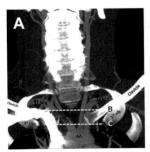
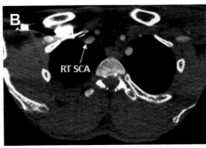
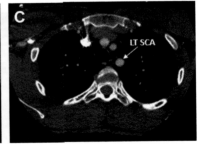

Fig. 5. CT Coronal oblique maximum intensity projection (MIP) (A) and axial (B, C) CT angiogram of the neck images showing the classic anatomy of the subclavian arteries (SCA) with the left SCA (LT SCA) arising at a lower level directly from the aortic arch (AA) (A, C) and the right SCA (RT SCA) arising at a higher level from the brachiocephalic trunk (BCT) (A, B). Both SCAs course superiorly and laterally posterior to the medial end of the clavicle and superior to the first ribs (A), passing through the interscalene triangle (Please see Figs. 2, 3, and 5), and terminating at the lateral borders of the 1st rib (A) as the axillary arteries (AXA). Note the horizontal dashed lines in Fig A delineate the levels of the axial images (B, C).

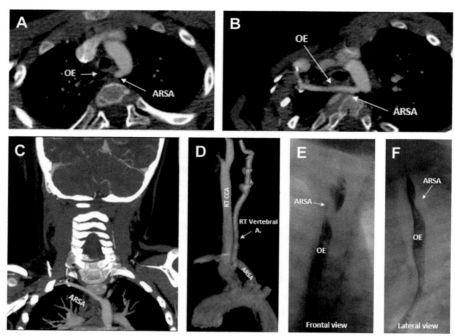

Fig. 6. CT Angiogram of the neck in axial (*A*), oblique axial (*B*), coronal oblique maximum intensity projection (MIP) (*C*), and volume rendered orientations (*D*) sowing an aberrant right subclavian artery (ARSA) arising as the most distal branch of the aortic arch and coursing to the right posterior to the esophagus. Note the right vertebral artery commonly arises from the common carotid artery instead of the right subclavian artery (*D*). Frontal (*E*) and lateral (*F*) barium esophagogram of a similar case showing the characteristic posterior indentation of the contrast-filled esophagus by the ARSA; frequently termed the bayonet deformity.

neck of the 1st 2 ribs and pleura dividing into 2 posterior intercostal arteries supplying the corresponding intercostal spaces. It may also arise from the thyrocervical trunk or any of its branches or even directly from the aorta.[41]

- o Deep cervical artery:

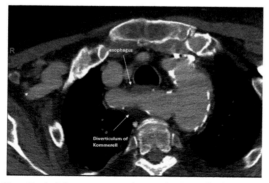

Fig. 7. Axial contrast-enhanced CT of the neck showing a left-sided aorta with a diverticulum of Kommerell of the proximal aberrant right subclavian artery passing posterior to the esophagus.

Passes posteriorly, above the 8th cervical nerve and between the C7 transverse process and the neck of the 1st rib whereby it passes cranially up to C2 vertebra between the semispinalis capitis and semispinalis cervicis to anastomose with the deep division of the descending branch of the occipital artery and branches of the VA. It supplies the adjacent cervical muscles and gives off a spinal twig that passes through the C7 intervertebral foramen to enter the spinal canal.[42]

Branches of the 3rd part:

- o Dorsal scapular artery (DSA). There is disagreement in the literature regarding the origin of the DSA, with variable citation describing an origin from the 3rd part of the SCA, branching off the thyrocervical trunk, branching off the transverse cervical artery, and less likely from the 2nd part of the SCA.[43–46] Occasionally 2 DSA arteries can be seen, arising from different origins.[43] The DSA passes posteriorly supplying the rhomboid and levator scapulae and terminates as part of the scapular arterial anastomosis.[47]

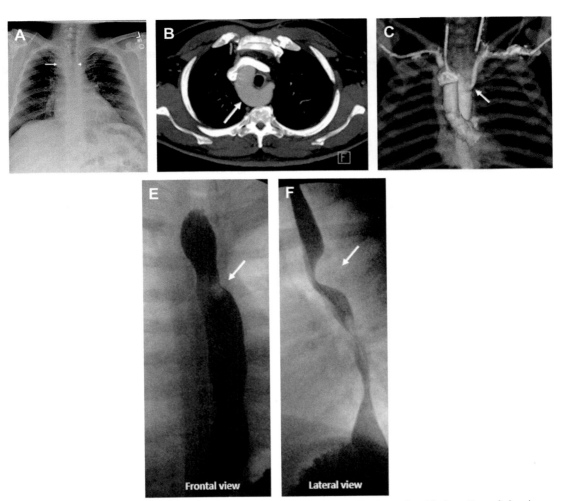

Fig. 8. Chest X-ray PA view (*A*) could be the first clue for the presence of a right-sided aortic arch by demonstrating the right aortic arch opacity (*arrow*) indenting the right aspect of the trachea and displacing it to the left (*arrowhead*). Axial maximum intensity projection (MIP) of CT angiogram of the neck (*B*) showing an ALSA arising from a retroesophageal diverticulum of Kommerell (*arrow*) without tracheal compression. Frontal volume rendered images (*C*) showing the right-sided aorta with the ALSA arising as the most distal of the arch branches. Frontal (*D*) and lateral (*E*) barium esophagogram of a similar case showing the characteristic oblique filling defect at proximal esophagus coursing from right inferior to left superior, with a large posterior indentation on the lateral view of the diverticulum of Kommerell.

There is also great variability in the relationship between the DSA and the brachial plexus; this is a clinically important relationship that could explain thoracic outlet syndrome and is important in performing surgery or nerve blocks in the posterior triangle. Verenna and colleagues reported the most typical DSA path as a subclavian artery origin before passing between upper and middle brachial plexus trunks (40% of DSAs), and less commonly between middle and lower trunks (23%), or inferior (4%) or superior to the plexus (1%). When the DSA branches from the TCT, the DSA tends to pass most frequently superior to the plexus (23%), less likely between the middle and lower trunks (6%), and least likely between the upper and middle trunks (4%).[43]

Finally, it is important to note that the 3 craniocaudally oriented longitudinal subclavian artery branches; the vertebral artery (VA), the ascending cervical artery (AsCA), and the deep cervical artery (DCA), together with their transversely oriented intercostal or cervical muscular branches, form a highly interconnected grid-like network (Fig. 14), which is pivotal in bypassing occlusions of any of

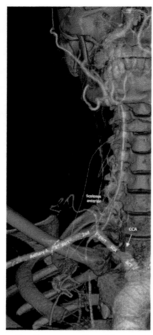

Fig. 9. Coronal volume rendered images of CT angiogram of the neck demonstrating the 3 parts of the right subclavian artery (SCA), with the first part from the SCA origin from the brachiocephalic trunk (BCT) to the medial border of the scalenus anterior muscle (green outline), 2nd part deep to the scalenus anterior muscle insertion into the first rib, and the third part from the lateral border of the scalenus anterior muscle to the lateral border of the 1st rib (*yellow curved dashed line*) at which the SCA continues as the axillary artery to the upper limb. The CCAs are segmented out of the image for clarity.

these 3 longitudinal oriented vessels, for example, occlusion of the VA is almost always reconstituted via the DCA.[48] Together with the occipital division of the external carotid artery, the network is also pivotal in bypassing common carotid artery occlusions via the occipito-carotid anastomoses.[49]

• Subclavian Vein (SCV):

The SCV is the proximal continuation of the axillary vein as it crosses the lateral border of the first rib. The vein then arches superiorly behind the medial end of the clavicle, and then caudally, receiving its only tributary, the external jugular vein at the lateral border of the scalenus anterior muscle. The vein continues to run medially anterior to the scalenus anterior muscle, separating it from the SCA, to join the IJV behind the sternoclavicular joint, forming the brachiocephalic vein. The SCV/IJV junction receives the thoracic duct on the left and the right lymphatic duct on the right. The most central venous valve lies at the lateral SCV,

thus medial to this valve the veins are considered central veins.[50]

The SCVs are readily visualized on cross-sectional imaging (Fig. 15) and can be visualized on ultrasound by inferior tilting of the transducer in the supraclavicular fossa.[51]

• Common carotid artery (CCA):

The left CCA arises directly from the aorta, while the right CCA arises as the medial terminal branch of the BCT. The arteries are contained in the carotid sheath/space, medial and slightly anterior to the internal jugular veins (Fig. 16), with the vagus trunk lying in the gap between the CCA and IJV posteriorly (Fig. 17). Both CCAs course superiorly in the neck posterior to the sternoclavicular joints and on both sides of the visceral space that contains the trachea, esophagus, and thyroid gland and more superiorly the larynx and pharynx.[52] The CCA arteries terminate by bifurcating into the external and internal carotid arteries, between the hyoid bone and the thyroid cartilage, usually at the C3/C4 level.[53] The CCA does not usually have any branches in the neck.

The CCAs are covered only by skin and superficial fascia at the carotid triangle bounded by the sternocleidomastoid, omohyoid, and posterior belly of digastric muscles, and covered by the omohyoid, sternohyoid, sternothyroid, sternocleidomastoid, and platysma elsewhere in the neck.

Variant Anatomy

• The left CCA and the brachiocephalic artery arise with a common origin from the aorta (~7.2–21.1%, so-called bovine arch) (Fig. 18).[54] It is mostly asymptomatic; however, awareness of the variant anatomy is important for the safe planning of surgical and vascular interventions in the neck. For example, some authors recommended using a transbrachial or transradial access instead of the transfemoral approach for carotid stenting of patients with this arch variant.[55,56]

• The LCCA arising from the BCT occurs in ~9% of cases and is referred to as "truncus bicaroticus," which is an inaccurate name as the right SCA also arises from the trunk. Awareness of this variant is important as it may be inadvertently injured during surgery (Fig. 19).

• Vertebral artery arising from the CCA (see Fig. 6): The incidence of anomalous origin of the right VA from the right CCA is 0.18%[57] and is invariably associated with an aberrant right subclavian artery. The Left VA arising from the left CCA is even rarer.[58] In both

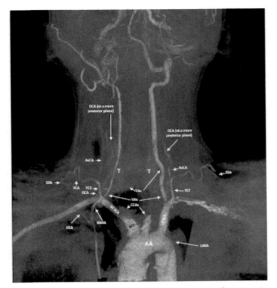

Fig. 10. Coronal volume rendered images of CT angiogram of the neck demonstrating the subclavian artery branches (A). The CCAs are segmented out of the image for clarity. On the right side, the RT SCA arises as the lateral terminal branch of the BCT. Branches of the 1st part of the SCA: The right VA arises as the first cranially directed branch (VAs), The RIMA arises as the 1st caudal branch of the SCA. the TCT arises as the 2nd cranially directed branch, dividing into the ITA branch which runs medially to supply the inferior thyroid gland, the AsCA which runs cranially, and the SSA and TCA arteries which generally run posteriorly and seen here arising from a common origin (normal variant known as cervicoscapular trunk). Branches of the 2nd part of the SCA: the costocervical trunk gives the DCA which passes posteriorly at first and then turns about the neck of the 1st rib to run caudocranially in the deep cervical musculature up to the C2 level. The 2nd branch of the costocervical trunk; the supreme (superior) intercostal artery is beyond the resolution of these reformats. Branches of the 3rd part of the SCA: The DSA most commonly arsis from the 3rd part of the SCA, but here it is seen arising as a branch of the RIMA (normal variant). On the left side, the LT SCA arsis directly from the aorta; only the left VA, LIMA, TCT, ITA, AsCA, DCA, and the SSA branches could be seen on this reformat. AA, Aortic arch; AsCA, ascending cervical artery; BCT, brachiocephalic trunk; CCA, common carotid artery; DCA, deep cervical artery; DSA, dorsal scapular artery; ITA, inferior thyroid artery; LIMA, left internal mammary artery; LT, left; RIMA, right internal mammary artery; RT, right; SCA, subclavian artery; SSA, suprascapular artery; TCA, transverse cervical artery; TCT, thyrocervical trunk; VA, vertebral artery.

cases, patients are usually asymptomatic; however, knowledge of this variant is important for preoperative surgical and endovascular planning and could potentially explain the

occurrence of posterior circulation insults with anterior circulation pathology.[10]

- Agenesis/Hypoplasia of the CCA:
A handful of CCA agenesis cases have been reported; in most patients, the ICA and ECA will form independently from the aortic arch or its branches, as the development of the CCA is from the third branchial arch, while the ECA and ICA develop from the first to third branchial arches. That said, there are case reports of CCA, ECA, and ICA agenesis. Mural calcification or arterial remnant with no contrast opacification is an important diagnostic clue differentiating congenital CCA agenesis versus acquired chronic occlusion.[59]

- Right common carotid gives rise to thyroidea ima artery (~7.5%). Often replacing the inferior thyroid artery in supplying the inferior aspect of the thyroid gland and trachea. Recognition of this variant is important to avoid damage during surgery (eg, thyroidectomy), as the artery could retract behind the sternum.[60,61]

- Internal jugular vein:

The IJV courses caudally in the carotid sheath as the continuation of the sigmoid sinus, posterolateral to the carotid arteries, and with the vagus nerve in between (see Fig. 17). At the root of the neck, it passes into the thorax posterior to the space between the 2 heads of the sternocleidomastoid muscle, anterior to the scalenus anterior muscle and pleura, to end by joining the subclavian vein to form the brachiocephalic vein.[62] The veins are often asymmetric in size (~80.5%).[62] Lim and colleagues, reported variable position of the IJV in relation to the CCA, with 85.2% of the IJVs found in the lateral position in relation to the CCA, 12.5% anteriorly, 1.1% medially and 1.1% posteriorly.[62] JV duplications and fenestrations are rare variants with reported prevalence of 0.4% to 3.3%.[63–65]

Nerves

Cervical sympathetic trunk

The cervical sympathetic trunk runs craniocaudally on both sides of the neck related to the prevertebral fascia and carotid sheath, with considerable variation in their reported locations. Two of the 3 interconnected cervical sympathetic ganglia lie at the root of the neck: the middle and the inferior (stellate) cervical ganglia.[66,67] The 3rd and most cranial of the cervical ganglia (superior cervical sympathetic ganglion) lies at the C2 level.

Familiarity and knowledge of the location of these ganglia is pivotal in avoiding surgical iatrogenic injury (eg, anterior approach spinal and

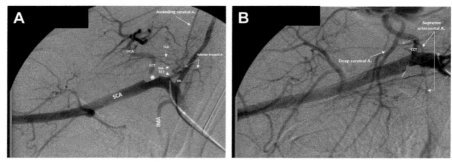

Fig. 11. Digital subtraction angiogram of the right subclavian artery (SCA) (*A, B*) showing branches of the first part of the SCA including the right vertebral artery (VA), internal mammary artery (IMA), and thyrocervical trunk (TCT). TCT branches into the inferior thyroid artery (ITA) coursing medially to supply the inferior thyroid gland, the suprascapular artery running laterally toward the superior scapula, the ascending cervical artery running cranially medial to the phrenic nerve, and the transverse cervical artery (TSA) coursing laterally. The 2nd part of the SCA gives the costocervical trunk (CCT) which typically branches into the supreme (*superior*) intercostal artery coursing inferiorly and the deep cervical artery passing posteriorly. Note a bullet fragment is lodged adjacent to the distal right subclavian artery (*). The Third part of the SCA typically gives origin to the dorsal scapular artery running posteriorly to supply the levator scapulae muscle and the rhomboid muscle.

thyroid gland surgeries), understanding the effects of trauma (eg, Horner's syndrome), guiding percutaneous nerve blocks[68] and avoiding misinterpretation as malignant lymph nodes, especially after radiation therapy for patients with head and neck cancer.[69] In addition to their location, suggested MRI criteria differentiating the cervical sympathetic ganglia from lymph nodes include spindle shape of the ganglia with tapering superior and/ or inferior poles on the craniocaudal axis and the central intraganglionic hypointense dot on axial T2-weighted and postcontrast T1-weighted

images.[70] Chaudhry and colleagues, were able to readily demonstrate the stellate ganglia in all 29 subjects who underwent high-resolution 3D-CISS MR imaging of the thoracic spine for reasons unrelated to sympathetic nervous system pathology.[71]

Middle cervical ganglion (MCG): The MCG is usually anterior to the longus colli muscle (LCM) and posterior to the carotid sheath at C3–C7 level. The MCG was reported mostly at the C6 level by Yinn and colleagues,[67] Civelek and colleagues and Shin and colleagues,[72,73] at the C6–C7 disc by Kiray and colleagues[74] and at the C3 and C4

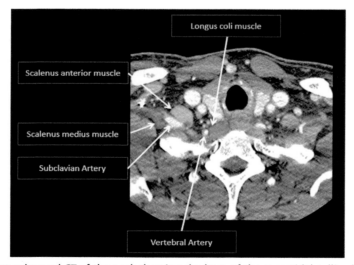

Fig. 12. Axial contrast-enhanced CT of the neck showing the base of the pyramidal colliscalene triangle formed between the scalenus anterior muscle (*shaded green*) and the longus colli muscle (*shaded red*), containing the vertebral artery. The subclavian artery forms the base of this pyramidal space, and it continues laterally with the brachial plexus (not shown) through the interscalene triangle bounded by the scalenus anterior and medius/posterior muscles (*shaded blue*).

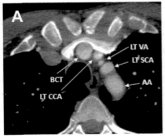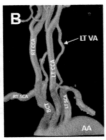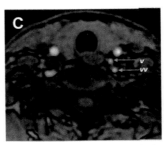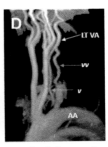

Fig. 13. CT angiogram of the neck in axial (A) and volume illumination rendering (B) showing the left vertebral artery arising directly from the aortic arch. Axial 3D TOF MRA of the neck (C) and coronal oblique maximum intensity projection (MIP) rendering of contrast-enhanced MRA of the neck showing partial duplication of the proximal left vertebral artery with the minor limb arising directly from the aorta (V) and the dominant limb arising from the left SCA (vv). AA, Aortic arch; BCT, brachiocephalic trunk; CCA, common carotid artery; LT, left; RT, right; SCA, subclavian artery; VA, vertebral artery.

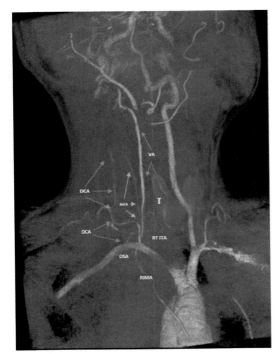

Fig. 14. Oblique coronal volume rendered images of CT angiogram of the neck. This orientation better demonstrates the DCA (gray arrows), and delineates the 3 craniocaudally oriented longitudinal subclavian artery branches; the vertebral artery (VA, green arrows), the ascending cervical artery (AsCA, orange arrows), and the deep cervical artery (DCA, gray arrows) which together with their transversely oriented intercostal or cervical muscular branches, form a highly interconnected grid-like network; playing a pivotal role in bypassing occlusions of any of these 3 longitudinal oriented vessels and in supplying the spinal cord. Abbreviations: AsCA, Ascending cervical artery; DCA, Deep cervical artery; ITA, inferior thyroid artery; RIMA, right internal mammary artery; RT, right; VA, vertebral artery.

levels by Ünsal and colleagues[70] A meta-analysis by Park and colleagues[75] found that the most typical site for the MCG was the lateral type, with the MCG located lateral and posterior to the common carotid artery (CCA) and anterior to the LCM, with variations including medial type, with the MCG located between the thyroid gland and the CCA, a double MCG, and MCG in the posterior wall of the carotid sheath.[75]

The MCG is also closely related to the inferior thyroid artery with the ganglion lying posterior (~25–75% of cases) or anterior to the artery, ultrasound evaluation of this relationship may minimize inadvertent arterial injury and hemorrhage during ganglion block.[75]

Inferior (stellate) cervical ganglion (Fig. 20): The first thoracic and the inferior cervical ganglion are fused in 80% of the cases forming the stellate ganglion, which is typically located anterior to the C7 transverse process or neck of the first rib, inferior to the subclavian artery, posterior or medial to the vertebral artery, lateral to the longus colli and medial to the superior intercostal artery.[71] Essentially all of the sympathetic innervations of the head, neck, and upper extremities relay in the stellate ganglion, and its damage has been implicated in multiple sympathetic nerve pathologies including reflex sympathetic dystrophy, Raynaud phenomenon, Horner's syndrome, and primary hyperhidrosis, among others.[76]

Phrenic Nerve

The paired phrenic nerves arise predominantly from the ventral ramus of C4 with contributions from the C3 and C5 ventral rami. The nerve descends anterior to the scalenus anterior muscle toward the thoracic inlet. On the left, the nerve crosses anterior to the left subclavian artery and posterior to the SCV and thoracic duct. It

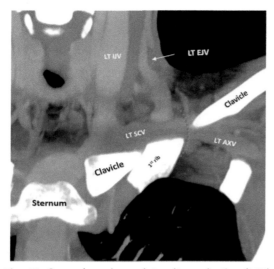

Fig. 15. Coronal maximum intensity projection (MIP) reformats of CT angiogram of the neck showing the left subclavian vein (SCV) arising as the continuation of the axillary vein (AXV) at the lateral border of the 1st rib (*red dashed line*). The SCV arches superiorly and then inferiorly posterior to the medial end of the clavicle, receiving its only tributary, the external jugular vein (EJV). It then joins the internal jugular vein posterior to the sternoclavicular joint to form the left brachiocephalic vein.

frequently passes anterior to the ITA origin, then descends along the lateral margin of the left SCA into the middle mediastinum. On the right, the phrenic nerve also enters the thorax sandwiched between the subclavian vein anteriorly and SCA posteriorly. It crosses from lateral to medial near the origin of the ITA descending into the middle mediastinum following the lateral margin of the brachiocephalic vein and superior vena cava.[42,77,78] In the thorax the nerves travel anteriorly along the anterior surface of the pericardium to reach the diaphragm, whereby they arborize on the superior and inferior surfaces of the diaphragm providing motor and sensory innervation to the diaphragm and the parietal pleura and peritoneum covering the diaphragm (**Fig. 21**).[79]

Variations in the phrenic nerve origin and course are common[80] as the nerve can descend anterior to the subclavian vein, or the phrenic nerve may arise entirely from the brachial plexus or receive branches from it. Cranial nerves XI or XII may also contribute branches to the phrenic nerve, or an accessory phrenic nerve may arise from roots C5 and C6 or from the nerve to the subclavius muscle.[78]

The phrenic nerve in the neck can be followed on MR neurography examinations aided by curved multiplanar maximum intensity projection reformates, as well as with ultrasound, as the nerve courses anterior to the scalenus anterior muscle.[81,82]

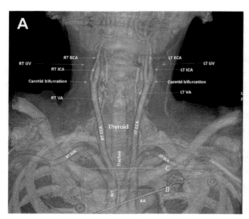
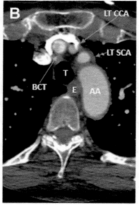
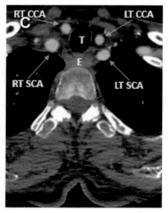

Fig. 16. Coronal volume render reformatted images from a CT angiogram of the neck (*A*) showing the classic origin of the left common carotid artery (LT CCA) directly from the aortic arch (AA), while the right common carotid artery (CCA) arises as the medial terminal branch of the brachiocephalic trunk (BCT). Both CCA ascend posterior to the sternoclavicular joint within the carotid sheath medial to the internal jugular veins (IJV) and on both sides of the visceral space containing the trachea, esophagus, and thyroid gland and more superiorly the larynx and pharynx. The CCA terminates approximately at C3/C4 level by dividing into the internal (ICA) and external carotid arteries (ECA). Axial CT angiogram of the neck at the level of the LT CCA origin from the aortic arch (*B*) and the right CCA from the BCT at a slightly higher level (*C*). Dashed lines on (*A*) show the location of the axial cuts.

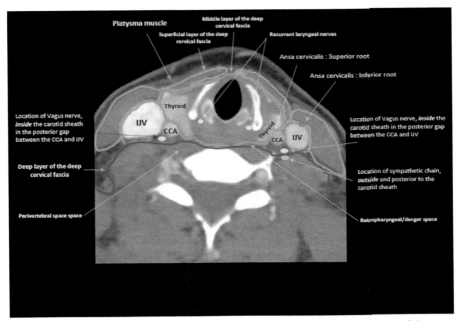

Fig. 17. Axial contrast-enhanced CT of the infrahyoid neck at the level of the lower border of the cricoid cartilage showing the common carotid arteries (CCA) ascending in the carotid sheath formed by the 3 layers of the deep cervical fascia (*red highlight on the left*). The CCA ascend medial to the internal jugular vein (IJV), with the vagus nerve (*yellow*) inside the carotid sheath in the posterior gap between the 2 vessels. The sympathetic trunk (*green*) also lies posterior but outside the carotid sheath. The superior and inferior roots of the ansa cervicalis are embedded in the anterior wall of carotid sheath (*light and dark pink, respectively*). Medially the CCA are related to the visceral space and its contents including the thyroid gland, larynx, and hypopharynx superiorly and trachea and esophagus inferiorly. Note the location of the recurrent laryngeal nerve at the cricothyroid joint.

Vagus Nerve

In the neck, the vagus nerves travel inferiorly in the carotid sheath posterolateral to the internal and common carotid arteries, to enter the thorax anterior to the aortic arch on the left and the SCA on the right (see Fig. 17). The right recurrent laryngeal nerve (RLN) branches off the vagus nerve and recurs at the cervicothoracic junction, passing posteriorly around the right SCA; while the left RLN recurs in the mediastinum passing posteriorly

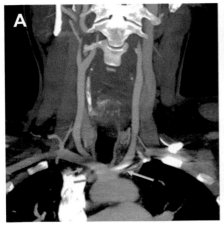
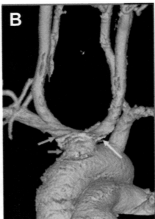
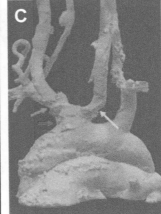

Fig. 18. Coronal MIP reconstruction (*A*), 3D volume rendering (*B*), and 3D STL Model (*C*) of CT Angiography of the neck showing the common origin (*red arrow*) of the brachiocephalic/innominate arterial trunk (*green arrow*) and left common carotid artery (*orange arrow*); a normal variant frequently named the "bovine arch" which is a misnomer.

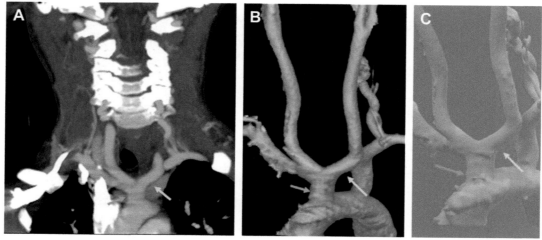

Fig. 19. Coronal MIP reconstruction (*A*), 3D volume rendering (*B*), and 3D STL Model (*C*) of CT angiography of the neck, showing the and left common carotid artery (*orange arrow*) arising from the brachiocephalic/innominate arterial trunk (*green arrow*) a normal variant frequently named the "truncus bicaroticus" which is a misnomer.

under the aorta at the aortopulmonary window. Both RLNs will then ascend through the root of the neck in the tracheoesophageal groove, posteromedial to thyroid lobe (see **Fig 17**) to enter the larynx at the level of the cricothyroid joint, providing motor supply to all laryngeal muscles except the cricothyroid muscle, and sensory supply to the intraglottic mucosa.[81]

Brachial Plexus

The interscalene segment of the brachial plexus lies at the root of the neck. The interscalene triangle could be readily identified on sagittal cross-sectional images of the root of the neck. The triangle is formed anteriorly by the anterior scalene muscle, posteriorly by the middle and posterior scalene muscles, which cannot be distinguished on imaging, and inferiorly by the first rib.[1,83,84]

The subclavian artery (SCA) traverses the lower part of the triangle and can be used as a landmark to identify the remainder of the relevant structures The upper (C5–C6) and middle (C7) trunks of the brachial plexus pass superior to the SCA, in the superior part of the triangle, while the lower trunk (C8–T1) passes posterior to the SCA in the lower part of the triangle. The dorsal scapular artery can be frequently seen between the middle and

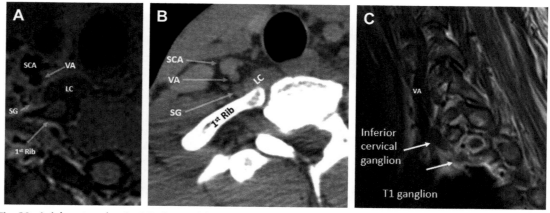

Fig. 20. Axial proton density MRI image (*A*) demonstrating how to locate the stellate ganglion (SG). At the C7–T1 level, the stellate ganglion (SG) is located just anterior to the neck of the first rib, lateral to the longus colli muscle (LC) and posterior to the vertebral artery (VA) as it is branching from the subclavian artery (SCA). Axial CT neck with contrast (*B*) of the same patient identifying the stellate ganglion (SG) using the same concept. Sagittal T2 WI of the cervical spine (*C*) in a different patient showing the inferior cervical ganglion just anterior to the neck of the first rib fused with the T1 ganglion to form the stellate ganglion just posterior to the VA origin.

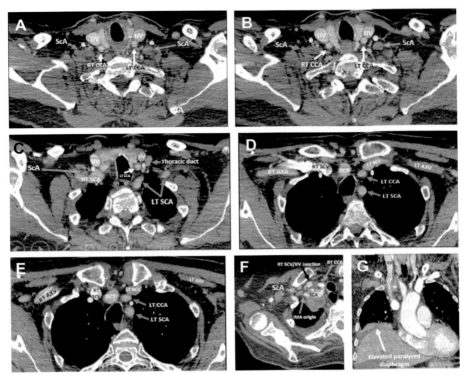

Fig. 21. Axial contrast-enhanced CT of the neck (*A–E*) showing the expected location of the phrenic nerves in the root of the neck region (yellow dots). Axial and contrast-enhanced CT of the chest (*F*) with coronal reformats (*G*), showing the involvement of the right phrenic nerve region posterior to the SCV and anterior to the SCA at the origin of the IMA by metastatic superior mediastinal lymph (*) node resulting in the elevated paralyzed right diaphragm. Level VII (superior mediastina) LNs lie at or below the manubrium, distinguishing this level from level VI LNs. Abbreviations: AXA, Axillary artery; AXV, Axillary vein; BCT, Brachiocephalic trunk; BCV, Brachiocephalic vein; CCA, Common carotid artery; IJV, Internal jugular vein; IMA, Internal mammary artery; LT, left; RT, right; SCA, subclavian artery; ScA, Scalenus anterior muscle; SVC, Subclavian vein; VA, vertebral artery.

the lower trunks.[85] The subclavian vein (SCV) lies outside of the interscalene triangle in the prescalene space, running anterior to the anterior scalene muscle, which separates it from the SCA (Figs. 22 and 23).[1,83,84]

Other Structures in the Root of the Neck

Thoracic duct and the right lymphatic duct

The lymphatic drainage of the right side of the head and neck, right arm, and right thorax gathers into the RLD, which terminates into the junction of the right internal jugular and right subclavian veins. The lymphatic drainage of the rest of the body drains via the left-sided TD into the junction of the left internal jugular and subclavian veins.[86]

The thoracic duct arises from the cisterna chyli entering the neck on the left side, passing posterior to the carotid sheath but anterior to the left SCA, phrenic nerve, and scalenus anterior muscle. At the root of the neck, the TD arches forwards and to the left, posterior to the carotid sheath, crossing

over the dome of the pleura and left SCA, terminating with a single trunk at the left SCV/IJV junction.[87]

For many decades, lymphography using lipiodol and lymphoscintigraphy were the sole methods to examine the thoracic duct, but these techniques had limitations, including patient discomfort, long examination time, invasive techniques, and technical difficulties. Recently, many studies have shown that both CT and MR imaging yielded the visualization of the cervical thoracic duct comparable to lymphography.[88]

On cross-sectional imaging, the TD and RLD can be visualized as continuous nonvenous, nonarterial vessels draining into the SCV/IJV junctions on both sides of the neck. Kammerer and colleagues classified the ducts into tubular, sacciform, or dendritic configurations based on duct morphology.[86] Seeger and colleagues, were also able to visualize the thoracic duct in 96% of their subjects using the high-resolution US with linear probes.[88]

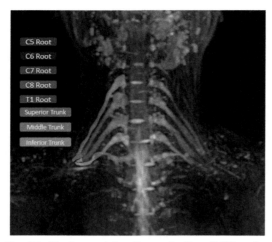

Fig. 22. Maximum intensity projection (MIP) reformats of coronal 3D T2-STIR-SPACE images of the brachial plexus (BP) demonstrating the C5–T1 nerve roots with the C5–C6 roots forming the superior trunk of the BP, the C7 root forming the middle trunk (can be used as a landmark as it is the only root that does not unite with another nerve root), and C8–T1 forming the inferior trunk.

Variant Anatomy

Typical thoracic duct anatomy described earlier is only present in 50% of the population. The duct empties on the right side in 2% to 3% of cases and bilaterally in up to 1.5% of cases. In over 95% of cases, the thoracic duct terminates in the internal jugular vein, the subclavian vein, or the angle between the 2 in 95% of the cases. In the remaining 5% the duct could terminate in the external jugular vein, vertebral vein, brachiocephalic vein, suprascapular vein, and transverse cervical vein. The thoracic duct terminates as a single vessel in up to 87.5%, bilateral ducts in up to 25%, or several terminal branches in up to 7% of the cases.[89]

Thyroid and Parathyroid glands

The thyroid gland is an endocrine gland that secretes 3 hormones: the 2 thyroid hormones triiodothyronine (T3) and thyroxine (T4) that influence metabolic rate and protein synthesis, and in children, growth, and development; and the peptide hormone calcitonin that plays a role in calcium homeostasis.

In adults, the normal thyroid gland is about 5 cm in greatest cranio-caudad dimension. It lies immediately caudad to the larynx, encircling the anterolateral portion of the trachea, and bordered by the trachea and esophagus medially and the carotid sheath laterally. The sternocleidomastoid muscle and the 3 strap muscles (sternohyoid, sternothyroid, and the superior belly of the omohyoid) border the gland anteriorly and laterally. The outer layer of its fibrous capsule is continuous with the pretracheal fascia, attaching the gland to the cricoid and thyroid cartilages by a posterior suspensory ligament of the thyroid gland. Hence, the thyroid moves up and down with the movement of these cartilages during swallowing.[90]

There are many anatomic variations in the basic butterfly-like shape of the thyroid gland. It has 2 lobes, with superior and inferior poles, and is connected by the thyroid isthmus. The thyroid lobes can be flat or globular but always have a three-dimensional shape as they curve around the trachea posteriorly. The isthmus is a narrow band of thyroid tissue overlying the second and third tracheal rings and connecting the 2 thyroid lobes. The thyroid isthmus can be wide, long, or absent. It may also have a pyramidal lobe that extends superiorly to the midthyroid cartilage (but can reach the level of the hyoid bone) and laterally to the common carotid arteries. It is found in 55% of individuals and in men more than women. The pyramidal lobe can be long, short and stumpy, bifid, or absent. A bifid lobe occurs as paired structures just to the right and left of the midline. A fibrous tract,

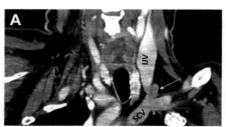
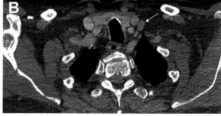

Fig. 23. Contrast-enhanced CT of the neck in the coronal (*A*) and axial planes (*B*), showing a tubular cystic structure posterior to the carotid sheath terminating with a single trunk at the left subclavian vain (SCV)/Internal jugular vein (IJV) junction consistent with the thoracic duct (*arrows*).

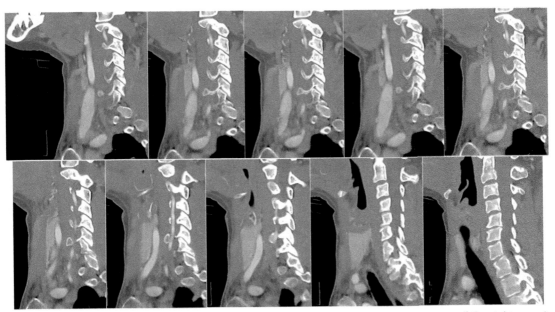

Fig. 24. Contiguous sagittal 2 mm slices from a CT angiogram of the neck to show the course of the right superior thyroid artery (*red arrow*) from its origin as the first branch of the external carotid artery (*top left panel of upper row*) sequentially to the right panel, then from the left panel of the lower row sequentially to the right panel whereby the artery merges with the right superior pole of the thyroid gland.

the obliterated thyroglossal duct, can extend from the pyramidal lobe to the hyoid bone and may harbor a thyroglossal duct cyst.[90,91] The tubercle of Zuckerkandl is a pyramidal extension of the thyroid gland located on the posterior aspect of each thyroid lobe.[92] The recurrent laryngeal nerve usually traverses the posterior aspect of the tubercle, which can help to find and identify the nerve during surgery.

Abnormalities in development during embryogenesis may result in ectopic thyroid tissue. A lingual thyroid tissue along the path of the thyroglossal duct is the most common site of thyroid ectopy. Ectopic tissue may also be present in the superior mediastinum/thymus. Rarely, thyroid tissue may be found in the lateral cervical lymph nodes (lateral aberrant thyroid)[90]

The arterial blood supply to the thyroid gland is primarily from the right and left superior (Fig. 24) and inferior (Fig. 25) thyroid arteries, derived from the external carotid arteries and thyrocervical trunk, respectively. In addition to supplying the thyroid, the superior thyroid artery is the primary blood supply to approximately 15% of superior parathyroid glands. The inferior thyroid artery also supplies the inferior parathyroid glands and approximately 85% of superior parathyroid glands. A thyroidea ima artery is found in approximately 3% of individuals and arises from the aortic

arch or innominate artery and courses to the inferior portion of the isthmus or inferior thyroid poles. The thyroidea ima artery can enlarge in patients with thyroid goiters or hyperthyroidism. The venous drainage consists of the superior, middle, and inferior (Fig. 26) thyroid veins that drain into the internal jugular vein and innominate vein.[90]

The right and left superior laryngeal nerves originate from the right and left vagus nerves as they exit the base of the skull. The superior laryngeal nerve courses with the superior thyroid artery until approximately 1 cm before the artery enters the capsule of the superior pole of the thyroid. The superior laryngeal nerve consists of 2 primary branches: The external branch is primarily motor in function, innervating the inferior constrictor and cricothyroid muscles. A few smaller branches may be seen entering the superior thyroid. The internal branch of the superior laryngeal nerve is sensory to the larynx, entering the larynx through the thyrohyoid membrane superior to the external branch.

The parathyroid gland produces and secretes parathyroid hormone in response to low blood calcium, thus playing a key role in the regulation of blood and bone calcium levels. The parathyroid glands are usually 2 pairs of superior and inferior glands, usually closely positioned behind the left and right lobes of the thyroid gland underneath

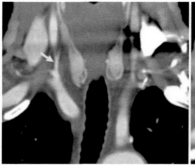
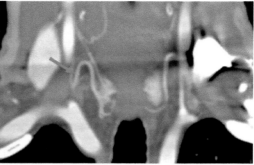

Fig. 25. Contiguous coronal 2 mm slices from a CT angiogram of the neck to show the course of the right inferior thyroid artery from its origin off the thyrocervical trunk (*yellow arrow*) in the left panel and more anteriorly to the right panel, showing the artery (*red arrow*) and its characteristic medial loop before merging with the right midpolar segment of the thyroid gland. A similar loop of the left inferior thyroid artery can be seen in the contralateral thyroid midpole.

the superficial thyroid fascia. The anatomic distribution of the glands is quite constant, with bilateral symmetry found in approximately 80% of cases. Each normal gland is about 6 mm long, 3 to 4 mm wide, and 1 to 2 mm anteroposteriorly. The normal glands are not visible on imaging. They are derived from the third and fourth pharyngeal pouches, with the superior glands arising from the fourth pouch and the inferior glands arising from the higher third pouch. Each parathyroid gland usually has its own end-artery.[93,94]

The parathyroid glands are variable in number: in 84% of individuals, there are 4 glands, in 13% there are supernumerary glands, and in 3% there are only 3 glands. Rarely, the parathyroid glands may be within the thyroid gland itself, the chest, or even the thymus. Indeed, a supernumerary

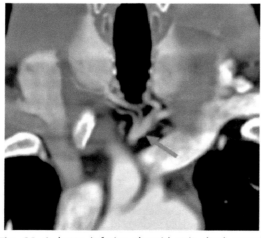

Fig. 26. A large inferior thyroid vein (*red arrow*) drains toward the right brachiocephalic vein.

gland is most often a fifth gland found in the thymus. Sometimes the lower parathyroid glands are situated higher up in the neck because of a failure of descent during embryologic development. These undescended or ectopic glands can be parapharyngeal, retropharyngeal, or retrotracheal within the middle cervical/mediastinal compartment. Enlarged parathyroid glands can also travel down the tracheoesophageal groove or the retropharyngeal space into the chest.[93,94]

Lymphatic Drainage

The following lymph node (LN) groups are related to the root of the neck (Figs. 27 and 28):

i. Level IV (low internal jugular chain, infracricoid) LNs: This group includes the low IJV and the prescalene LN groups. The level IV group starts superiorly at the lower border of the cricoid cartilage, distinguishing it from the level III group. It continues inferiorly along the IJV down to the level of the clavicle and is distinguished laterally from the level V LN group by laying anterior to an oblique line connecting the posterior border of the sternocleidomastoid muscle to the lateral posterior edge of the anterior scalene muscle. If this line transects an LN it is considered level IV if most of the nodal cross-sectional area lies anterior to this line. It is also distinguished medially from the level VI LN by being lateral to the medial margin of the CCA.[95]

ii. Level VB (posterior cervical space, transverse cervical) LNs: The VB level starts superiorly at the lower margin of the cricoid cartilage distinguishing it from the level VA LN group. This group extends inferiorly in the posterior triangle of the neck down to the level of the clavicle,

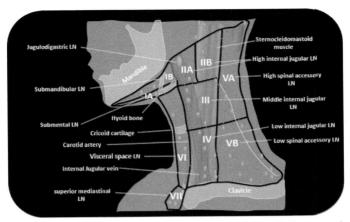

Fig. 27. Diagrammatic representation of the locations of the lymph node (LN) groups in the neck. The lower border of the hyoid bone separates level II (*above*) from level III IJV groups. The lower border of the cricoid carti-lage separates the level III (*above*) from level IV (*below*), and level VA (*above*) from VB (*below*). Level VI runs in the midline from the hyoid bone above to the clavicle below, medial to the medial border of the ICA/CCA. A line along the manubrium separates level VI (*above*) from level VII (*below*).

distinguished from the level IV group medially, by lying posterior to an oblique line connecting the posterior border of the sternocleidomas-toid muscle to the lateral posterior edge of the anterior scalene muscle. If this line tran-sects an LN it is considered level V if most of the nodal cross-sectional area lies posterior to this line. Laterally, it is distinguished from the supraclavicular nodes by lying above the level of the clavicle as seen on axial images.[95]

iii. Level VI (visceral) LNs. These include the prel-aryngeal, pretracheal, and paratracheal sub-groups. This group runs in the midline between the medial margins of the CCA/ICA, extending from the lower margin of hyoid bone superiorly to top of manubrium inferiorly.

It is distinguished from level IV LNs by lying medial to the medial margin of CCA/ICA.[95]

iv. Level VII (superior mediastinal) LNs. These lie caudal to the top of the manubrium, separating it from level VI LNs. They extend in the superior mediastinum between carotid arteries down to the top of the BCV.[95]

v. Supraclavicular nodes LN (ie, Virchow lymph node if enlarged on the left): Found in the supraclavicular fossa, lateral to the medial margin of the common carotid artery. To differ-entiate the supraclavicular LNs from the level IV/V group, if an LN lies at or below a portion of the clavicle as visualized on axial images it is considered a supraclavicular LN.[95]

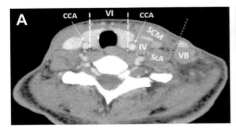
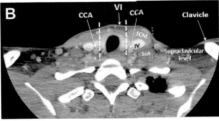

Fig. 28. Axial contrast-enhanced CT of the neck below the level of the lower border of the cricoid cartilage showing the lymph node levels at the root of the neck. In Fig A, an oblique line is drawn along posterior border of sternocleidomastoid (SCM) & posterolateral border of anterior scalene muscle (ScA) (*red dotted line*), sepa-rating the level IV and level V LNs which lie anterior and posterior to this line, respectively. A vertical line drawn along the medial border of the CCA (*white dashed line*) would separate the level IV (*lateral to this line*) from the level VI LNs (*medial to this line*). In Fig. B, when a segment of the clavicle is seen on axial images, LNs at this loca-tion are considered supraclavicular LNs (as opposed to level VB). Level VII (superior mediastina) LNs lie at or below the manubrium, distinguishing this level from level VI LNs (Please see Fig. 26).

CLINICS CARE POINTS

- The root of the neck, also defined as the thoracic outlet, is an important anatomic structure as it connects the thorax to the neck and the upper limbs, therefore, impacting a number of critical bodily systems.

- Familiarity with the anatomy of the root of the neck is crucial for neuroradiologists regardless of their area of interest within the subspecialty, whether neurologic, vascular, oncologic, functional, and so forth.

- Perhaps more than for any other anatomic areas of the human body, proper recognition of normal and abnormal muscles, nerves, bones, blood vessels, lymph nodes, and knowledge of major embryologic variations are key.

DISCLOSURE

The authors have no disclosures to declare in relation to this article.

REFERENCES

1. Demondion X, Herbinet P, Van Sint Jan S, et al. Imaging assessment of thoracic outlet syndrome. Radiographics 2006;26(6):1735–50. https://doi.org/10.1148/rg.266055079.

2. Kanzaria H, Stein JC. A severe sore throat in a middle-aged man: calcific tendonitis of the longus colli tendon. J Emerg Med 2011;41(2):151–3. https://doi.org/10.1016/j.jemermed.2008.01.016.

3. McDavid LJ, Khan YS. Anatomy, head and neck, prevertebral muscles. . In: StatPearls [Internet]. Treasure Island (FL): StatPearls Publishing; 2021.

4. Boardman J, Kanal E, Aldred P, et al. Frequency of acute longus colli tendinitis on CT examinations. Emerg Radiol 2017;24(6):645–51. https://doi.org/10.1007/s10140-017-1537-z.

5. Mayoux-Benhamou MA, Revel M, Vallée C, et al. Longus colli has a postural function on cervical curvature. Surg Radiol Anat 1994;16(4):367–71. https://doi.org/10.1007/BF01627655.

6. Ochoa VM, Yeghiazarians Y. Subclavian artery stenosis: a review for the vascular medicine practitioner. Vasc Med 2011;16(1):29–34. https://doi.org/10.1177/1358863X10384174.

7. Jones J, Hacking C. Subclavian artery. Reference article. Radiopaedia.org. 2021. https://doi.org/10.53347/rID-24579. Accessed 26 November, 2021.

8. Myers PO, Fasel JH, Kalangos A, et al. Arteria lusoria: developmental anatomy, clinical, radiological and surgical aspects. Ann Cardiol Angeiol (Paris) 2010;59(3):147–54. https://doi.org/10.1016/j.ancard.2009.07.008.

9. Epstein DA, Debord JR. Abnormalities associated with aberrant right subclavian arteries-a case report. Vasc Endovascular Surg 2002;36(4):297–303. https://doi.org/10.1177/153857440203600408.

10. Ali A, Sedora Roman NI, Cox M, et al. Anomalous Origin of the Right Vertebral Artery from the Right Common Carotid Artery. Cureus 2018;10(11):e3602. https://doi.org/10.7759/cureus.3602.

11. Donnelly LF, Fleck RJ, Pacharn P, et al. Aberrant subclavian arteries: cross-sectional imaging findings in infants and children referred for evaluation of extrinsic airway compression. AJR Am J Roentgenol 2002;178(5):1269–74. https://doi.org/10.2214/ajr.178.5.1781269.

12. Amini B, Sheikh Y. Aberrant right subclavian artery. Reference article, Radiopaedia.org. 2021. https://doi.org/10.53347/rID-831. Accessed on 29 Nov 2021.

13. Mahmodlou R, Sepehrvand N, Hatami S. Aberrant Right Subclavian Artery: A Life-threatening Anomaly that should be considered during Esophagectomy. J Surg Tech Case Rep 2014;6(2):61–3. https://doi.org/10.4103/2006-8808.147262.

14. Fisher RG, Whigham CJ, Trinh C. Diverticula of Kommerell and aberrant subclavian arteries complicated by aneurysms. Cardiovasc Intervent Radiol 2005;28(5):553–60. https://doi.org/10.1007/s00270-003-0229-0.

15. Cinà CS, Althani H, Pasenau J, et al. Kommerell's diverticulum and right-sided aortic arch: a cohort study and review of the literature. J Vasc Surg 2004;39(1):131–9. https://doi.org/10.1016/j.jvs.2003.07.021.

16. Chai OH, Han EH, Kim HT, et al. Right-sided aortic arch with the retroesophageal left subclavian artery as the fourth branch. Anat Cell Biol 2013;46(2):167–70. https://doi.org/10.5115/acb.2013.46.2.167.

17. Luetmer PH, Miller GM. Right aortic arch with isolation of the left subclavian artery: case report and review of the literature. Mayo Clin Proc 1990;65(3):407–13. https://doi.org/10.1016/s0025-6196(12)62540-3.

18. Panakkal BJ, Rajesh GN, Parakkal HB, et al. Saje18 - ev CG. Bilateral variant origin of subclavian artery branches. BJR Case Rep 2016;2(3):20150429. https://doi.org/10.1259/bjrcr.20150429.

19. Satti SR, Cerniglia CA, Koenigsberg RA. Cervical vertebral artery variations: an anatomic study. AJNR Am J Neuroradiol 2007;28(5):976–80.

20. Yuan SM. Aberrant Origin of Vertebral Artery and its Clinical Implications. Braz J Cardiovasc Surg 2016;31(1):52–9. https://doi.org/10.5935/1678-9741.20150071.

21. Ranganatha Sastry V, Manjunath K. The course of the V1 segment of the vertebral artery. Ann Indian Acad Neurol 2006;9(4):223–6.

22. Kalia J, Hussain S, Wolfe T, et al. Prevalence of co-dominance in vertebral arteries: A CT angiographic assessment. J NeuroInterventional Surg 2009;1:98.

23. Turan-Ozdemir S, Yıldız C, Cankur NS. Evaluation of vertebral artery system in a healthy population by using colour duplex Doppler ultrasonography. (in Turkish). Uludag Univ Tıp Fak Derg 2002;28:95–9.

24. Schmitto JD, Rajab TK, Cohn LH. Prevalence and variability of internal mammary graft use in contemporary multivessel coronary artery bypass graft. Curr Opin Cardiol 2010;25(6):609–12. https://doi.org/10.1097/HCO.0b013e32833f0498.

25. Paraskevas G, Natsis K, Tzika M, et al. Abnormal origin of internal thoracic artery from the thyrocervical trunk: surgical considerations. J Cardiothorac Surg 2012;7:63. https://doi.org/10.1186/1749-8090-7-63.

26. Andreou AY, Iakovou I, Vasiliadis I, et al. Aberrant left internal thoracic artery origin from the extrascalenic part of the subclavian artery. Exp Clin Cardiol 2011;16(2):62–4.

27. Noussios G, Chatzis I, Konstantinidis S, et al. The Anatomical Relationship of Inferior Thyroid Artery and Recurrent Laryngeal Nerve: A Review of the Literature and Its Clinical Importance. J Clin Med Res 2020;12(10):640–6. https://doi.org/10.14740/jocmr4296.

28. Hacking C, MacManus D. Thyrocervical trunk. Radiopaedia.org. 2021. Available at: https://doi.org/10.53347/rID-49096. Accessed 02 December, 2021.

29. Toni R, Casa CD, Castorina S, et al. A meta-analysis of inferior thyroid artery variations in different human ethnic groups and their clinical implications. Ann Anat 2005;187(4):371–85. https://doi.org/10.1016/j.aanat.2005.04.004.

30. Krudy AG, Doppman JL, Brennan MF. The significance of the thyroidea ima artery in arteriographic localization of parathyroid adenomas. Radiology 1980;136(1):45–51. https://doi.org/10.1148/radiology.136.1.7384523.

31. Yurasakpong L, Nantasenamat C, Janta S, et al. The decreasing prevalence of the thyroid ima artery: A systematic review and machine learning assisted meta-analysis. Ann Anat 2022;239:151803. https://doi.org/10.1016/j.aanat.2021.151803.

32. Naidoo N, Lazarus L, De Gama BZ, et al. The variant course of the suprascapular artery. Folia Morphol (Warsz) 2014;73(2):206–9. https://doi.org/10.5603/FM.2014.0030.

33. Tountas C, Bergman R. Arteries. In: Tountas C, Bergman R, editors. Anatomic variations of the upper extremity. Churchill Livingstone; 1993. p. 190–2. chap Churchill Livingstone.

34. Singh R. Variations in the origin and course of the suprascapular artery: case report and literature review. J Vasc Bras 2018;17(1):61–5. https://doi.org/10.1590/1677-5449.008117.

35. Lippert H, Reinhard P. Arterial variations in man: classification and frequency. Springer Verlag; 1985.

36. Saadeh FA. The suprascapular artery: case report of an unusual origin. Anat Anz 1979;145(1):83–6.

37. Karsonovich TW, Hawkins JC, Gordhan A. Traumatic Pseudoaneurysm of the Ascending Cervical Artery Treated with N-butyl Cyanoacrylate Embolization: A Case Report and Review of the Literature. Cureus 2019;11(12):e6276. https://doi.org/10.7759/cureus.6276.

38. Munger D, O'Neill B, Priest R. Embolization of Basilar Tip Aneurysm via Ascending Cervical Artery. World Neurosurg 2020;140:262–6. https://doi.org/10.1016/j.wneu.2020.04.163.

39. Tessler O, Gilardino MS, Bartow MJ, et al. Transverse Cervical Artery: Consistent Anatomical Landmarks and Clinical Experience with Its Use as a Recipient Artery in Complex Head and Neck Reconstruction. Plast Reconstr Surg 2017;139(3):745e–51e. https://doi.org/10.1097/PRS.0000000000003085.

40. Alabduladhem T, Lasrado S. Costocervical trunk arteries. StatPearls [Internet]. StatPearls Publishing; 2021. chap Anatomy, Head and Neck.

41. Granger C, Martin A. Superior intercostal arteries. StatPearls [Internet]. StatPearls Publishing; 2021. chap Anatomy.

42. Standring S. Gray's anatomy: the anatomical basis of clinical practice. Elsevier Limited; 2016.

43. Verenna AA, Alexandru D, Karimi A, et al. Dorsal Scapular Artery Variations and Relationship to the Brachial Plexus, and a Related Thoracic Outlet Syndrome Case. J Brachial Plex Peripher Nerve Inj 2016;11(1):e21–8. https://doi.org/10.1055/s-0036-1583756.

44. Huelke DF. A study of the transverse cervical and dorsal scapular arteries. Anat Rec 1958;132(3):233–45. https://doi.org/10.1002/ar.1091320302.

45. Chaijaroonkhanarak W, Kunatippapong N, Ratanasuwan S, et al. Origin of the dorsal scapular artery and its relation to the brachial plexus in Thais. Anat Sci Int 2014;89(2):65–70. https://doi.org/10.1007/s12565-013-0200-3.

46. Read WT, Trotter M. The origins of transverse cervical and of transverse scapular arteries in American Whites and Negroes. Am J Phys Anthropol 1941;28(2):239–47.

47. Jin L, Fitzgerald A. Delayed diagnosis of dorsal scapular artery pseudoaneurysm following blunt chest trauma. Trauma Case Rep 2021;35:100521. https://doi.org/10.1016/j.tcr.2021.100521.

48. Deep Cervical Artery. 2021. Available at: http://neuroangio.org/anatomy-and-variants/deep-cervical-artery/. Accessed 29 December 2021.

49. Kajikawa R, Fujinaka T, Nakamura H, et al. Carotid artery stenting for patients with occipital-vertebral anastomosis. Interv Neuroradiol 2019;25(2):212–8. https://doi.org/10.1177/1591019918802924.

50. Capobianco SM, Fahmy MW, Sicari V. Anatomy, thorax, subclavian veins. In: StatPearls [Internet]. Treasure Island (FL): StatPearls Publishing; 2021. Available at: https://www.ncbi.nlm.nih.gov/books/NBK532885/.

51. Sidoti A, Brogi E, Biancofiore G, et al. Ultrasound-versus landmark-guided subclavian vein catheterization: a prospective observational study from a tertiary referral hospital. Sci Rep 2019;9(1):12248. https://doi.org/10.1038/s41598-019-48766-1.

52. Chengazi HU, Bhatt AA. Pathology of the carotid space. Insights Imaging 2019;10(1):21. https://doi.org/10.1186/s13244-019-0704-z.

53. Barral J, Coribier A. 14-The common carotid artery. In: Barral J, Coribier A, editors. Visceral vascular manipulations. Churchill Livingstone; 2011. p. 133–8. https://doi.org/10.1016/B978-0-7020-4351-2.00014. ISBN 9780702043512.

54. Clerici G, Giulietti E, Babucci G, et al. Bovine aortic arch: clinical significance and hemodynamic evaluation. J Matern Fetal Neonatal Med 2018;31(18):2381–7. https://doi.org/10.1080/14767058.2017.1342807.

55. Gan HW, Bhasin A, Wu CJ. Transradial carotid stenting in a patient with bovine arch anatomy. Catheter Cardiovasc Interv 2010;75(4):540–3. https://doi.org/10.1002/ccd.22350.

56. Montorsi P, Galli S, Ravagnani P, et al. Carotid stenting through the right brachial approach for left internal carotid artery stenosis and bovine aortic arch configuration. Eur Radiol 2009;19(8):2009–15. https://doi.org/10.1007/s00330-009-1355-0.

57. Palmer FJ. Origin of the right vertebral artery from the right common carotid artery: angiographic demonstration of three cases. Br J Radiol 1977;50(591):185–7. https://doi.org/10.1259/0007-1285-50-591-185.

58. Troutman DA, Bicking GK, Madden NJ, et al. Aberrant origin of left vertebral artery. J Vasc Surg 2013;58(6):1670. https://doi.org/10.1016/j.jvs.2012.08.101.

59. Maybody M, Uszynski M, Morton E, et al. Absence of the common carotid artery: a rare vascular anomaly. AJNR Am J Neuroradiol 2003;24(4):711–3.

60. Chen L, Liu JM, Zhou D. Congenital absence of the right common carotid artery, internal carotid artery and external carotid artery associated with anterior communicating artery aneurysm: a rare case. Neurol Sci 2008;29(6):485–7. https://doi.org/10.1007/s10072-008-1030-2.

61. Saran S, Rajagopal R, Khera PS, et al. Nonvisualization of the Internal Carotid Artery on Computed Tomography Angiography: Discussion of Two Cases with Review of Literature. Case Rep Neurol Med 2016;2016:7584384. https://doi.org/10.1155/2016/7584384.

62. Lim CL, Keshava SN, Lea M. Anatomical variations of the internal jugular veins and their relationship to the carotid arteries: a CT evaluation. Australas Radiol 2006;50(4):314–8. https://doi.org/10.1111/j.1440-1673.2006.01589.x.

63. Hashimoto Y, Otsuki N, Morimoto K, et al. Four cases of spinal accessory nerve passing through the fenestrated internal jugular vein. Surg Radiol Anat 2012;34(4):373–5. https://doi.org/10.1007/s00276-011-0875-x.

64. Prades JM, Timoshenko A, Dumollard JM, et al. High duplication of the internal jugular vein: clinical incidence in the adult and surgical consequences, a report of three clinical cases. Surg Radiol Anat 2002;24(2):129–32. https://doi.org/10.1007/s00276-002-0020-y.

65. Contrera KJ, Aygun N, Ward BK, et al. Internal jugular vein duplication and fenestration: Case series and literature review. Laryngoscope 2016;126(7):1585–8. https://doi.org/10.1002/lary.25743.

66. Yokota H, Mukai H, Hattori S, et al. MR Imaging of the Superior Cervical Ganglion and Inferior Ganglion of the Vagus Nerve: Structures That Can Mimic Pathologic Retropharyngeal Lymph Nodes. AJNR Am J Neuroradiol 2018;39(1):170–6. https://doi.org/10.3174/ajnr.A5434.

67. Yin Z, Yin J, Cai J, et al. Neuroanatomy and clinical analysis of the cervical sympathetic trunk and longus colli. J Biomed Res 2015;29(6):501–7. https://doi.org/10.7555/JBR.29.20150047.

68. Lee JY, Lee JH, Song JS, et al. Superior Cervical Sympathetic Ganglion: Normal Imaging Appearance on 3T-MRI. Korean J Radiol 2016;17(5):657–63. https://doi.org/10.3348/kjr.2016.17.5.657.

69. Ravanelli M, Tononcelli E, Leali M, et al. Magnetic resonance imaging features of the superior cervical ganglion and expected changes after radiation therapy to the head and neck in a long-term follow-up. Neuroradiology 2020;62(4):519–24. https://doi.org/10.1007/s00234-020-02373-4.

70. Ünsal Ü, Şentürk S, Aygün S. Radiological evaluation of the localization of sympathetic ganglia in the cervical region. Surg Radiol Anat 2021;43(8):1249–58. https://doi.org/10.1007/s00276-021-02705-w.

71. Chaudhry A, Kamali A, Herzka DA, et al. Detection of the Stellate and Thoracic Sympathetic Chain Ganglia with High-Resolution 3D-CISS MR Imaging. AJNR Am J Neuroradiol 2018;39(8):1550–4. https://doi.org/10.3174/ajnr.A5698.

72. Civelek E, Karasu A, Cansever T, et al. Surgical anatomy of the cervical sympathetic trunk during anterolateral approach to cervical spine. Eur Spine J 2008;17(8):991–5. https://doi.org/10.1007/s00586-008-0696-8.

73. Shin JE, Baek JH, Ha EJ, et al. Ultrasound Features of Middle Cervical Sympathetic Ganglion. Clin J Pain 2015;31(10):909–13. https://doi.org/10.1097/AJP.0000000000000184.

74. Kiray A, Arman C, Naderi S, et al. Surgical anatomy of the cervical sympathetic trunk. Clin Anat 2005;18(3):179–85. https://doi.org/10.1002/ca.20055.

75. Park C, Suh CH, Shin JE, et al. Characteristics of the Middle Cervical Sympathetic Ganglion: A Systematic Review and Meta-Analysis. Pain Physician 2018;21(1):9–18.

76. Hogan QH, Erickson SJ. MR imaging of the stellate ganglion: normal appearance. AJR Am J Roentgenol 1992;158(3):655–9. https://doi.org/10.2214/ajr.158.3.1739014.

77. Cummings KW, Sridhar S, Parsons MS, et al. Cross-sectional Imaging Anatomy and Pathologic Conditions Affecting Thoracic Nerves. Radiographics 2017;37(1):73–92. https://doi.org/10.1148/rg.2017160071.

78. Bigeleisen PE. Anatomical variations of the phrenic nerve and its clinical implication for supraclavicular block. Br J Anaesth 2003;91(6):916–7. https://doi.org/10.1093/bja/aeg254.

79. Nason LK, Walker CM, McNeeley MF, et al. Imaging of the diaphragm: anatomy and function. Radiographics 2012;32(2):E51–70. https://doi.org/10.1148/rg.322115127.

80. Bergman R, Thompson S, Afifi A, Saadeh F. Compendium of human anatomic variation. Urban & Schwarzenberg; 1988.

81. Krishnan KR, Wolfe SW, Feinberg JH, et al. Imaging and treatment of phrenic nerve hourglass-like constrictions in neuralgic amyotrophy. ' Muscle Nerve; 62(5):E81-E82. doi: 10.1002/mus.27049. .

82. Harnsberger H, Osborn AG, MacDonald A, et al. Diagnostic and Surgical Imaging Anatomy: Brain, Head & Neck, Spine. Amirsys 2006.

83. Khalilzadeh O, Glover M, Torriani M, et al. Imaging Assessment of Thoracic Outlet Syndrome. Thorac Surg Clin 2021;31(1):19–25. https://doi.org/10.1016/j.thorsurg.2020.09.002.

84. Raptis CA, Sridhar S, Thompson RW, et al. Imaging of the Patient with Thoracic Outlet Syndrome. Radiographics 2016;36(4):984–1000. https://doi.org/10.1148/rg.2016150221.

85. Demondion X, Boutry N, Drizenko A, et al. Thoracic outlet: anatomic correlation with MR imaging. AJR Am J Roentgenol 2000;175(2):417–22. https://doi.org/10.2214/ajr.175.2.1750417.

86. Kammerer FJ, Schlude B, Kuefner MA, et al. Morphology of the distal thoracic duct and the right lymphatic duct in different head and neck pathologies: an imaging based study. Head Face Med 2016;12:15. https://doi.org/10.1186/s13005-016-0108-y.

87. Liu ME, Branstetter BF, Whetstone J, et al. Normal CT appearance of the distal thoracic duct. AJR Am J Roentgenol 2006;187(6):1615–20. https://doi.org/10.2214/AJR.05.1173.

88. Seeger M, Bewig B, Günther R, et al. Terminal part of thoracic duct: high-resolution US imaging. Radiology 2009;252(3):897–904. https://doi.org/10.1148/radiol.2531082036.

89. Ilahi M, St Lucia K, Ilahi T. Thoracic Duct. StatPearls [Internet]. StatPearls Publishing; 2021:chap Anatomy, Thorax.

90. Lyden ML, Wang TS, Sosa JA. Surgical anatomy of the thyroid gland. Available at: https://www.uptodate.com/contents/surgical-anatomy-of-the-thyroid-gland. Accessed 21 November 2022.

91. Sinos G, Sakorafas GH. Pyramidal Lobe of the Thyroid: Anatomical Considerations of Importance in Thyroid Cancer Surgery. Oncol Res Treat 2015;38:309–10. https://doi.org/10.1159/000430894.

92. Won H-J, Won H-S, Kwak D-S, et al. Zuckerkandl Tubercle of the Thyroid Gland: Correlations between Findings of Anatomic Dissections and CT Imaging. AJNR Am J Neuroradiol 2017;38(7):1416–20. https://doi.org/10.3174/ajnr.A5172.

93. Lyden ML, Wang TS, Sosa JA. Surgical anatomy of the parathyroid glands. Available at: https://www.uptodate.com/contents/surgical-anatomy-of-the-parathyroid-glands. Accessed 21 November 2022.

94. Itani M, Middleton WD. Parathyroid Imaging. Radiol Clin North Am 2020;58(6):1071–83. https://doi.org/10.1016/j.rcl.2020.07.006.

95. Som PM, Curtin HD, Mancuso AA. An imaging-based classification for the cervical nodes designed as an adjunct to recent clinically based nodal classifications. Arch Otolaryngol Head Neck Surg 1999;125(4):388–96. https://doi.org/10.1001/archotol.125.4.388.

Craniocervical Junction and Cervical Spine Anatomy

Curtis Edward Offiah, BSc, MB, ChB, FRCS, FRCR[a,b,*]

KEYWORDS

- Craniocervical • Craniovertebral • Cervical • Vertebra • Ligaments • Subaxial

KEY POINTS

- The craniocervical junction is a critical osseo-ligamentous anatomic structure that serves vital motor and sensory functions.
- A knowledge and understanding of the embryology and anatomy of the craniocervical junction may prevent erroneous radiological evaluation.
- The anatomy of the craniocervical junction is central to the understanding of pathomechanisms associated with disorders of this structure.
- The subaxial cervical spine is frequently affected by pathologic processes, in particular, trauma and infection, and neoplastic disease—a firm basis of the anatomy of this region is vital for radiological evaluation.
- Familiarity with the osseo-ligamentous anatomy of the subaxial cervical spine allows a clear dialogue between radiologist and spinal surgeon/neurosurgeon.

INTRODUCTION

The craniocervical (craniovertebral) junction represents the complex transitional zone between the cranium and the spine and comprises a complex balance of different elements: it should be considered anatomically and radiologically a distinct entity from both the cranium and, in particular, the cervical spine. It is composed of osseous structures articulated with synovial joints, intrinsic ligaments and membranes, and muscles. In addition to housing the spinal cord and multiple cranial nerves, it is also approximated by critical vasculature supplying both the brain and the cervical spinal cord parenchyma. The physiologic requirements placed on the craniocervical junction are onerous—not only must it house, protect, and support structures critical for function (and ultimately evolutionary survival), but it must also simultaneously provide significant mobility.

The subaxial cervical spine refers to that part of the cervical spine below the craniocervical junction, that is, C3 to C7 although from a clinical radiological perspective, particularly when evaluating the subaxial cervical spine for trauma, T1 level must also be considered otherwise the radiological evaluation is not complete. Anatomically, not only must the subaxial cervical spine provide vital mobility for the sensory pathways that have proved critical for the survival and evolution of the species, but it must also provide protection for the cervical spinal cord and nerve roots exiting and entering the spinal canal and is juxtaposed to the arterial vessels responsible for the anterior and posterior intracranial circulation. The large strap muscles of the neck and the smaller paraspinal

Financial disclosure statement: The author has no commercial or conflicts of interest to declare.
[a] Department of Radiology and Imaging, Royal London Hospital, Barts Health NHS Trust, Whitechapel E1 1FR, London; [b] William Harvey Research Institute, Barts and The London School of Medicine and Dentistry, Queen Mary University, London
* Department of Radiology and Imaging, Royal London Hospital, Barts Health NHS Trust, Whitechapel E1 1FR, London.
E-mail address: c.offiah@nhs.net

muscles play an evolutionary role in facilitating vital sensory pathway function and response and likely have significant causation in common twenty-first-century pathologies such as "whiplash" type injuries. An anatomic knowledge of these muscles is therefore significant to the Radiologist.

Embryology of the Craniocervical Junction

Embryology is the essential starting point in our understanding of all anatomy, both in the maturing specimen such as the infant as well as in the mature adult and in relation to normal-variant anatomic appearances. An awareness of such embryologic derivation is particularly relevant in understanding the craniocervical junction anatomy. It is useful to visualize the craniocervical junction as composed of two components: the first is a central pillar consisting of the central basiocciput (even though it is anatomically part of the skull base), odontoid process (dens or peg), and the C2 vertebral body; the second component consists of the two-ringed structures surrounding the central pillar—these are the ring of the foramen magnum including the lateral portions of the basiocciput, the exocciput incorporating the occipital condyles and the opisthion (the posterior margin of the foramen magnum), and the ring of the C1 vertebra (atlas) consisting of the anterior and posterior arches and lateral masses of the atlas[1-9] (Figs. 1 and 2). Functionally, the latter stacked two-ringed component allows limited rotation around the central pillar as well as intrinsic limited flexion extension. Ligaments bind these two structural components of the craniocervical junction providing stability. Knowledge of the embryology of the craniocervical junction is germane to this analogy of a two-component structure and also helps to confidently distinguish developmental anomalous/normal variant appearances of the imaged osseous craniocervical junction from genuine traumatic injury. Although a detailed description of the embryologic development of the craniocervical junction is beyond the scope of this review, a brief summary of selected aspects will be given.

The craniocervical junction is of mesodermal origin and appears in the third gestational week. During gastrulation, cells from the embryonic plate condense to form the parachordal mesoderm on each side of the notochord. This mesoderm eventually separates into segmental clusters called somites. These paired somites the number of which is species-specific (42 pairs in humans) will eventually give rise to the smooth muscle of the dermis, axial skeletal musculature, and the vertebral column (amongst other structures). Once mature, somites differentiate into ventromedial sclerotomes and dorsolateral dermomyotomes. The sclerotomes eventually develop into vertebral bodies, neural arches, ligaments, and membranes.[1-11]

The craniocervical junction develops from the four occipital somites and the first three cervical somites (Fig. 3). The first three occipital somites will give rise to the rostral basiocciput. The fourth occipital somite combines with the cranial part of the first cervical somite to form the sclerotome called the proatlas which is the precursor of the craniocervical junction. The cranial part of the axial region of this sclerotome fuses with sclerotome segments of the first three occipital somites to form the basion of the basiocciput. The caudal part of the axial region of the proatlas derived from the first cervical somite gives rise to the apical segment of the dens. The lateral region of the proatlas eventually gives rise to the occipital condyles and the remainder of the anterolateral foramen magnum[1,3-11] (see Fig. 3).

The caudal half of somite five and the cranial half of somite six combine to form the first cervical sclerotome. Similarly, the caudal half of somite six and the cranial half of somite seven combine to form the second cervical sclerotome. Part of the first cervical sclerotome gives rise to the basal part of the odontoid peg (dens), whereas part of the second cervical sclerotome gives rise to the body of the axis (C2 vertebra). A distinct feature of the first and second cervical sclerotomes compared with the more caudal sclerotomes is the absence of the conversion of part of the sclerotomes to the annulus fibrosus and nucleus pulposus of the intervertebral disks. Instead, this tissue disappears and the mesenchyme at these junctional sites turns into the upper dental synchondrosis between the apical dens and basal dens and the lower dental synchondrosis between the basal dens and the body of the axis. Hence, the C2 vertebra is distinctive in that it is derived from three adjacent sclerotomes that ultimately give rise to cranial as well as vertebral elements and this vertebra is the true embryologic juncture of the cranium and the spine, and, therefore, must, somewhat challengingly, serve the biomechanical requirements of both.[1,3-14]

The lateral zone of the first cervical sclerotome develops into the posterior arch of the C1 vertebra, whereas the lateral zone of the second cervical sclerotome develops into the arch of the axis (C2 vertebra; see Fig. 3). The anterior arch of the C1 vertebra develops from a small mesenchymal off-shoot ventral to both the notochord and the axial segment of first cervical sclerotome called

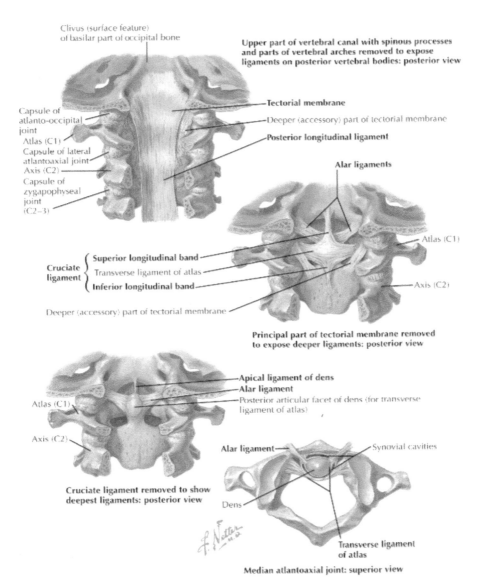

Clivus (surface feature) of basilar part of occipital bone

Upper part of vertebral canal with spinous processes and parts of vertebral arches removed to expose ligaments on posterior vertebral bodies: posterior view

Capsule of atlanto-occipital joint
Atlas (C1)
Capsule of lateral atlantoaxial joint
Axis (C2)
Capsule of zygapophyseal joint (C2–3)

Tectorial membrane
Deeper (accessory) part of tectorial membrane
Posterior longitudinal ligament
Alar ligaments
Atlas (C1)
Axis (C2)

Cruciate ligament
{ Superior longitudinal band
  Transverse ligament of atlas
  Inferior longitudinal band }

Deeper (accessory) part of tectorial membrane

Principal part of tectorial membrane removed to expose deeper ligaments: posterior view

Atlas (C1)
Axis (C2)

Apical ligament of dens
Alar ligament
Posterior articular facet of dens (for transverse ligament of atlas)

Alar ligament
Synovial cavities

Cruciate ligament removed to show deepest ligaments: posterior view

Dens

Transverse ligament of atlas

Median atlantoaxial joint: superior view

Fig. 1. Illustrative anatomy of the craniocervical junction osseous and ligamentous structures: top left—posterior view with posterior arches of the upper cervical vertebrae and occiput removed to expose ligaments; top right—posterior view with tectorial membrane removed to expose deeper ligaments of the craniocervical junction; bottom left—posterior view with cruciate ligament removed to reveal alar and apical ligament; and bottom right—superior view of the C1–C2 articulation demonstrating alar and transverse ligaments. (*From* Rubin M, Safdieh JE. Bone coverings of brain and spinal cord. In: Rubin M, Safdieh JE, editors. Netter's Concise Neuroanatomy - UPDATED EDITION. Philadelphia: Elsevier; 2017. p. 24.)

the hypochordal bow. The hypochordal bow of the proatlas gives rise to a small osseous midline tubercle attached to the ventral surface of the basiocciput below the anterior margin of the foramen magnum (basion) and is frequently visible on CT (and MRI) of the mature normal craniocervical junction.

The apical ligament is derived from the axial proatlas. The alar ligaments and the transverse ligamentous component of the cruciform (cruciate) ligament develop from the axial component of the first cervical sclerotome.

ANATOMY

The craniocervical junction is composed of two major joints: the atlantooccipital joint and the atlantoaxial joint (see **Figs. 1** and **2**; **Fig. 4**). These two joints are responsible for the majority of the movement available in the entire cervical spine.

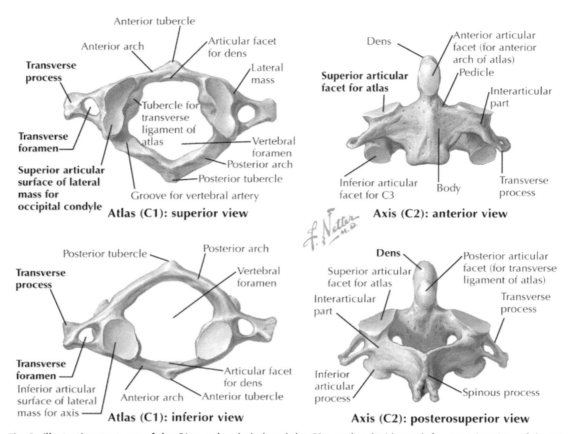

Fig. 2. Illustrative anatomy of the C1 vertebra (atlas) and the C2 vertebra (axis): top left—superior view of the C1 vertebra; bottom left—inferior view of the C1 vertebra—note the articular facet for the dens on the posterior median surface of the anterior arch of C1 synovium is located at this articular interface; top right—anterior view of the C2 vertebra; and bottom right—posterior view of the C2 vertebra—articular facets are present on the anterior and posterior surfaces of the dens with synovium will be located at these facets. (*From* Rubin M, Safdieh JE, editors. Netter's Concise Neuroanatomy - UPDATED EDITION. Philadelphia: Elsevier; 2017. p. 19.)

The Occipital Bone

The occipital bone encompasses the foramen magnum and extends from the clivus anteriorly to the lambdoid suture posteriorly. Embryologically it develops from four cartilaginous centers around the foramen magnum within the chondrocranium and from a fifth membranous component. The foramen magnum is a critical component of the occipital bone and is composed of a squamosal component forming the posterior aspect of the foramen magnum, the basal or clival portion contributing to the anterior component of the foramen magnum and the condylar portions which connect the squamosal and clival portions. The anterior margin of the foramen magnum is called the basion and the diametrically opposite posterior margin of the foramen magnum is called the opisthion. The occipital condyles angle medially and inferiorly from the posterior to anterior: this

angulation limits the mobility of the atlantooccipital joints (ie, C0–C1 joints), particularly in axial rotation compared with the atlantoaxial joint (ie, C1–C2 joint).[15–17]

The Atlas (C1 Vertebra)

The atlas or C1 vertebra originates from the fourth occipital and first cervical sclerotomes. It is unique in that it lacks a vertebral body and is formed from three ossification sites—the anterior arch (also called the centrum) and a left and right neural arch (which fuse to form a single posterior arch). The atlas also develops lateral masses. The anterior arch has an anterior tubercle in the midline that provides attachment for the anterior longitudinal ligament and the longus colli muscles. The atlas articulates with the odontoid process (also called the dens or peg) which is the bony superior extension. There is synovium located between the

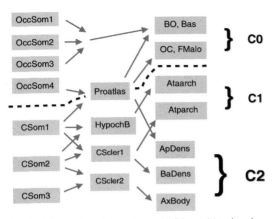

Fig. 3. Schematic of craniocervical junction developmental segmentation and resegmentation during embryogenesis. OccSom1, occipital somite 1; Occ-Som2, occipital somite 2; OccSom3, occipital somite 3; OccSom4, occipital somite 4; CSom1, cervical somite 1; CSom2, cervical somite 2; CSom3, cervical somite 3; CScler1, cervical sclerotome 1; CScler2, cervical sclerotome 2; BO- basiocciput; Bas, basion; OC, occipital condyles; FMalp, anterolateral foramen magnum and opisthion; Ataarch, anterior arch of C1 vertebra (atlas); Atparch, posterior arch of C1 vertebra (atlas); ApDens, apical segment of the dens; BaDens, basal segment of the dens; body of C2 vertebra (axis). Severed black line denotes the embryologic separation between the cranial skull base and cervical spine during craniocervical junction development.

anterior surface of the dens and the posterior surface of the median anterior arch of the C1 vertebra. The atlas also articulates inferiorly with the axis through flat wide articular facets.[12-13]

The Axis (C2 Vertebra)

The axis or C2 vertebra was historically termed the *epistropheus* which is derived from the Latin meaning "to twist" and is indicative of the role of the axis in craniocervical junction biomechanics—it is the pivot around which the atlas and therefore the head "twist" or rotate. It is formed from five ossification centers—one in the body, one in each vertebral arch and two in the odontoid process. The odontoid process of the axis extends cranially from the body of the axis.[12-14]

The Craniocervical Ligaments

Alar ligaments
These paired ligaments attach the axis to the base of the skull (see Figs. 1, 2 and 4; Fig. 5) and originate from the posterior surface of the upper third of the dens and typically travel caudocranially (in 50% of cadaveric dissections) or horizontally (in

50% of subjects); the exact insertion point of the alar ligaments has been subject to some contention with researchers variably describing insertion on the medial aspect of the occipital condyles or the anterolateral aspect of the foramen magnum.[17-24] Each ligament is narrowest at its origin and comparatively wider at its insertion giving it a "V-shaped" configuration.[23]

Cruciform ligament (cruciate ligament)
The cruciform ligament is composed of transverse and vertical parts which form a cross behind the odontoid peg (see Figs. 1, 2, and 4; Figs. 6 and 7).[17-22] The vertical component inserts onto the upper surface of the clivus between the apical ligament and tectorial membrane and a caudally directed band that inserts onto the posterior surface of the body of the axis.

Transverse ligament
The transverse ligament (sometimes termed the transverse atlantal ligament) of the cruciform ligament complex arches behind the odontoid peg attaching to a tubercle arising from the medial aspect of each lateral mass of the atlas[17-24] (see Figs. 1, 2, 4, 6 and 7). There is synovium located between the posterior surface of the dens and the anterior surface of the median region of the transverse ligament.

Tectorial membrane
This thin structure represents an upward extension of the posterior longitudinal ligament (see Figs. 1 and 7; Fig. 8). It forms the posterior border to the supraodontoid space or "apical cave"[17,21,25-28] and runs posterior to the cruciform ligament. It extends cranially to the clivus (as far cranially as the spheno-occipital synchondrosis) and caudally to the posterior surface of the body of the axis. It attaches as far laterally as the hypoglossal canals and, at the level of C0–C1, merges with the atlanto-occipital capsular ligaments (Arnold's ligaments). The cranial portion of the membrane is adherent to and anatomically indistinguishable from dura.[17,25-28]

Apical ligament
This ligament extends from the tip of the odontoid process to the basion and is situated between the anterior atlantooccipital membrane and the cruciform ligament (see Figs. 1, 7, and 8); it is surrounded by fat, connective tissue and a venous plexus which accounts for the slightly variable signal characteristics of this supraodontoid space or "apical cave" on MR imaging. It may be absent in up to 20% of subjects based on cadaveric dissections undertaken by Tubbs and colleagues.[17,21,22,25-28]

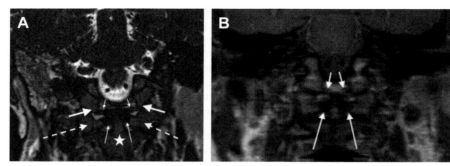

Fig. 4. (A): Coronal three-dimensional T2 SPACE (sampling perfection with application-optimized contrast using different flip-angle evolutions) sequence image through normal craniocervical junction demonstrating normal MRI appearances of the transverse ligament (*long thin arrows*) and alar ligaments (*short thin arrows*); occipital condyle attachment of the alar ligaments are shown (*thick white arrows*) as well as C1 vertebra (*broken white arrows*) and body of C2 vertebra (*white star*). (B) Coronal isovolumetric T1-weight image through normal craniocervical junction demonstrating alar ligaments (some partial volume averaging is present) shown by short thin arrows and transverse ligament (*long thin arrows*).

Anterior atlantooccipital membrane

This structure consists of a thinner superficial component (sometimes referred to as the superficial anterior atlantooccipital ligament) and a thicker deeper component and attaches the anterior aspect of the atlas to the anterior rim of the foramen magnum (see **Figs. 1** and **8**) and is located immediately posterior to the prevertebral muscles.[17],[21–23],[28] It forms the anterior wall of the supraodontoid space (which is very discernible on MRI assessment owing to its contents of fat

and veins), which also houses the alar and apical (and Barkow) ligaments.

Anterior atlantoaxial ligament

This thin ligament extends from the anterior tubercle on the anterior arch of the atlas to the axis inferiorly[17],[22] (see **Fig. 8**).

Posterior atlantooccipital membrane

This is highly visible on MRI assessment. This ligament attaches the posterior arch of the atlas to the posterior margin of the foramen magnum and

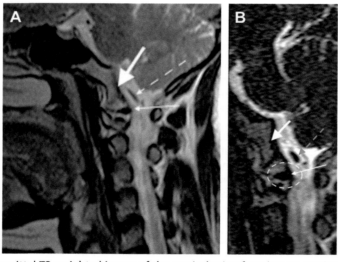

Fig. 5. (A): Right parasagittal T2-weighted image of the cervical spine focusing on craniocervical junction shows the right alar ligament (*long thin white arrow*) between its attachments to the dens and the right occipital condyle—the right vertebral artery flow void (*broken long thin white arrow*) and the right basiocciput (*thick white arrow*); (B): right parasagittal multiplanar reconstructed T2 SPACE image of the craniocervical junction at the same level as 5a showing the right alar ligament (*long thin white arrow*) between its attachments to the dens and the right occipital condyle, the right vertebral artery flow void (*broken red arrow*) and the right basiocciput (*thick white arrow*).

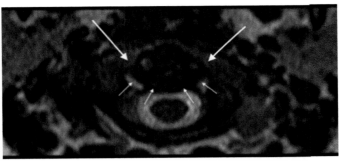

Fig. 6. Axial multi-planar reconstruction of coronal three-dimensional T2 SPACE sequence image through normal craniocervical junction demonstrating normal MRI appearances of the transverse ligament (*short thin white arrows*) and attachment to the medial tubercles (*long white arrows*) of the anterior arch of the C1 vertebra.

is continuous with the posterior atlantoaxial membrane and, subsequently, the ligamentum flavum[17,21–23,28] (see Fig. 1; Fig. 9). Laterally, it may extend over the capsules of the atlantooccipital joints. Posteriorly, it is related to the rectus capitis posterior minor muscle and, anteriorly, to the dura mater which lies immediately deep into the membrane. Interdigitations with both the dura mater and the related rectus capitis posterior minor muscle parenchyma may be present in this ligament. An important consideration in the trauma of this component of the craniocervical junction is the

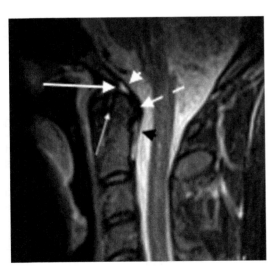

Fig. 7. Sagittal midline STIR (short tau inversion recovery) sequence image of the cervical spine demonstrating normal high signal synovial capsule anterior to the dens on the pre-dental (anterior atlantodental) interval (*long thin solid arrow*); the transverse ligament posterior to the dens is shown (*broken white arrow*); the tectorial membrane is discernible (*short white arrow*) as well as the posterior longitudinal membrane (*short black arrow*) and the apical ligament in the "apical cave" (supraodontoid space).

vertebral artery which pierces the posterior atlantooccipital membrane and then the dura mater before entering the posterior fossa.

Capsular ligaments
The synovial joints of the paired atlantooccipital and atlantoaxial joints are bound by capsules, that is, capsular ligaments that span the joint margins. The joint spaces should be less than 2 mm. Fluid within these joint spaces can indicate capsular strain injury at which point these capsular ligaments become much more discernible radiologically (Fig. 10).

Ligamentum nuchae
This is a cephalic extension of the supraspinous ligament and extends from the spinous process of the C7 vertebra attaching to the inion of the occipital bone.[17,22,29]

Normal variant craniocervical anatomy
There are several developmental anomalies of the craniocervical junction that, although uncommon, can be misinterpreted as fractures but their appearance (including radiological features) can be better understood if the embryologic derivations of the craniocervical junction are considered. Such developmental anomalies include:

- *Condylus tertius*: the hypochondral bow of the fourth occipital sclerotome or proatlas fails to integrate and will be evident as an ossified remnant at the caudal end of the basiocciput (immediately below the basion) and may be single or multiple.
- *Posterior rachischisis*: developmental cleft in the posterior arch of the atlas and are predominantly (but not always) midline but may be posterolateral through the region of the sulcus of the vertebral artery.
- *Anterior rachischisis or split atlas*: an anterior developmental cleft is rare and may be

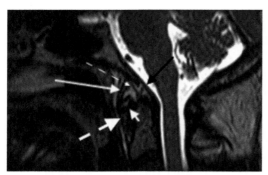

Fig. 8. Sagittal multi-planar reconstruction of coronal three-dimensional T2 SPACE sequence image through normal craniocervical junction demonstrating anterior atlanto-occipital membrane (*long solid white arrow*) and anterior atlanto-axial membrane (*broken thick white arrow*) and the relationship to the anterior arch of the C1 vertebra (*short solid white arrow*). The tectorial membrane is evident (*long thin black arrow*) and the apical ligament (*long thin broken white arrow*) in the "apical cave".

associated with a posterior rachischisis when it is then termed a "split" atlas.

- The dens fuses to the C2 body at the subdental synchondrosis, with the latter persisting into adulthood as a sclerotic line that can be confused for a fracture.
- *Os terminale*: this is a small secondary ossification center cranial to the odontoid process tip that may fail to fuse appropriately with the rest of the dens by adulthood.

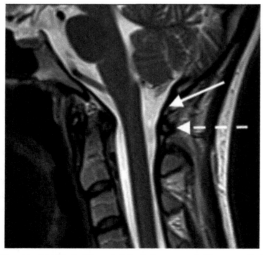

Fig. 9. Sagittal T2-weighted image of the cervical spine. The posterior atlanto-occipital membrane is demonstrated (*white solid arrow*) intimately related to the underlying dura and the overlying myofascial soft tissues as well as the posterior arch of the C1 vertebra (*broken white arrow*).

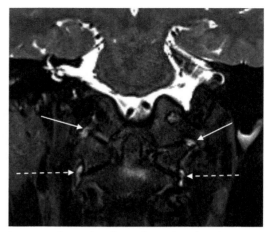

Fig. 10. Coronal three-dimensional T2 SPACE sequence image through normal craniocervical junction demonstrating traumatic effusions distending the joint capsules of the paired atlanto-occipital and atlanto-axial joints rendering the capsular ligaments of each (*solid arrows* and *broken arrows*, respectively) discernible.

- *Os odontoideum*: this may mimic a type II odontoid process fracture but in fact represents a separate well-corticated ossicle superior to a hypoplastic odontoid process and larger than an os terminale. It can be in a similar location as the os terminale (ie, orthotopic os odontoideum) or more displaced (ie, dystopic os odontoideum). The adjacent anterior arch of the atlas may be hypertrophic.

THE SUBAXIAL CERVICAL SPINE
Embryologic Derivation

The notochord plays a central role in coordinating the maturation of the vertebral column. The notochord is formed following the cephalad movement of invaginating intraembryonic mesoderm cells that attach to embryonic endoderm. The notochord induces the overlying ectoderma cells to proliferate and thicken to form the neural plate and, at approximately 19 days, this neuroectodermal tissue will curl to form the neural groove and eventually close to from the neural tube. Invaginating cells that migrate more laterally develop into mesodermal precursors called paraxial mesoderm, intermediate mesoderm, and lateral plate mesoderm. These mesoderm precursors will develop to form the spinal column, the urogenital system, and the alimentary cavity.[4,5,29] This close developmental relationship presumably is the reason for the significant association of vertebral anomalies and genitourinary anomalies (eg, VATER syndrome).

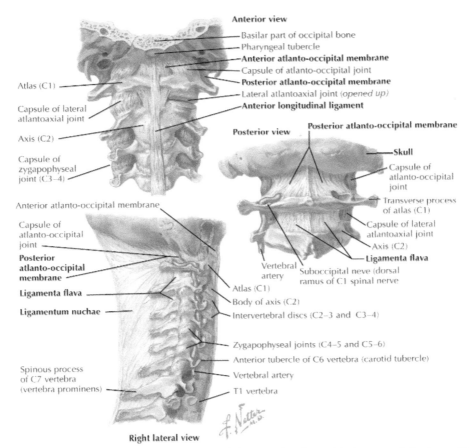

Anterior view

—Basilar part of occipital bone
—Pharyngeal tubercle
—**Anterior atlanto-occipital membrane**
—Capsule of atlanto-occipital joint
—**Posterior atlanto-occipital membrane**
—Lateral atlantoaxial joint (*opened up*)
—**Anterior longitudinal ligament**

Atlas (C1)

Capsule of lateral
atlantoaxial joint

Axis (C2)

Capsule of
zygapophyseal
joint (C3–4)

Anterior atlanto-occipital membrane

Capsule of
atlanto-occipital
joint
**Posterior
atlanto-occipital
membrane**
Ligamenta flava
Ligamentum nuchae

Spinous process
of C7 vertebra
(vertebra prominens)

Posterior view

Posterior atlanto-occipital membrane

—Skull
—Capsule of
atlanto-occipital
joint
—Transverse process
of atlas (C1)
—Capsule of lateral
atlantoaxial joint
—Axis (C2)
—**Ligamenta flava**

Vertebral
artery   Suboccipital neve (dorsal
ramus of C1 spinal nerve

Atlas (C1)
Body of axis (C2)
Intervertebral discs (C2–3 and C3–4)

Zygapophyseal joints (C4–5 and C5–6)
Anterior tubercle of C6 vertebra (carotid tubercle)
Vertebral artery
T1 vertebra

Right lateral view

Fig. 11. Illustrative anatomy of the cervical spine: top left—anterior view with the prevertebral muscles removed depicting the anterior ligaments of the craniocervical junction and the upper subaxial cervical spine; top right— posterior view of the craniocervical junction and relationship of the vertebral artery as it pierces the posterior atlanto-occipital membrane and overlying myofascia; and bottom left—lateral view of the cervical spine. (*From* Rubin M, Safdieh JE. Bone coverings of brain and spinal cord. In: Rubin M, Safdieh JE, editors. Netter's Concise Neuroanatomy - UPDATED EDITION. Philadelphia: Elsevier; 2017. p. 22.)

The paraxial mesoderm develops into 42 to 44 pairs of somites in a cranial to caudal direction. Each individual somite further differentiates into two parts—the dorsolateral area of the somite made up of the myotome and dermatome will eventually form the spinal musculature and the overlying dermis of the skin; the ventromedial region—the sclerotome of the somite—is the precursor for the vertebral column. The neural tube differentiates to form the spinal cord.[5,29]

By 4 to 5 weeks gestation, individual vertebral bodies form from the somites. In a process called resegmentaion, each sclerotome divides into a rostral and a caudal half and each vertebra is formed from the caudal half of one sclerotome and the rostral half of the adjacent sclerotome. The fusion of these two sclerotome parts forms the centrum that will become and individual

vertebral body. The notochord may play a part in coordinating resegmentation. Mesodermal cells adjacent to the neural tube develop into pedicles and lamina. The notochord eventually disintegrates between the vertebrae but enlarges at the intervertebral disk to form the nucleus pulposus while cells of the sclerotome proliferate to from the surrounding annulus fibrosus.[4,5,29]

During week 6, factors released by the notochord and neural tube prompt vertebral chrondrification: two chondrification centers in the centrum fuse to form one large chondrification segment while a single chondrification center is formed in each neural arch which subsequently fuse. Ossification of these chondrification centers begins at around week 9. As a result, each vertebra shows three ossification centers, one located in the centrum and one located in each half of the

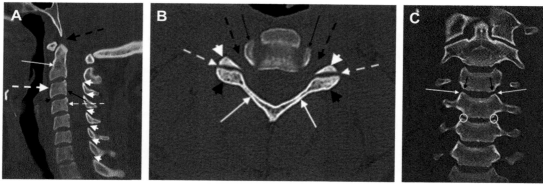

Fig. 12. (A): Sagittal multiplanar reconstructed CT image of the cervical spine on bone windows: demonstrating the region of the tectorial membrane (*long broken black arrow*), the remnant of the lower dental synchondrosis of dens with the body of the C2 vertebra (*long thin solid white arrow*), the location of the anterior longitudinal ligament at the C3 level (*broken thick white arrow*), the location of the posterior longitudinal ligament at the C3 level (*long solid thin black arrow*), the C3–C4 disk space (*short solid black arrow*), basivertebral canal of the C4 vertebral body (*broken long thin white arrow*) and the location of the ligamentum flavum (*short solid white arrows*); (B): Axial CT image of C4 vertebra on bone windows demonstrates lamina of the C3 vertebra (*solid white arrows*), the inferior articular processes of the C3 vertebra (*short black arrows*), superior articular processes of the C4 vertebra (*short white arrows*), uncinate processes of the C4 vertebral body (*long thin solid black arrows*) and neural foramina (exiting foramina) (*broken long black arrow*). (C): coronal multiplanar reconstructed CT image of the cervical spine on bone windows demonstrates uncinate processes of the C4 vertebra (*white arrows*) and the uncus of the C3 vertebra (*black arrows*) and the locations of the intervening uncovertebral "joints" at the C4–C5 level (*white ovals*).

vertebral arch. Ossification begins in the lower thoracic spine and proceeds cranially and caudally; the fusion of each vertebral arch may not be completed until around 6 years of age.[4,5,29]

Anatomy of the Mature Subaxial Cervical Spine

The subaxial cervical spine is lordotic and consists of the C3 to the C7 vertebrae (**Fig. 11**). The first and

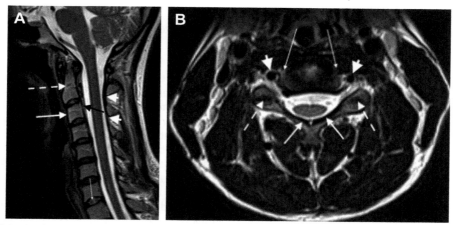

Fig. 13. (A) Sagittal T2 weighted image of the cervical spine demonstrating the remnant of the lower dental synchondrosis (*thick broken white arrow*), the posterior longitudinal ligament (*thin solid black arrow*), the anterior longitudinal ligament (*thick solid white arrow*), the ligamentum flavum at the C2–C3 and C3–C4 levels and the low signal nucleus pulposis within the non-degenerative C7-T1 disk. (There is some calcification/ossification of the posterior longitudinal ligament at the C2 level). (B) Axial T2-weighted image through the C3–C4 level demonstrates the ligamentum flavum (*solid white arrows*), the facet joints (*broken white arrows*), the uncinate processes of the uncovertebral "joints" (*long thin arrows*) and the flow voids of the vertebral arteries (*short solid white arrowheads*).

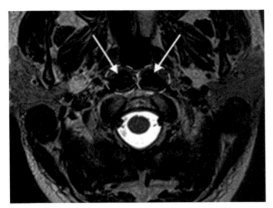

Fig. 14. Axial three-dimensional T2 SPACE image through the atlanto-occipital level demonstrates the longus capitis muscles (*white arrows* within the *broken ovals*).

second cervical vertebrae are unique—the C1 vertebra lacks a central vertebral body; the C2 vertebra has an odontoid process. All of the vertebrae of the subaxial cervical spine are similar with only slight variations in size and configuration and consist of an anteriorly located vertebral body attached to a left and right lateral mass and the posterior elements consisting of, from anterior to posterior, a left and a right pedicle, a left and right lamina and a midline spinous process. The pedicles and laminae are connected by an articular pillar or pars interarticularis on each side that possess a superior articular process and facet and an inferior articular process and facet that form the articular surfaces of the facet joints (also called zygoapophyseal joints) (see Figs. 1, 2, 11; Fig. 12).[29–33]

Unique to the subaxial cervical spine are the bilateral uncovertebral joints or neurocentric joints also referred to as the joints of Luschka (see Figs. 1, 2, and 12). These synovial joints are formed by articulation of the uncinate process of the inferior vertebral body with the uncus (which is groove-shaped) of the adjacent superior vertebral body; it remains the subject of debate whether these represent true joints or articulation points related to degenerative hypertrophy associated with aging. The neural foramen is located posterior to the uncovertebral joint. The subaxial cervical vertebrae (as well as the C1 and C2 vertebrae) also show foramina transversaria (transverse foramina) through which the vertebral arteries course (see Figs. 11 and 12). Although the C7 vertebra shows foramina transversaria, the vertebral arteries do not normally traverse the C7 foramina transversaria but, rather, enter the foramina transversria of the C6 vertebra.

The vertebral body ligaments of the subaxial cervical spine include the anterior longitudinal ligament which lies on the anterior surface of the vertebral bodies and resists excessive extension of the subaxial cervical spine and the posterior longitudinal ligament which is an extension of the tectorial membrane and is located on the posterior surface of the vertebral bodies and provides stability in flexion (Figs. 7, 8, and 12; Fig. 13). The vertebral arch ligaments are more numerous and comprise the posterior ligamentous complex: the ligamentum flavum derives its name from the Latin ("flavum" meaning "yellow") because it is yellow in color owing to its high content of elastin, which allows it to endure greater elastic deformation under tension (see Figs. 1, 11 and 13); the ligamentum nuchae extends from the tip of the C2 spinous

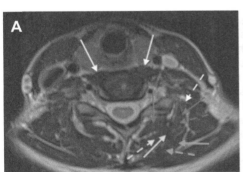
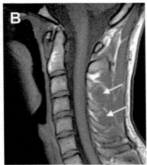
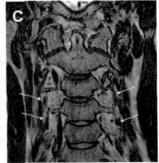

Fig. 15. (A) Axial T2-weighted image of the lower cervical spine demonstrates the prevertebral and paraspinal muscles: longus colli (*solid white arrow*), iliocostalis cervicis (*broken white arrow*), longissimus cervicis (*solid red arrow*), longissimus capitis (*broken red arrow*), splenius cervicis (*solid green arrow*), splenius capitis (*broken green arrow*), semispinalis capitis (*solid yellow arrow*), semispinalis cervicis (*broken yellow arrow*), multifidus-rotatores (*solid pink arrow*). (B) Sagittal T1 weighted image of the cervical spine demonstrates interspinales muscles (*white arrows*); (C): coronal three-dimensional T2 SPACE sequence of the cervical spine demonstrates the intertransversarii muscles (*arrows*).

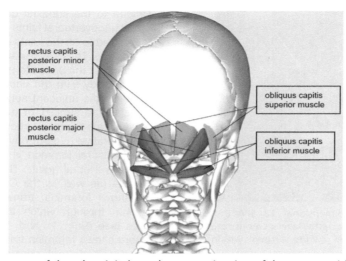

rectus capitis
posterior minor
muscle

obliquus capitis
superior muscle

rectus capitis
posterior major
muscle

obliquus capitis
inferior muscle

Fig. 16. Illustrative anatomy of the suboccipital muscles—posterior view of the rectus capitis and obliquus capitis muscles.

process to the tip of the C7 spinous process; the interspinous ligament connects adjacent spinous processes; the intertransverse ligaments connect the transverse processes and limit lateral flexion.[29–33]

THE PARAVERTEBRAL AND PREVERTEBRAL MUSCLES
Anterior Vertebral/Prevertebral Muscles

The *longus capitis* muscle is most easily identifiable at the level of the C1 vertebra in front of the anterior arch of the C1 vertebra and attaches cranially to the basiocciput; caudally, the muscle can be followed lateral to the longus colli muscle and attaches to the anterior tubercles of the transverse processes of the C3 to C6 vertebrae[33–35] (Figs. 14 and 15).

The *longus colli* muscle is most easily identifiable anterior and lateral to the vertebral bodies of the C6 and C7 vertebrae; it ascends medial to the longus capitis muscle and can be observed at all levels up to the C1 vertebral level (see Figs. 14 and 15).

The Paravertebral Muscles

The muscles related to the cervical spine have served critical evolutionary function and continue to do so allowing precise positioning of the cranium. Despite the importance of these muscles, they have been poorly detailed in the literature. However, the identification of all 27 muscles may also serve little purpose given that these muscles are also individually poorly recognized by clinicians. Nevertheless, the close anatomic

relationship of these muscles to the cervical spine and the upper aerodigestive tract, and therefore salient pathology with significant morbidity, justifies some knowledge of these muscles. For ease, these muscles may be grouped into anterior vertebral muscles, lateral vertebral muscles and posterior vertebral muscles.[33–35]

These intrinsic muscles of the spine include the extensors and rotators of the head and neck (splenius capitis, splenius cervicis muscles), the extensors and rotators of the spine (erector spinae, transversospinalis and rotatores-multifidus muscles) and the short segmental spinal muscles (interspinales and intertransversarii muscles) (see Fig. 15).

The individual components of the extensors and rotators of the spine include: the erector spinae muscles which consist of 3 columns of muscles—the iliocostalis cervicis and capitis muscles in the neck, the longissimus cervicis and capitis muscles in the neck and spinalis cervicis and capitis muscles in the neck; the transversospinalis muscles which consist of semispinalis cervicis and capitis muscles in the neck and multifidus muscles and the rotatores cervicis muscles in the neck; the multifidus muscle and rotatores muscle are difficult to differentiate anatomically and on cross-sectional imaging (see Fig. 15).

The individual components of the short segmental spinal muscles include: the interspinales muscles that extend from the tips and bodies of the spinous processes of contiguous vertebrae; the intertransversarii muscles extend between the transverse processes of contiguous vertebrae (see Fig. 15).

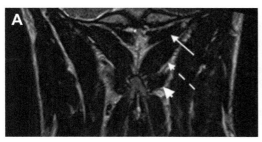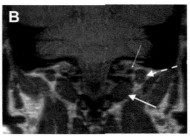

Fig. 17. (A) Coronal T2 image through posterior suboccipital region demonstrating the rectus capitis posterior minor (*solid white arrow*), rectus capitis posterior major (*broken white arrow*) and the origin of obliquus capitis inferior (*short arrow*). (B) Coronal isovolumetric T1 image through posterior suboccipital region demonstrating the obliquus capitis superior muscle (*broken thick white arrow*), obliquus capitis inferior muscle (*solid thick white arrow*) and the flow void of the V3 segment of the left vertebral artery (*thin white arrow*) as it extends anteriorly toward the posterior atlanto-occipital membrane and the underlying dura.

The Suboccipital Muscles

These short posteriorly located nuchal muscles and cranioveretebral muscles are central to extension and rotation and lateral bending of the head. They include the rectus capitis posterior major and minor muscles and the obliquus capitis superior and inferior muscles (Figs. 16 and 17). The muscles are the boundaries of the suboccipital triangle, across the floor of which the vertebral artery courses and through the floor of which the suboccipital (C1) nerve emerges and across the roof of which run the greater occipital (C2) nerve and the occipital artery. *Rectus capitis posterior major* is in fact oblique despite its name ("rectus" is Latin for "straight"). It arises from the spinous process of the C2 vertebra and extends obliquely upwards and outwards to attach to the lateral part of the inferior nuchal line. *Obliquus capitis inferior* arises from the spinous process of the C2 vertebra (below the origin of rectus capitis posterior major) and attaches to the posterior aspect of the lateral mass of the C1 vertebra. *Obliquus capitis superior* arises from the posterior aspect of the lateral mass of the C1 vertebra and attaches to the lateral part of the occipital bone between the superior and inferior nuchal lines. *Rectus capitis posterior minor* is the only muscle attached the posterior arch of the C1 vertebra and extends vertically upwards to insert into the medial part of the area below the inferior nuchal line.[33,34,36]

CLINICS CARE POINTS

- Knowledge of the anatomy of the craniocervical junction is important in identifying sites of innate vulnerability and potential sites of injury in the event of trauma.

- Developmental normal-variants of the craniocervical junction are derived from its embryological development, some of which can mimic fractures. Awareness of these will prevent false-positive reporting of fractures and unnecessary further imaging and treatment.

- There are critical vessels intimately related to the craniocervical junction and sub-axial cervical spine which may sustain traumatic vascular injury in the event of blunt trauma or penetrating trauma to these sites.

- Increased fluid signal related to the synovium atlanto-dental articulation and the atlanto-occipital and atlanto-axial joints can indicate major or mnor ligamentous strain injury, tear or rupture of the associated ligaments.

- Cervical spine joints/articulations and prevertebral and paraspinal musculature may be significant "pain-generators" in musculoskeletal neck pain pathologies such as longus colli tendonitis and "whiplash" injury: familiarity with the relevant anatomy will assist the radiological interpretation of pertinent imaging assessment of such clinical presentations.

REFERENCES

1. Offiah CE, Day E. The craniocervical junction: embryology, anatomy, biomechanics and imaging in blunt trauma. Insights Imaging 2017;8:29–47.
2. Müller F, óRahilly R. Segmentation. In staged human embryos: the occipitocervical region revisited. J Anat 2003;203(3):297–315.
3. Shoja MM, Ramdhan R, Jensen CJ, et al. Embryology of the craniocervical junction and posterior cranial fossa, part II: Embryogenesis of the hindbrain. Clin Anat 2018;31(4):488–500.
4. Jinkins JR. Atlas of neuroradiological embryology, anatomy and variants. Philadelphia, PA: Lippincott Williams & Wilkins; 2000. p. 1–60.

5. Benjamin C, Pascione D. Anatomy and embryology of the skull base and cervical spine. In: Passias P, editor. Cervical myelopathy. 1st edition. Jaypee Brother Medical Publishers; 2015. p. 1–17.

6. Menezes AH. Craniocervical developmental anatomy and its implications. Childs Nerv Syst 2008; 24(10):1109–22.

7. Junewick JJ. Pediatric craniocervical junction injuries. Am J Roentgenol 2011;196(5):1003–10.

8. Prescher A. The craniocervical junction in man, the osseous variations, their significance and differential diagnosis. Ann Anat 1997;179(1):1–19.

9. Pang D, Thompson DN. Embryology and bony malformations of the craniovertebral junction. Childs Nerv Syst 2011;27(4):523–64.

10. Pang D, Thompson DN. Embryology, classification, and surgical management of bony malformations of the craniovertebral junction. Adv Tech Stand Neurosurg 2014;40:19–109.

11. Akobo S, Rizk E, Loukas M, et al. The odontoid process: a comprehensive review of its anatomy, embryology, and variations. Childs Nerv Syst 2015; 31(11):2025–34.

12. Karwacki GM, Schneider JF. Normal ossification patterns of atlas and axis: a CT study. AJNR Am J Neuroradiol 2012;33(10):1882–7.

13. Arvin B, Fournier-Gosselin MP, Fehlings MG. Os odontoideum: etiology and surgical management. Neurosurgery 2010;66(3 Suppl):22–31.

14. O'Brien WT Sr, Shen P, Lee P. The dens: normal development, developmental variants and anomalies, and traumatic injuries. J Clin Imaging Sci 2015;5:38.

15. Panjabi M, Dvorak J, Crisco J 3rd, et al. Flexion, extension, and lateral bending of the upper cervical spine in response to alar ligament transections. J Spinal Disord 1991;4(2):157–67.

16. Steinmetz MP, Mroz TE, Benzel EC. Craniovertebral junction: biomechanical considerations. Neurosurgery 2010;66(3 Suppl):7–12.

17. Tubbs RS, Hallock JD, Radcliff V, et al. Ligaments of the craniocervical junction. J Neurosurg Spine 2011; 14(6):697–709.

18. Martin MD, Bruner HJ, Maiman DJ. Anatomic and biomechanical considerations of the craniovertebral junction. Neurosurgery 2010;66(3 Suppl):2–6.

19. Pang D, Li V. Atlantoaxial rotatory fixation: Part 1– Biomechanics of normal rotation at the atlantoaxial joint in children. Neurosurgery 2004;55(3):614–25.

20. Dvorak J, Schneider E, Saldinger P, et al. Biomechanics of the craniocervical region: the alar and transverse ligaments. J Orthop Res 1988;6(3): 452–61.

21. Tubbs RS, Dixon J, Loukas M, et al. Ligament of Barkow of the craniocervical junction: its anatomy and potential clinical and functional significance. J Neurosurg Spine 2010;12(6):619–22.

22. Debernardi A, D'Aliberti G, Talamonti G, et al. The craniovertebral junction area and the role of the ligaments and membranes. Neurosurgery 2015; 76(Suppl 1):S22–32.

23. Krakenes J, Kaale BR, Rorvik J, et al. MRI assessment of normal ligamentous structures in the craniovertebral junction. Neuroradiology 2001;43(12): 1089–97.

24. Vetti N, Kråkenes J, Eide GE, et al. MRI of the alar and transverse ligaments in whiplash- associated disorders (WAD) grades 1–2: high-signal changes by age, gender, event and time since trauma. Neuroradiology 2009;51(4):227–35.

25. Haffajee MR, Thompson C, Govender S. The supraodontoid space or Bapical cave at the craniocervical junction: a microdissection study. Clin Anat 2008;21(5):405–15.

26. Tubbs RS, Kelly DR, Humphrey ER, et al. The tectorial membrane: anatomical, biomechanical, and histological analysis. Clin Anat 2007;20(4):382–6.

27. Tubbs RS, Grabb P, Spooner A, et al. The apical ligament: anatomy and functional significance. J Neurosurg 2000;92(2 Suppl):197–200.

28. Krakenes J, Kaale BR, Moen G, et al. MRI of the tectorial and posterior atlanto-occipital membranes in the late stage of whiplash injury. Neuroradiology 2003;45(9):585–91.

29. Aarabi B, Agarwala A, Alanay A, et al. Spinal Embryology and Anatomy of the Pediatric and Adult Spine. In: Vaccaro AR, Fehlings MG, Dvorak MF, editors. Spine and spinal cord trauma. 1st edition. Verlagsgruppe: Thieme; 2011. p. 39–50.

30. Shanechi AM, et al. Spine anatomy imaging: an update. Neuroimaging Clin N Am 2019;29(4):461–80.

31. Au J, Perriman DM, Pickering MR, et al. Magnetic resonance imaging atlas of the cervical spine musculature. Clin Anat 2016;29(5):643–59.

32. Girolami M, Ghermandi R, Ghirelli M, et al. Anatomy of the subaxial cervical spine. In: Boriani S, Presutti L, Gasbarrini A, et al. Atlas of craniocervical junction and cervical spine surgery.1st edition. Springer International Publishing; Switzerland: 17-26.

33. McMinn RMH. Head and neck and spine. In: Last RJ, McMinn RMH.Last's anatomy, regional and applied, 9th edition.Churchill Livingstone; Edinburgh;1994:535-574.

34. Mekonen, et al. Development of the epaxial muscles in the human embryo. Clin Anat 2016;29(8): 1031–45.

35. Osborn AG, et al. Computed tomography of the paraspinal musculature: normal and pathologic anatomy. Am J Roentgenol 1982;138(1):93–8.

36. Alicandri-Ciufelli M, Menichetti M, Alberici MP, et al. Anatomy of the craniocervical junction. In: Boriani S, Presutti L, Gasbarrini A, et al. Atlas of craniocervical junction and cervical spine surgery. 1st edition. Springer International Publishing; Switzerland:3-15.

Thoracic and Lumbosacral Spine Anatomy

Syed S. Hashmi, MD*, Kimberly D. Seifert, MD, MS, Tarik F. Massoud, MD, PhD

KEYWORDS

- Thoracic and lumbar spine anatomy • Morphometry • Transitional and variant anatomy
- Spine metabolic imaging • Bone marrow • Intervertebral disc • Advanced spine imaging

KEY POINTS

- Knowledge of normal anatomy and normal variants is important when reviewing imaging of the spine.
- Familiarity of the normal appearance of the spine using different imaging techniques allows for easier detection of abnormal findings.
- CT and MR imaging are complementary in the evaluation of the spinal axis.

INTRODUCTION

Understanding thoracolumbar spine anatomy is important for the diagnosis and treatment of spinal diseases. This understanding includes spine biomechanics, normal variants, differences between genders, and expected changes related to aging. A 3-dimensional (3D) understanding of the anatomy is required, with knowledge of the imaging techniques and limitations involved. Given the rapid development and advancement of imaging, it is imperative to stay up to date on these techniques and best ways to assess the spine. Although radiographs are still obtained for a basic evaluation of the spine, the principal spinal imaging techniques include computed tomography (CT) and MR imaging.

SPINAL COMPUTED TOMOGRAPHIC IMAGING TECHNIQUES

CT imaging provides a comprehensive assessment of the spinal osseous structures and is often the first-line modality for evaluating patients, especially in the setting of trauma.[1,2] Compared with MR imaging, CT is faster, less expensive, and provides superior-quality osseous detail, which allows for better evaluation of the bone cortex,

calcifications, and cortical osteophytes. The development of multidetector CT with large numbers of detector arrays has allowed for thinner sections, and acquisition by helical rotation has shortened scan times. Imaging data can be displayed in multiple planes, in bone and/or soft tissue algorithms, and can be formatted into 3D models (Fig. 1). CT is based on the differences in attenuation of tissues, measured as Hounsfield units (HU), based on a normalized index of X-ray attenuation. Although dual X-ray absorptiometry scan (DEXA) has been used for the routine evaluation of bone density, a correlation has been found between bone density and CT HU, suggesting that bone marrow density can be evaluated on CTs performed for other indications.[3] Texture analysis can also be performed, evaluating skeletal integrity, and was found to be superior to DEXA in patients with low body mass index.[4] For presurgical evaluation, increased HU may predict implant success, as both hard and soft bone are associated with a higher risk of implant failure, and HU in the normal bone density range correlates with primary implant stability. In addition to evaluating the expected postoperative healing, CT can also assess implant malposition, disruption, and loosening.[5] A limitation of CT spinal imaging is the relative

Funding Information: None.

Department of Radiology, Stanford University School of Medicine, Center for Academic Medicine (CAM), 453 Quarry Road, Room 325B, Palo Alto, CA 94304, USA

* Corresponding author.

E-mail address: hashmi@stanford.edu

Neuroimag Clin N Am 32 (2022) 889–902

https://doi.org/10.1016/j.nic.2022.07.024

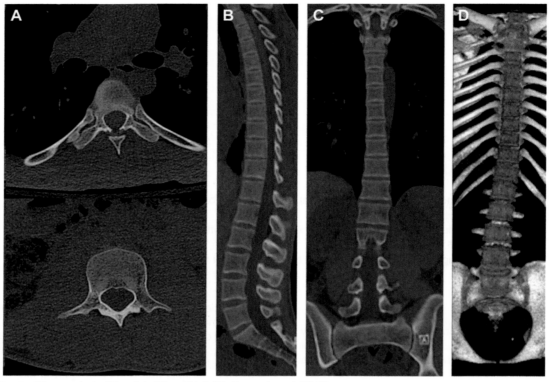

Fig. 1. CT example in (*A*) axial, (*B*) sagittal, (*C*) Coronal, and (*D*) 3D.

suboptimal evaluation of soft tissues structures when compared with MR imaging.

SPINAL MR IMAGING TECHNIQUES

The main advantages of MR imaging over CT include high-contrast resolution and the absence of ionizing radiation.[2,6] Given the superior evaluation of soft tissues as well as marrow changes, MR imaging can help diagnose bony contusions, ligamentous injuries, and disc herniations; and distinguish between acute and chronic fractures.

MR imaging is based on the varying relaxivity of hydrogen atoms, which are placed in a static field, while gradient magnetic fields are applied during specific timepoints. Common spine sequences include T1, T2, and fat saturation short-tau inversion recovery (STIR) imaging (Fig. 2). T1 fluid-attenuated inversion recovery (FLAIR) demonstrates superior image contrast over fast spin echo, including improved lesion-to-background contrast, as well as improved cerebrospinal fluid (CSF) nulling.[7,8] Postcontrast T1 imaging may be included, based on the indication; fat saturation aids in lesion detection. Although STIR is the most common fat suppression technique of the spine, other techniques may have additional benefits. For example, T2 Dixon has a more uniform fat suppression, and spectral

attenuated inversion recovery is relatively insensitive to field inhomogeneity with a higher signal-to-noise ratio (SNR) when compared with STIR.[9] Other imaging techniques may be advantageous in specific circumstances: high-resolution 3D heavily weighted T2 imaging should be considered to evaluate small structures in or containing CSF; gradient-recalled echo (GRE) better defines the cortex, disc margins, and neural foramina; proton density (PD) can further characterize abnormal pathologic condition; and diffusion weighted imaging (DWI), in addition to detecting abscesses, can differentiate an acute osteoporotic compression fracture from a pathologic fracture from a malignant lesion that will demonstrate diffusion restriction.[10,11]

MR spine imaging is obtained in at least 2 planes, commonly done in the axial and sagittal planes. Axial imaging oriented to the disc may be useful when assessing degenerative changes. Slice thickness of approximately 3 to 4 mm is generally optimal for spine imaging.[11] Spine imaging is commonly performed at either 1.5 T or 3 T, with 7 T magnets predominantly performed in the research setting.[12] With increasing magnetic field strength, there is an increase in the SNR and decreased scan time, to the detriment of increasing artifacts.[6]

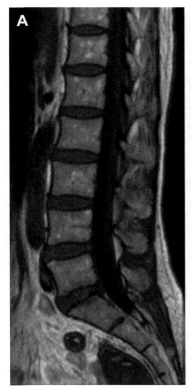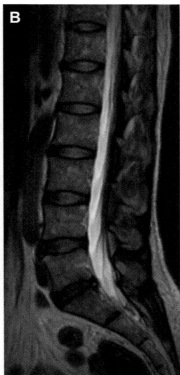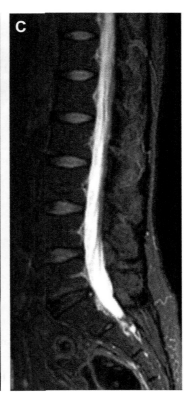

Fig. 2. MR spine using (*A*) T1, (*B*) T2, and (*C*) STIR techniques.

THORACIC AND LUMBAR SPINE ANATOMY

The normal thoracic spine consists of 12 rib-bearing vertebrae, and the normal lumbar spine consists of 5 nonrib-bearing vertebrae. The vertebrae are made up of a body and posterior elements: pedicles, transverse processes, superior and inferior articular processes, laminae, and spinous processes (Figs. 3A, B, 4A, B, 5A,B, and 6A, B). The basivertebral vein can be seen as a notch in the midposterior vertebral body and should not be confused with a fracture (Figs. 3–6C). On the posterior aspect of the thoracic vertebral bodies, the costal facets articulate with ribs (see Figs. 3A, B and 4A). The facet joints are located at the junction between the pedicles and laminae (Figs. 3–6D).

The neural foramina are formed between 2 vertebral bodies and contain the nerve root, dorsal root ganglion, fat, blood vessels, and ligaments (see Figs. 3D and 5D; Fig. 4D, E). [13] The anterior margin is the vertebral bodies and discs, the superior and inferior margins are the pedicles, and the posterior margin is the ligamentum flavum covered facets. CT and MR imaging can both be used to image the neural foramina, by viewing in a parasagittal plane. CT will detail any osseous impingement on the foraminal fat. MR imaging can better evaluate soft tissues, with the foraminal fat best evaluated using the sagittal T1 sequence. MR imaging can better visualize soft tissue impingement, such as an intervertebral disc.

THORACOLUMBAR MORPHOMETRY

Vertebral morphometry refers to the size and shape of the spine, which can be assessed at each vertebral level, spinal section, and the total spine. Each vertebral body varies slightly in height, anterior-posterior (AP) dimension, pedicle diameter, lamina width and length, and spinal canal diameter and shape. The endplates are asymmetric, with the cranial endplate more concave and denser than the corresponding caudal endplate. [14] Vertebral body height is affected by multiple intrinsic factors of the spine such as trabecular architecture, disc integrity, scoliosis, and bone density. [15] Patient factors contributing to alterations of vertebral body height include age, gender, smoking, alcohol intake, prior fracture, and corticosteroid use. [16,17] Pedicle length, width, and angle also fluctuate. In the thoracic spine, the pedicle length decreases and width increases moving caudally, whereas the pedicle length increases moving caudally in the lumbar spine. [18]

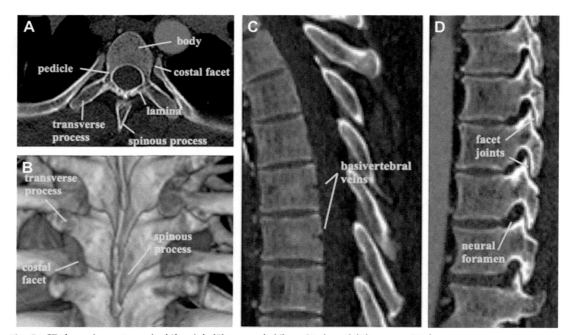

Fig. 3. CT thoracic anatomy in (A) axial, (B) coronal, (C) sagittal, and (D) parasagittal.

The anteroposterior diameter of the spinal canal, which is larger in women, gradually decreases from T12 to L4, minimally increases at L5, and subsequently decreases at L5 to S1, also changing shape from circular to oval.[17] The lateral recess and neural foramen diameter progressively decrease from T12 to S1.

In newborns, the entire spine is kyphotic (Fig. 7A). The cervical and lumbar lordosis (Fig. 7B) develops with age secondary to holding the head upright, and acquiring an erect posture.[19]

The overall curvature of the spine is more pronounced in thoracic kyphosis than lumbar lordosis.[20] However, the curvatures are not symmetric, thoracic kyphosis has an apex at T7, maximum progression in the middle, and smaller progression on the ends. Lumbar spine curvature is more important in respect to posture, stabilization of the upper body, and load bearing.[21] Lumbar lordosis depends mostly on the configuration of L4 to L5 and L5 to S1. With aging after 50 years, there is increased lordosis, related to posterior

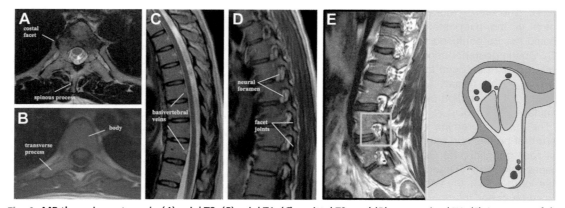

Fig. 4. MR thoracic anatomy in (A) axial T2, (B) axial T1, (C) sagittal T2, and (D) parasagittal T1. (E) Anatomy of the intervertebral foramen (IVF). Left panel. Parasagittal image from a T2-weighted spine MR imaging. Inset shows left L4-L5 IVF. Right panel. Inverted pear-shaped IVF, its bony and joint surroundings, and contents. Exiting ventral and dorsal nerve roots (*light orange*) are found in the superior aspect of the IVF, and radicular (or radiculomedullary) arteries (*red*) and foraminal veins (*blue*) are both in the superior and inferior aspects of the IVF, all surrounded by fat (*yellow*). (Reproduced with permission from reference [13].)

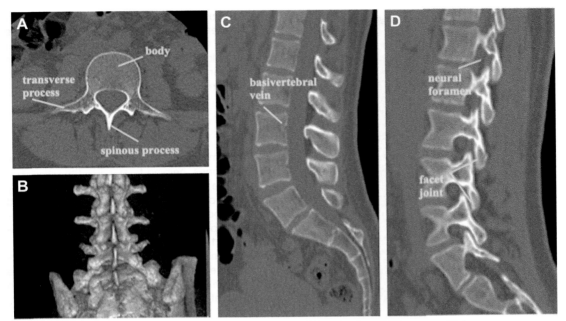

Fig. 5. CT anatomy of the lumbar spine in (A) axial, (B) 3D, (C) sagittal, and (D) parasagittal.

intervertebral disc and posterior vertebral body height loss.[22] Contact of the adjacent spinous processes can result, causing interspinous degenerative changes and may contribute to pain symptoms.[23] Finally, there is a relationship between lumbar lordosis and pelvic incidence, which should be within 11° because larger values correlate with standing and walking pain.[24] Vertebral bodies also demonstrate rotation in the transverse plane, changing with age.[25] In infancy, there is leftward rotation of the upper thoracic spine; there is no significant rotation in the juvenile spine; and

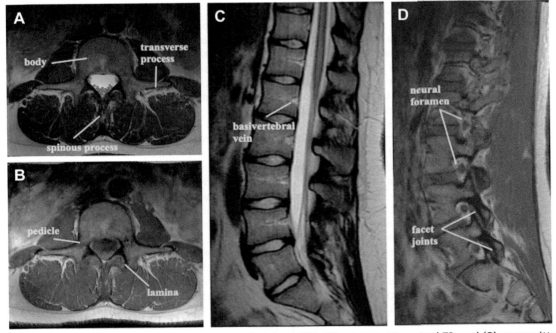

Fig. 6. MR imaging anatomy of the lumbar spine in (A) axial T2, (B) axial T1, (C) sagittal T2, and (D) parasagittal T1.

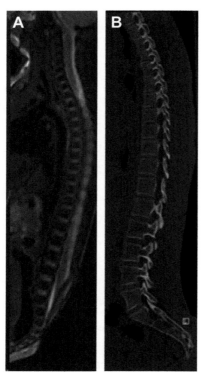

Fig. 7. (A) Newborn and (B) adult spine curvature.

rightward rotation of the mid-to-lower thoracic spine in adolescence.

Spinal alignment varies with age. In adolescents, the foundational plane is coronal, whereas in adults, it is sagittal.[26] For sagittal balance, the plumb line has shown to be reliable and valid and is a vertical line from the center of the C7 vertebral body that should pass within 2 cm from the posterosuperior corner of S1 on a sagittal view.[27] Obesity has been shown to affect sagittal balance, with an increased body mass index (BMI) correlating with an increased thoracic kyphosis.[28] Although surgery should aim to correct the spinal balance, it is important to understand that altering a portion of the curvature will affect the remaining spine because the body tries to maintain sagittal and coronal balances.[29]

Similar to the cervical spine, the thoracic and lumbar spine alignment can be evaluated using "spinal lines." The anterior vertebral line is formed by the anterior vertebral bodies, which are connected anteriorly by the anterior longitudinal ligament. The posterior vertebral line is formed by the posterior vertebral bodies, which are connected by the posterior longitudinal ligament. The posterior vertebral line is also the anterior border of the spinal canal. The posterior border of the spinal canal is termed the spinolaminar line. The spinal canal contains the thecal sac

surrounded by epidural space containing fat and venous plexus. Finally, the posterior spinous line is made of the tips of the spinous process. These lines should follow the normal thoracic kyphosis and lumbar lordosis, without stepoffs. Any malalignments may be evidence of injury.

SACRAL AND COCCYGEAL ANATOMY AND MORPHOMETRY

The sacrum provides a transition from the spine to the iliac bones, helping to stabilize the pelvis and hips.[30] The sacrum is a trilateral bone formed by the fusion of 5 vertebrae, which results in a fused vertebral body, and 2 lateral sacral alae. This results in 4 pairs of neural foramina, to accommodate the S1 to S4 nerve roots.

Sacral morphometry is notable for sex differences where female S1 vertebral bodies are smaller, with larger sacral alae compared with male counterparts. In addition, there are differences in the curvature of the sacrum with males demonstrating a greater degree of curvature, which is evenly distributed over the sacrum.

The coccyx consists of 4 rudimentary vertebral bodies that form the caudal aspect of the spine. The first segment is the largest, and the subsequent segments decrease in size. The coccyx in women is shorter, straighter, and are prone to retroversion.[31]

NORMAL SPINE BONE MARROW IMAGING

Bone marrow is easily visualized and distinguished from the proton-poor cortex on MR imaging. Bone marrow undergoes conversion from red to yellow marrow, usually complete by the age of 25. The red, hematopoetically active marrow, is composed of 40% fat, 40% water, and 20% protein. In contrast, yellow hematopoetically inactive marrow, is composed of 80% fat, 15% water, and 5% protein. Given the presence of fat, the T1 signal is hyperintense to muscle and intervertebral disc, and the differences in fat content results in relative hypointensity of red marrow compared with yellow marrow (Fig. 8).[32] Alternatively, abnormal bone marrow, such as with replacement or infiltration, will be hypointense to muscle and disc on T1. The normal T2 signal is also hyperintense secondary to the high fat content. STIR is a fat-saturation technique that is highly water sensitive that nulls fat and allows for the visualization of bone marrow edema, which can be seen in trauma, infection, inflammation, ischemia, and neoplasm. In-phase and out-of-phase sequences can help distinguish between benign edema with a signal drop of 20% at 1.5 T and 25% at 3T,

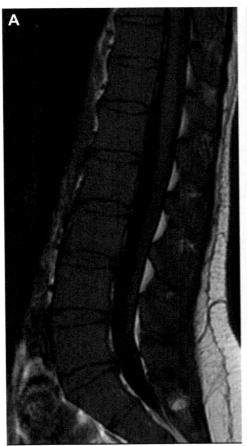
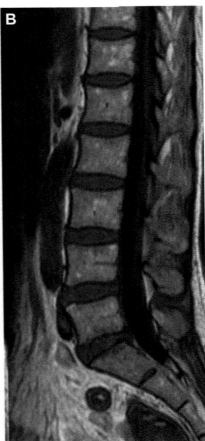

Fig. 8. (*A*) T1 red marrow and (*B*) T1 yellow marrow.

versus malignant edema with less signal drop. A newer technique, PD fat fraction, can evaluate the fat density of a lesion, with benign lesions, such as a vertebral hemangioma, demonstrating higher fat content (Fig. 9).[33,34]

Endplate changes occur with degenerative disease in 3 phases, which are recognizable on MR imaging.[35] Type 1 is associated with edema, visualized as decreased T1 signal and increased T2 signal. Type 2 is related to fatty changes, resulting in increased signal on both T1 and T2 sequences. Finally, Type 3 changes are associated with sclerosis, with decreased signal on both T1 and T2 (Fig. 10).

NORMAL IMAGING OF INTERVERTEBRAL DISCS AND SPINAL LIGAMENTS

Intervertebral discs are essential to the spine, making up the compliant flexible portions, absorbing the axial load, and providing mobility. In infants, the discs are more spherical in shape (Fig. 11A), and become flatter with increasing age and axial loading. Disc morphometry varies considerably with the level, sex, and age.[36] Men have larger discs than women; there is an increase in disc height and other dimensions caudally, with largest height at L4 to L5; and there is a decrease in disc height with age.[37] Moreover, the L5 to S1 disc is significantly different in terms of morphometry and deformation, because it is stiffer, and results in less compression and shear strain. Furthermore, the L5 to S1 disc has the smallest load-bearing surface, which may explain why it is the most common site of degeneration.[14]

MR imaging is the preferred modality for disc evaluation. The central nucleus pulposus is primarily composed of water, whereas the peripheral annulus fibrosus is made up of proton-poor lamellated collagen, and these are easily distinguished on MR imaging. A PD sequence provides the best SNR, and a T2 sequence provides the best contrast between tissue types.[38] An annular fissure incites edema and places the nucleus pulposus at a risk for herniation, both resulting in focal high intensity on T2 imaging (Fig. 11B).

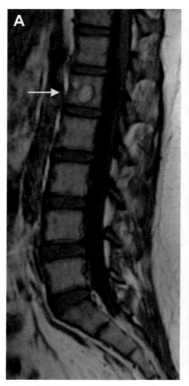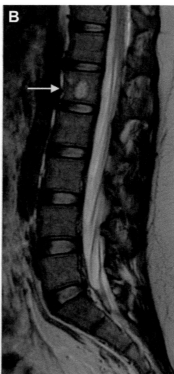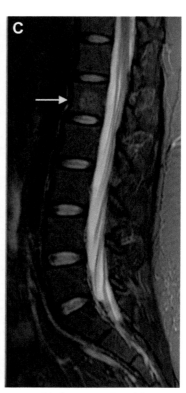

Fig. 9. (A) T1 and (B) T2 hyperintense lesion *(arrows)* that becomes hypointense with fat saturation (C).

Degeneration of the disc will cause decrease in fluid and an increase in collagen, resulting in a decrease in T2 signal (Fig. 11C; Figs. 12–14). Degenerative changes of the intervertebral discs also cause degenerative changes to the adjacent vertebral endplates, as mentioned above. Although a T2* sequence can be used to identify early degenerative changes, it is also sensitive to normal variations of the disc, with values that fluctuate related to axial loading throughout the day and unloading in the morning.[39]

Spinal imaging is generally performed in the supine position, limiting the evaluation of the natural disc position. Skeletal kinematics evaluation during a load-lifting motion has been proposed to better assess the true morphometry and deformation of the discs.[40] The anterior-posterior and medial-lateral radiographic disc spaces are measured during dynamic activities that include flexed and upright positions, and each disc space is reconstructed. A positional MR imaging (pMRI) is another technique that can evaluate discs in different positions.[41] However, pMRI is often limited owing to the open MR imaging technique with low field strength.

Degeneration of the intervertebral discs results in changes in disc height and mobility, causing stress to the other discs. A similar change in

biodynamics occurs with spinal fusion, which limits mobility. Hence, fusion should also include restoration of the disc height, with close attention to the normal morphology at that level.[42]

The main ligaments of the thoracic and lumbar spine include the anterior longitudinal ligament, posterior longitudinal ligament, ligamentum flavum, interspinous ligaments, and supraspinatus ligaments. CT poorly evaluates the spinal ligaments, which are soft tissue in density, and given their thin structure, the normal anterior and posterior longitudinal ligaments are generally not visualized. One advantage of CT is identifying and confirming calcified disc components.[43] MR imaging provides superior evaluation of the ligamentous structures and can even identify small ligamentous structures, such as the foraminal ligaments.[44] Because ligaments are proton poor, they normally seem hypointense on all sequences and T2-weighted sequences can show ligamentous edema, suggestive of injury.[10]

TRANSITIONAL ANATOMY OF THE THORACOLUMBAR AND LUMBOSACRAL SPINE

Transitional anatomy is a segmentation anomaly, with variation in the number of vertebral bodies

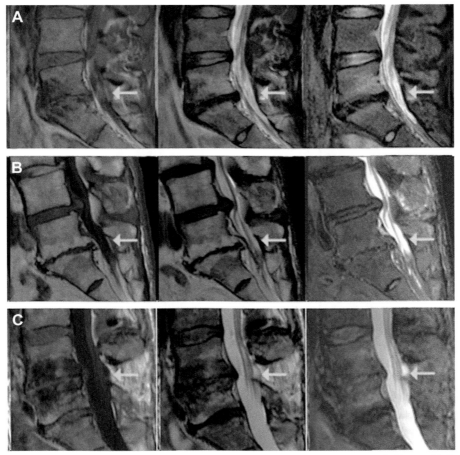

Fig. 10. Changes in T1, T2, and STIR signal *(left to right)* with *(A)* type I, *(B)* type II, and *(C)* type III degenerative endplate changes *(arrows)*.

and is one of the most common segmentation anomalies, occurring in approximately 10% of the population, more common in men.[45] There is no good consensus on how to define the transitional vertebrae. Landmarks, such as the aortic bifurcation, or iliolumbar ligament, have been suggested; however, these have been unreliable. Given the confusion around multiple classification schemes, once transitional anatomy is identified, presurgical workup should incorporate full spine imaging to document numbering from C2 to help avoid wrong level surgery. Transitional anatomy also causes confusion of the corresponding nerves, leading to poor correlation with patient symptoms. Innervation may result from an adjacent nerve than the typical distribution, or occur as an overlap of multiple nerves.

The most common finding of transitional thoracolumbar vertebra is the presence of hypoplastic ribs on the lowest rib-bearing vertebra, seen in approximately 4% of the population.[19] With respect to thoracolumbar variants, 13 rib-bearing with 4 nonrib-bearing vertebral bodies is more common than 11 rib-bearing with 6 nonrib-bearing vertebral bodies.

The prevalence of transitional lumbosacral anatomy ranges from 7% to 30%. The last lumbar body may show association with the sacrum, and is called sacralization, or the first sacral segment may morphologically seem as a lumbar vertebra, called lumbarization.[19] Enlarged lumbar transverse processes and variations of the S1-S2 disc also signal transitional lumbosacral anatomy. Although usually asymptomatic, an enlarged lumbar transverse process can cause compression symptoms of an adjacent nerve, resulting in radiculopathy. Additionally, transitional anatomy may result in altered biomechanics at the lumbosacral junction, predisposing the level to accelerated degenerative changes. The Castellvi classification has been used to describe the different morphologic appearances of sacralization. Type I

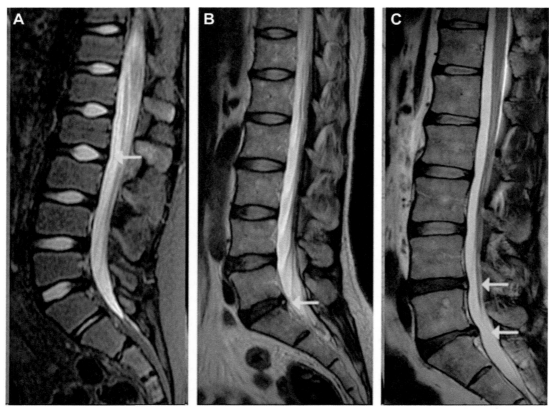

Fig. 11. (A) Spherical discs in young patient, (B) annular fissure, and (C) increased collagen with loss of T2 signal (arrows).

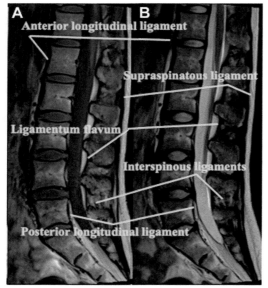

Fig. 12. Due to high-collagen content, ligaments show up dark in both (A) T1 and (B) T2 sequences.

describes a lumbar transverse process that is enlarged and dysplastic. Type II is an enlarged lumbar transverse process with pseudoarticulation with the sacrum. Transitional anatomy is labeled as type III secondary to fusion of the lumbar transverse process with the sacrum, and is the most common.[46] In types I, II, and III, the addition of "a" designates a unilateral process, and "b" designates bilateral. Type IV represents type IIa on one side and type IIIa on the contralateral side. Although not fully detailed in this article, transitional coccygeal sacralization may be clinically pertinent in the setting of coccydynia.

ANATOMIC VARIANTS OF THE THORACOLUMBAR AND LUMBOSACRAL SPINE

Anomalies can arise from the spinal development process. Asymmetric development can result in hemivertebra or butterfly vertebra.[30,35,47] Symmetric development may produce an altered number of vertebral bodies, a block vertebra when the intervertebral disc fails to form, and a unilateral

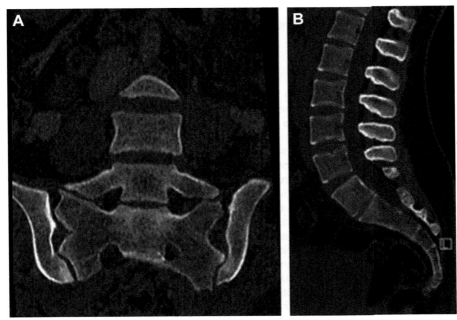

Fig. 13. Transitional lumbosacral anatomy with (A) enlarged L5 transverse processes that articulate with the sacrum bilaterally (Castellvi IIb) and (B) hypoplastic L5-S1 disc.

bar vertebra when only part of the disc forms.[19,47] Short pedicles can result in congenital narrowing of the spine. Less severe congenital abnormalities include partial hypoplasia or absence of a pedicle or pars interarticularis. A severe defect can occur in the sacrum, resulting in the complete absence of the sacrum, termed sacral agenesis, which typically occurs in the setting of caudal regression syndrome. This congenital disorder presents with anomalies of the rectum, urinary bladder, genital system, lumbosacral spine, and lower extremities.

Spinal dysraphism develops from incomplete posterior midline fusion, with a spectrum of severity. Variations of the sacral hiatus also occur, ranging from S2 to S5, with the most common location of S4. Rarely, there can be complete absence of the sacral hiatus, which is clinically significant in the setting of epidural anesthesia failure.

Other anomalies occur during the growing process. A limbus vertebra is focal herniation of disc into the adjacent endplate, usually occurring at the anterior-superior endplate, producing a wedge-shaped fragment that should not be mistaken for a fracture. In Scheuermann disease, there is uneven growth, where the posterior vertebral body grows more than the anterior aspect,

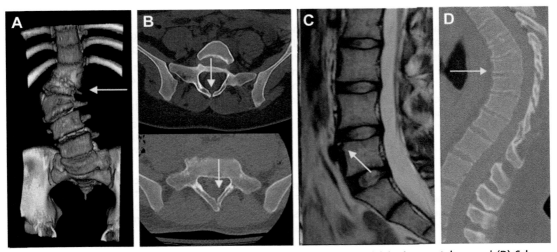

Fig. 14. Spine anomalies including (A) butterfly, (B) spina bifida occulta, (C) limbus vertebra, and (D) Scheuermann disease (arrows).

causing wedge shaped vertebral bodies and exaggerated kyphosis.

COMMON SPINE MR IMAGING ARTIFACTS

Artifacts may mimic pathologic condition on MR imaging; therefore, it is important to recognize them and ways to reduce them to ensure proper diagnosis.

Inhomogeneity of the magnetic field causes proton dephasing, resulting in spatial distortion, blurring, and intensity loss. Inhomogeneity is reduced with shim coils, by making small corrective field differences. Inhomogeneity contributes to T2*, which worsens with a large field of view, and use of GRE, planar, and fat suppression sequences.

Susceptibility artifacts creates local field inhomogeneities, causing distortion and a signal void surrounding the ferromagnetic object.[48] Susceptibility worsens with an increase in field strength, and GRE and planar sequences. To reduce susceptibility artifact, a spin echo sequence with a short echo time is preferred. Iterative decomposition of water and fat with echo asymmetry and the least-squares estimation is a newer technique that reduces metallic artifact, also producing fat saturation. Common implants causing susceptibility on spinal imaging are fusion hardware and aortic stent grafts.

Aliasing, also known as wraparound, is when an object outside the field of view projects on the opposite side of the image. To overcome this artifact, the field of view is increased to the detriment of lower resolution.[10]

Differences in resonance between fat and water cause spatial misregistration proportional to the magnetic field strength, resulting in chemical shift artifact. In the spine, this manifests as asymmetric end plate thickness.

Finally, motion artifact can happen with breathing, patient motion, cardiac movement, and swallowing, occurring in the phase-encoding direction, which is usually in the anterior-posterior direction. The result is blurring, decreased edge definition, and ghosting.[35] Motion artifact can be reduced by using a fast imaging technique.[48]

NORMAL METABOLIC IMAGING OF THE THORACOLUMBAR SPINE

PET imaging allows the assessment of spinal metabolism.[49] Fluorine-18-sodium fluoride (18F-NaF) can evaluate degeneration and osteoporosis. 18F-NaF imaging has shown a correlation between increased uptake with increased patient weight, likely related to increased degenerative changes owing to the increased mechanical load on the spine, with associated increased remodeling.

ADVANCED MR IMAGING TECHNIQUES OF THE THORACOLUMBAR SPINE

Several advanced MR techniques are available to image the spine.[6,50] Vascular time resolved imaging of contrast kinetics can identify vascular malformations in the spine, and localize specific vessels, such as the artery of Adamkiewicz. Dynamic MRA may be used to evaluate a dissection or a partially thrombosed aneurysm.

Back pain is a common indication for spine imaging, and it is often difficult to determine if the findings seen on imaging are the cause of the patient's symptoms. Studies have shown that atrophy and fatty infiltration of the paraspinal muscles is correlated with some forms of back and lower extremity pain. A newer technique that is being investigated in the laboratory setting, muscle functional MR imaging, can directly measure the muscular response to induced pain.[10,51]

Other nuclear medicine techniques can be used to evaluate the spine.[52] Bone scans can evaluate osteomyelitis using planar imaging with either Technicium-99, Gallium-67 and/or white blood cell labeling with indium-111 or technium-99m. PET imaging with FDG provides increased spatial resolution. Additional radiopharmaceuticals, such as antibodies and antimicrobial peptides, are less common and have not been studied in depth.

CLINICS CARE POINTS

- Principal spine-imaging techniques include computed tomography (CT) and MR imaging.

- CT imaging provides a comprehensive assessment of the spinal osseous structures and is often the first-line modality for evaluating patients, especially in the setting of trauma.

- MR imaging provides superior evaluation of the soft tissues, including bone marrow, ligaments, and intervertebral discs without ionizing radiation.

- The normal thoracic spine consists of 12 rib-bearing vertebrae, the normal lumbar spine consists of 5 nonrib-bearing vertebrae, and the normal sacrum consists of 5 fused vertebrae.

- Transitional anatomy occurs in approximately 10% of the population.

DISCLOSURE

The authors have nothing to disclose.

REFERENCES

1. Goldberg AL, Kershah SM. Advances in imaging of vertebral and spinal cord injury. J Spinal Cord Med 2010;33(2):105–16.
2.. Splendiani A, Bruno F, Patriarca L, et al. Thoracic spine trauma: advanced imaging modality. Radiol Med 2016;121(10):780–92.
3.. Schreiber JJ, Anderson PA, Rosas HG, et al. Hounsfield units for assessing bone mineral density and strength: a tool for osteoporosis management. J Bone Joint Surg Am 2011;93(11):1057–63.
4.. Tabari A, Torriani M, Miller KK, et al. Anorexia Nervosa: Analysis of Trabecular Texture with CT. Radiology 2017;283(1):178–85.
5.. Corona-Cedillo R, Saavedra-Navarrete M, Espinoza-Garcia J, et al. Imaging Assessment of the Postoperative Spine: An Updated Pictorial Review of Selected Complications. Biomed Res Int 2021; 2021:9940001.
6.. Vargas MI, Delattre BM, Boto J, et al. Advanced magnetic resonance imaging (MRI) techniques of the spine and spinal cord in children and adults. Insights Imaging 2018;9(4):549–57.
7.. Lavdas E, Vlychou M, Arikidis N, et al. Comparison of T1-weighted fast spin-echo and T1-weighted fluid-attenuated inversion recovery images of the lumbar spine at 3.0 Tesla. Acta Radiol 2010;51(3): 290–5.
8.. Lavdas E, Tsougos I, Arikidis N, et al. Evaluation of fat saturation and contrast enhancement on T1-weighted FLAIR sequence of the spine at 3.0 T. Clin Imaging 2014;38(4):428–33.
9.. Lee S, Choi DS, Shin HS, et al. FSE T2-weighted two-point Dixon technique for fat suppression in the lumbar spine: comparison with SPAIR technique. Diagn Interv Radiol 2018;24(3):175–80.
10.. Elliott JM, Flynn TW, Al-Najjar A, et al. The pearls and pitfalls of magnetic resonance imaging for the spine. J Orthop Sports Phys Ther 2011;41(11): 848–60.
11. Jindal G, Pukenas B. Normal spinal anatomy on magnetic resonance imaging. Magn Reson Imaging Clin N Am 2011;19(3):475–88.
12.. Grams AE, Kraff O, Umutlu L, et al. MRI of the lumbar spine at 7 Tesla in healthy volunteers and a patient with congenital malformations. Skeletal Radiol 2012;41(5):509–14.
13. Khalaf AM, Yedavalli V, Massoud TF. Magnetic resonance imaging anatomy and morphometry of lumbar intervertebral foramina to guide safe transforaminal subarachnoid punctures. Clin Anat 2020;33(3):405–13.

14.. Tang R, Gungor C, Sesek RF, et al. Morphometry of the lower lumbar intervertebral discs and endplates: comparative analyses of new MRI data with previous findings. Eur Spine J 2016;25(12): 4116–31.
15. Diacinti D, Guglielmi G. Vertebral morphometry. Radiol Clin North Am 2010;48(3):561–75.
16.. Alam MM, Waqas M, Shallwani H, et al. Lumbar morphometry: a study of lumbar vertebrae from a pakistani population using computed tomography scans. Asian Spine J 2014;8(4):421–6.
17.. Yadav U, Singh V, Bhargava N, et al. Lumbar Canal Diameter Evaluation by CT Morphometry-Study of Indian Population. Int J Spine Surg 2020;14(2): 175–81.
18.. Mohanty SP, Kanhangad PM, Bhat SN, et al. Morphometry of the lower thoracic and lumbar pedicles and its relevance in pedicle fixation. Musculoskelet Surg 2018;102(3):299–305.
19. Thawait GK, Chhabra A, Carrino JA. Spine segmentation and enumeration and normal variants. Radiol Clin North Am 2012;50(4):587–98.
20.. Ohlendorf D, Adjami F, Scharnweber B, et al. Standard values of the upper body posture in male adults. Adv Clin Exp Med 2018;27(11):1521–8.
21.. Been E, Barash A, Pessah H, et al. A new look at the geometry of the lumbar spine. Spine (Phila Pa 1976) 2010;35(20):E1014–7.
22. Yildiz HK, Ekin EE. Normal aging of the lumbar spine in women. J Back Musculoskelet Rehabil 2017; 30(5):1061–7.
23. Kwong Y, Rao N, Latief K. MDCT findings in Baastrup disease: disease or normal feature of the aging spine? AJR Am J Roentgenol 2011;196(5): 1156–9.
24. Celestre PC, Dimar JR 2nd, Glassman SD. Spinopelvic Parameters: Lumbar Lordosis, Pelvic Incidence, Pelvic Tilt, and Sacral Slope: What Does a Spine Surgeon Need to Know to Plan a Lumbar Deformity Correction? Neurosurg Clin N Am 2018;29(3):323–9.
25.. Janssen MM, Kouwenhoven JM, Schlosser TP, et al. Analysis of preexistent vertebral rotation in the normal infantile, juvenile, and adolescent spine. Spine (Phila Pa 1976) 2011;36(7):E486–91.
26.. Lafage R, Steinberger J, Pesenti S, et al. Understanding Thoracic Spine Morphology, Shape, and Proportionality. Spine (Phila Pa 1976) 2020;45(3): 149–57.
27.. Negrini A, Vanossi M, Donzelli S, et al. Spinal Coronal and Sagittal Balance in 584 Healthy Individuals During Growth: Normal Plumb Line Values and Their Correlation With Radiographic Measurements. Phys Ther 2019;99(12):1712–8.
28.. Valdovino AG, Bastrom TP, Reighard FG, et al. Obesity Is Associated With Increased Thoracic Kyphosis in Adolescent Idiopathic Scoliosis

Patients and Nonscoliotic Adolescents. Spine Deform 2019;7(6):865–9.

29.. Newton PO, Yaszay B, Upasani VV, et al. Preservation of thoracic kyphosis is critical to maintain lumbar lordosis in the surgical treatment of adolescent idiopathic scoliosis. Spine (Phila Pa 1976) 2010;35(14):1365–70.

30.. Nastoulis E, Karakasi MV, Pavlidis P, et al. Anatomy and clinical significance of sacral variations: a systematic review. Folia Morphol (Warsz) 2019;78(4):651–67.

31.. Woon JT, Perumal V, Maigne J-Y, et al. CT morphology and morphometry of the normal adult coccyx. Eur Spine J 2013;22(4):863–70.

32.. Chiarilli MG, Pizzi AD, Mastrodicasa D, et al. Bone marrow magnetic resonance imaging: physiologic and pathologic findings that radiologist should know. Radiol Med 2021;126(2):264–76.

33.. Schmeel FC, Luetkens JA, Enkirch SJ, et al. Proton density fat fraction (PDFF) MR imaging for differentiation of acute benign and neoplastic compression fractures of the spine. Eur Radiol 2018;28(12):5001–9.

34.. Nabavizadeh SA, Mamourian A, Schmitt JE, et al. Utility of fat-suppressed sequences in differentiation of aggressive vs typical asymptomatic haemangioma of the spine. Br J Radiol 2016;89(1057):20150557.

35. Tehranzadeh J, Andrews C, Wong E. Lumbar spine imaging. Normal variants, imaging pitfalls, and artifacts. Radiol Clin North Am 2000;38(6):1207–53. v-vi.

36.. Fletcher JG, Stringer MD, Briggs CA, et al. CT morphometry of adult thoracic intervertebral discs. Eur Spine J 2015;24(10):2321–9.

37.. Zhong W, Driscoll SJ, Wu M, et al. In vivo morphological features of human lumbar discs. Medicine (Baltimore) 2014;93(28):e333.

38.. Wijayathunga VN, Tanner SF, Ridgeway JP, et al. An In Vitro Study of the Intervertebral Disc Structure Using 3 T Magnetic Resonance Imaging. Spine (Phila Pa 1976) 2019;44(11):793–800.

39.. Kolf AK, Konieczny M, Hesper T, et al. T2* Mapping of the Adult Intervertebral Lumbar Disc: Normative Data and Analysis of Diurnal Effects. J Orthop Res 2019;37(9):1956–62.

40. Byrne RM, Aiyangar AK, Zhang X. A Dynamic Radiographic Imaging Study of Lumbar Intervertebral

Disc Morphometry and Deformation In Vivo. Sci Rep 2019;9(1):15490.

41.. Weber CI, Hwang C-T, van Dillen LR, et al. Effects of standing on lumbar spine alignment and intervertebral disc geometry in young, healthy individuals determined by positional magnetic resonance imaging. Clin Biomech (Bristol, Avon) 2019;65:128–34.

42.. Fyllos AH, Arvanitis DL, Karantanas AH, et al. Magnetic resonance morphometry of the adult normal lumbar intervertebral space. Surg Radiol Anat 2018;40(9):1055–61.

43.. Kalb S, Martirosyan NL, Perez-Orribo L, et al. Analysis of demographics, risk factors, clinical presentation, and surgical treatment modalities for the ossified posterior longitudinal ligament. Neurosurg Focus 2011;30(3):E11.

44.. Maric DL, Krstonosic B, Eric M, et al. An anatomical study of the lumbar external foraminal ligaments: appearance at MR imaging. Surg Radiol Anat 2015;37(1):87–91.

45.. Hu Z, Zhang Z, Zhao Z, et al. A neglected point in surgical treatment of adolescent idiopathic scoliosis: Variations in the number of vertebrae. Medicine (Baltimore) 2016;95(34):e4682.

46.. Tatara Y, Niimura T, Sekiya T, et al. Changes in Lumbosacral Anatomy and Vertebral Numbering in Patients with Thoracolumbar and/or Lumbosacral Transitional Vertebrae. JB JS Open Access 2021;6(3):1–7.

47.. Hiremath SB, Boto J, Regnaud A, et al. Incidentalomas in Spine and Spinal Cord Imaging. Clin Neuroradiol 2019;29(2):191–213.

48. Krupa K, Bekiesinska-Figatowska M. Artifacts in magnetic resonance imaging. Pol J Radiol 2015;80:93–106.

49.. Ayubcha C, Zadeh MZ, Stochkendahl MJ, et al. Quantitative evaluation of normal spinal osseous metabolism with 18F-NaF PET/CT. Nucl Med Commun 2018;39(10):945–50.

50. Vargas MI, Boto J, Meling TR. Imaging of the spine and spinal cord: An overview of magnetic resonance imaging (MRI) techniques. Rev Neurol (Paris) 2021;177(5):451–8.

51.. Hiepe P, Gussew A, Rzanny R, et al. Age-related structural and functional changes of low back muscles. Exp Gerontol 2015;65:23–34.

52. Love C, Palestro CJ. Nuclear medicine imaging of bone infections. Clin Radiol 2016;71(7):632–46.

Anatomy of the Spinal Cord, Coverings, and Nerves

Syed S. Hashmi, MD*, Eric K. van Staalduinen, DO,
Tarik F. Massoud, MD, PhD

KEYWORDS

• Spinal cord • Thecal sac and nerve anatomy • Embryology and morphometry • Spinal MR imaging
• Myelography • Dura • Meninges

KEY POINTS

- This article reviews and illustrates normal spinal cord anatomy as defined by MR imaging, with complementary diagrams and CT myelography images.
- Knowledge of normal spinal cord anatomy and familiarity with common imaging artifacts improves recognition of spinal cord pathologic condition.
- The spinal cord is best evaluated on spine MRI imaging.

INTRODUCTION

The spinal cord serves as a conduit for the transfer of information between the brain and the peripheral nervous system. It is an elegant structure with a complex arrangement of patterns and connections that are challenging to visualize because of its small cross-sectional area and location in the body. However, significant advances in imaging techniques, hardware, and software have occurred during the last decade that allow for better evaluation of this anatomy, with improved resolution and greater detail.

This article will focus primarily on the anatomy of the spinal cord, with attention also given to its coverings and nerves. We will discuss basic anatomy of the cord, its gross and structural features, as well as its microscopic organization. We will also review how this anatomy seems on current neuroimaging techniques, with an emphasis on MR imaging.

Our goal for this article is to provide a framework for understanding this complex anatomy while also serving as a reference for practicing radiologists, clinicians, and scientists.

EMBRYOLOGY OF THE SPINAL CORD, COVERINGS, AND NERVES

A brief understanding of spinal cord development is vital to understanding its anatomy. The initial phase of neural tube formation commences from the end of the third week of gestation to the eighth week of gestation and can be divided into 3 stages: neurulation, caudal differentiation, and retrogressive differentiation.[1] Neurulation is characterized by the formation of the neural groove from the cephalic end of the primitive streak, which progresses to form the neural tube. The cephalic and caudal ends of the neural tube are called the anterior and posterior neuropores, with closure occurring anteriorly during the middle of the fourth gestational week and posteriorly at the end of the same week. The stage of caudal differentiation occurs from the fifth week of gestation to the end of the seventh week. During this stage, a cell mass originates

Funding Information: None.
Department of Radiology, Stanford University School of Medicine, Center for Academic Medicine (CAM), 453 Quarry Rd Room 325B, Palo Alto CA 94304
* Corresponding author.
E-mail address: hashmi@stanford.edu

near the caudal end of the neural tube, initially forming small vacuoles, before eventually coalescing into a large vacuole and connecting to the neural tube. This process results in the formation of the lower part of the spinal cord. The stage of retrogressive differentiation is characterized by differential vertebral column and neural tube development rates, with slower rate of development for the cord compared with the spinal canal. During the first 3 months of embryonic development, the spinal cord and spinal canal grow at the same rate, with the spinal cord spanning the length of the spinal canal. Subsequently, the cord grows at a slower rate than the canal, which results in the lower parts of the cord being displaced cranially relative to the canal.[2]

BASIC ANATOMY OF THE SPINAL CORD, COVERINGS, AND NERVES

The spinal cord is contained in the thecal sac, which lies in the vertebral canal of the vertebral column. It extends from below the foramen magnum to the tip of the conus medullaris and has a tubular shape that is elliptical in the cervical region and round in the thoracic region. It is focally enlarged at the cervical and lumbar levels secondary to innervation of the extremities (termed *intumescentia cervicalis and lumbalis*).[3] The caudal tip of the spinal cord tapers into the conus medullaris and continues as a thread, known as the filum terminale, to the level of the sacrum, where it attaches to the first coccygeal segment. A bundle of lumbar, sacral, and coccygeal roots surrounds the filum terminale caudal to the cord, known as the *cauda equina* (or horse tail).

The gray matter in the spinal cord is located centrally and surrounded by white matter columns, which contrasts with the gray–white matter organization of the brain. The gray matter appears as an H- or butterfly-shaped region in the center of the cord, which is secondary to the arrangement of the dorsal horns, the ventral horns, and the commissures that connect them. The white matter is composed of long projections of myelinated axons and is organized into 3 main columns or *funiculi*, known as the ventral, lateral, and dorsal columns. There is extensive compartmentalization of the information that travels through these pathways, with ascending sensory and descending motor impulses.

Thirty-one neuronal segments divide the spinal cord along its length, including 8 cervical, 12 thoracic, 5 lumbar, 5 sacral, and 1 coccygeal segment(s). At each segmental level, ventral and dorsal rootlets give rise to pairs of ventral and dorsal roots. The ventral nerve roots emerge from the spinal cord along the anterior cord surface at the ventrolateral sulci, whereas the dorsal nerve roots enter the spinal cord along the posterior surface through dorsolateral sulci. Together, the ventral and dorsal roots combine to form pairs of spinal nerves. The dorsal roots also contain the spinal ganglia, which are located in the intervertebral foramina.

On MR imaging, the central gray matter seems hypointense on T1-weighted images and hyperintense on T2/fluid-sensitive sequences. In contrast, the peripheral white matter columns seem hyperintense to gray matter on T1-weighted images. Gradient echo sequences such as multiple echo recombined gradient echo and multiecho data image combination (MEDIC) demonstrate excellent contrast between spinal cord, cerebrospinal fluid (CSF), and disc as well as reduced CSF pulsation artifact. On these sequences, the central gray matter seems hyperintense while the peripheral white matter is hypointense. Examples depicting these anatomic relationships are seen in Figs. 1–4.

All segments of the spinal cord are supplied by 3 longitudinal spinal arteries. The *anterior spinal artery* is ventral and runs in the anterior median fissure, whereas paired *posterior spinal arteries* run along the dorsal root entry zones. The anterior spinal artery is formed by the fusion of vertebral artery branches, whereas the posterior spinal arteries originate from either the posterior inferior cerebellar arteries or the vertebral arteries. The spinal arteries are supplied by segmental anterior and posterior radicular arteries, which originate from vertebral, intercostal, and lumbar arteries. Segmental arteries are only present in about half of spinal segments because there is usually one prominent radicular artery supplying the rest, known as the *arteria radicularis magna of Adamkiewicz*, which is an intersegmental branch from the aorta at the lower thoracic or upper lumbar level, usually off the left side of the aorta between the T9 and L2 vertebral levels.[3] Tiny branch arteries enter the cord from these longitudinal spinal arteries, where they supply specific territories. The anterior spinal artery supplies the anterior two-thirds of the spinal cord, whereas the posterior spinal arteries supply the posterior third. Watershed regions in the middle to lower thoracic cord are susceptible to ischemia during hypoperfusion states.[4]

The veins show a distribution pattern comparable to that of the arterial supply; however, only one spinal vein is present on the dorsal side. This is termed the posterior spinal vein, and it is situated in the posterior median sulcus. There are also fewer segmental veins than arteries and there is no single, prominent draining vein among them.

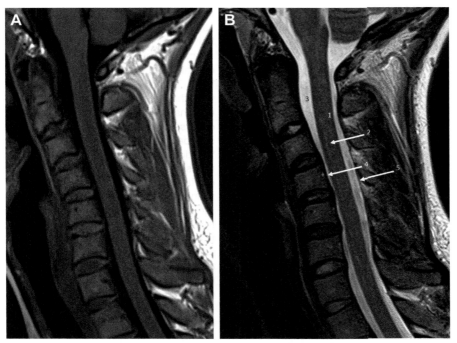

Fig. 1. Sagittal (*A*) T1-weighted and (*B*) T2-weighted MR images of the cervical spine at 3T. 1, spinal cord; 2, gray matter along central canal; 3, subarachnoid space; 4, posterior longitudinal ligament/anterior thecal sac dura; 5, posterior dural sac.

Segmental veins also communicate with the internal spinal venous plexus (which is located in the epidural space), the vertebrae, and the external spinal venous plexus.[4]

The meninges of the spine are a continuation of those of the brain, consisting of dura, arachnoid, and pia mater. The dura extends beyond the spinal cord in the spinal canal to the lower sacral levels and forms the thecal or dural sac. This sac is traversed by the anterior and posterior roots of the cauda equina at various segmental levels. The cord is surrounded by cerebrospinal fluid and attached to the dura by the triangular denticular ligaments along the lateral aspect of the cord.[4] As the meninges extend along the spinal nerves, the dura mater is contiguous with the epineurium and the arachnoid mater is contiguous with the perineurium of the nerves.[5]

MICROSCOPIC AND GROSS ANATOMY OF THE SPINAL CORD

The spinal cord demonstrates a deep anterior median fissure along the ventral surface as well as shallow median and dorsolateral sulci along the

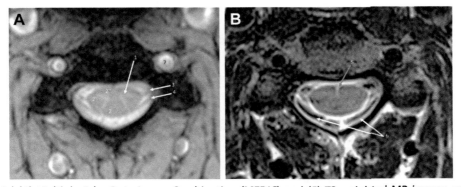

Fig. 2. Axial (*A*) Multiple Echo Data Image Combination (MEDIC) and (*B*) T2-weighted MR images, midcervical spine at 3T. 1, central gray matter; 2, white matter, dorsal column; 2', white matter, lateral column; 2", white matter, ventral column; 3, ventral rootlet; 4, dorsal rootlet; 5, anterior median fissure; 6, CSF pulsation artifact; 7, vertebral artery.

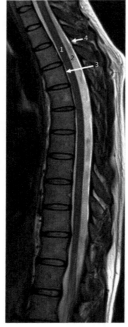

Fig. 3. Sagittal T2-weighted MR image of the thoracic spine at 3T. 1, thoracic spinal cord; 2, subarachnoid space; 3, posterior longitudinal ligament/anterior thecal sac dura; 4, posterior dural sac/ligamentum flavum.

dorsally from the central canal to the median dorsal sulcus, thus dividing the cord into 2 symmetric halves.

The central gray matter can be subdivided into a dorsal horn, an intermediate zone, and a ventral horn. The dorsal horn is laminated and derived from the alar plate.[3] It is covered by a bundle of unmyelinated fibers, known as the *dorsolateral tract of Lissauer*, which is mostly derived from the dorsal roots and reaches the meningeal surface at the dorsolateral sulcus.[3] The ventral horn originates from the basal plate of the neural tube and contains groups of large motoneurons.[3] It is surrounded by the ventral and lateral white matter of the cord. The intermediate zone is located between the 2 horns, serving as an intermediary between the motoneurons and many of their afferent systems. There are also anterior and posterior gray commissures, which represent unmyelinated fibers that cross the midline, ventral and dorsal to the central canal.[3]

Lamination of human spinal cord gray matter has been largely inferred based on the study of Rexed, who studied spinal cord gray matter in cats.[6] In general, there are 10 described layers, for which a brief review is presented. Laminae I–IV are in the dorsal horn while laminae V–X occupy the base of the dorsal horn and the central region of the ventral horn.[3] Laminae V and VI represent the intermediate zone and cannot be separated in the human cord.[3] Many neurons in this region give rise to *propriospinal neurons*, which are axons that terminate within the cord itself.[3] Lamina VIII is

dorsal cord. A central canal is present in the central portion of the cord, which is often obliterated and represents the ventricular portion of the spinal cord. A glial posterior median septum extends

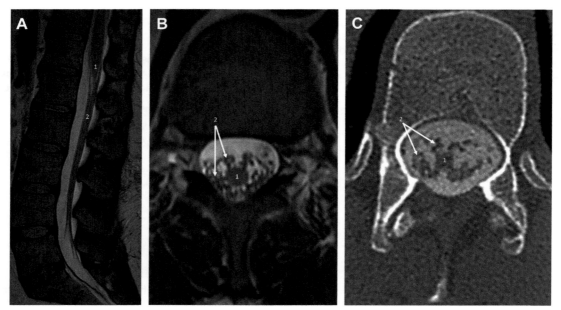

Fig. 4. (A) Sagittal and (*B*) axial T2-weighted MR images at 3T and (*C*) axial CT-myelographic image through the conus medullaris. 1, conus medullaris; 2, cauda equina nerve roots.

in the ventromedial aspect of the ventral horn and consists of *commissural neurons*, which send axons into the ventral white commissure.[3] Lamina IX is in the ventrolateral aspect of the ventral horn and consists of large groups of motoneurons that give rise to the ventral roots.[3] Lamina X consists of small, densely packed neurons surrounding the central canal.[3]

Several other nuclei are present at certain levels of the cord. These include the *central cervical nucleus*, located centrally in the intermediate zone of the upper cervical cord and caudal brainstem; *Clarke's dorsal column*, which is a discrete collection of large neurons in the medial base of the dorsal horn at thoracic and high lumbar levels; *spinal border cells* are medial in the lumbar ventral horn. These nuclei receive dorsal root afferents and give rise to spinocerebellar pathways.[3]

Additionally, the gray matter of the thoracic cord between the ventral and dorsal horns protrudes laterally as the *intermediate horn*. This contains visceromotor neurons (*nucleus intermediolateralis*), which gives rise to preganglionic axons that leave the cord via ventral thoracic roots.[3]

As mentioned earlier, there are 3 primary white matter columns, or *funiculi*. The dorsal white matter contained between the dorsal horn and the dorsal median septum is known as the *posterior funiculus*. It consists mainly of primary afferent fibers that ascend without synaptic interruption to the dorsal column nuclei.[3] The ventral rootlets, which emerge from the ventral horn, represent the arbitrary border between the *anterior* and *lateral funicular* tracts. The lateral funiculus is between the dorsal and ventral rootlets and can be subdivided into anterolateral and posterolateral funiculi. The white matter of the anterior and lateral funiculi contains propriospinal fibers (those that originate and terminate within the cord), as well as long ascending and descending pathways that cross the border with the brainstem.[3] The propriospinal fibers surround the gray matter as the *ground bundles* (or *fasciculi propria*) of the spinal cord.[3] Myelinated fibers that traverse the midline ventral to the central canal are known as *commissura alba*. These fibers serve as the decussation for short and long pathways of the spinal cord.[3]

Descending pathways include long tracts that extend from the cerebral cortex as the *pyramidal* or *corticospinal tract*, from the contralateral red nucleus as the *rubrospinal tract*, from the lateral vestibular nucleus as the *lateral vestibulospinal tract*, and from various regions of the brainstem as the *medial longitudinal fasciculus*.[3] The pyramidal tract partially decussates at the border of the brainstem and spinal cord. The crossed fibers then descend in the dorsal half of the lateral funiculus as the lateral corticospinal tract while the uncrossed fibers of the anterior corticospinal tract are located in the anterior funiculus, adjacent to the anterior median fissure.[3] The medial longitudinal fascicle is in the anterior funiculus, adjacent to the uncrossed fibers of the pyramidal tract. These descending fibers enter the gray matter of the spinal cord from their position in the anterior and lateral funiculi, with most terminating on interneurons in the intermediate zone.[3]

Ascending pathways transmit sensory information and include the *fasciculus gracilis* and *cuneatus* in the dorsal columns, the ventral and dorsal spinocerebellar tracts in the superficial lateral columns, and the spinothalamic, spinoreticular, and spino-olivary tracts in the deeper aspect of the lateral columns.

Although this microstructural anatomy is appreciated histologically, imaging methods cannot reliably differentiate individual or specific tracts with accuracy. However, applied clinical anatomy related to this knowledge can be put to great use when cord imaging is directed at interpretation of patients with neurologic syndromes of the cord (eg, anterior, posterior, central, and Brown-Séquard syndromes). See **Figs. 5** and **6** for detailed diagrams and MR images of this anatomy.

MORPHOMETRY OF THE SPINAL CORD, COVERINGS, AND NERVES

The spinal cord is approximately 45 cm in length and extends from C1 to the level of the L1 vertebra.[1] It is cylindrical in shape but tapers caudally and demonstrates 2 areas of focal enlargement in the cervical and lumbar region. Based on postmortem studies that rely on the spinal rootlets to determine spinal cord neuronal segmental levels, and not based on vertebral column levels, the largest transverse diameter is.....etc etc. The largest transverse diameter is at C5 (13.3 ± 2.2 mm), with decrease at T8 (8.3 ± 2.1 mm), and increase again at L3 (to 9.4 ± 1.5 mm).[7] The anteroposterior diameter demonstrates less variation at C5 (7.4 ± 1.6 mm), T8 (6.3 ± 2.0 mm), and L3 (7.5 ± 1.6 mm).[7] The number of myelinated axons decreases monotonically when extending caudally from the brain down the spine, which is owing to the ingress (sensory) and egress (motor) branching at successive nerve root levels that continues while descending the spine. This decrease in the number of fibers correlates with the reduction in cross-sectional area.[8] It also corresponds with an increasing ratio of gray matter area to total transverse area as we progress from cervical cord to conus.[1] However, the myelin volume fraction is relatively constant along the spinal cord and spinal cord microstructure is highly

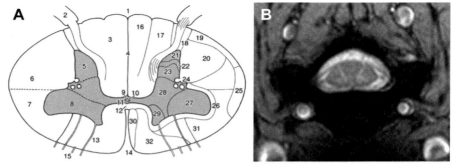

Fig. 5. Axial diagram of gray and white matter in the spinal cord (*A*) with corresponding axial MEDIC MR image (*B*) at 3T. Please note that the MR image has been rotated 180° to mirror the diagram. 1, posterior median sulcus; 2, dorsal root; 3, dorsal column; 4, posterior median septum; 5, dorsal horn; 6, posterolateral column; 7, antero-lateral column; 8, ventral horn; 9, posterior gray commissure; 10, central canal; 11, anterior gray commissure; 12, ventral (*white*) commissure; 13, anterior column; 14, anterior median fissure; 15, ventral root; 16, fasciculus gracilus; 17, fasciculus cuneatus; 18, dorsolateral tract of Lissauer; 19, dorsal spinocerebellar tract; 20, lateral pyramidal tract; 21, dorsal horn, marginal cells (lamina I); 22, dorsal horn, substantia gelatinosa (laminae II and III); 23, dorsal horn, nucleus proprius (lamina IV); 24, intermediate zone, processes reticularis; 25, ventral spinocerebellar tract; 26, ground bundles (fasciculi proprii); 27, lateral motor column (lamina IX); 28, intermediate zone (laminae V–VIII); 29, medial motor zone (lamina IX); 30, anterior pyramidal tract; 31, anterolateral fasciculus; 32, medial longitudinal fasciculus. (*From* Nieuwenhuys R, Voogd J, van Huijzen C. Topography of Spinal Cord, Brain Stem and Cerebellum. In: *The Human Central Nervous System*. 4th ed. Springer, Berlin, Heidelberg; 2008.)

symmetric.[8] Spinal cord total cross-sectional area, gray matter area, and white matter area show age-dependency, with smaller values in the elderly.[9] Men generally demonstrate larger total cross-sectional area and gray matter area compared with women, and a trend toward larger white matter area. However, the ratio of gray matter to total cord area is not influenced by age and gender.[9]

ANATOMIC VARIANTS OF THE SPINAL CORD, COVERINGS, AND NERVES

The presence of lumbosacral transitional vertebrae affects the termination level of the conus medullaris. In normal individuals, it is usually at the mid-L1 level, whereas it is at the upper third in individuals with sacralization of L5, and at the lower third in individuals with lumbarization of the sacrum.[10]

The central canal of the spinal cord runs from the obex at the cervicomedullary junction to the conus medullaris and is lined by ependymal cells, similar to the ventricular surfaces within brain. It serves as a conduit for CSF flow, although it is often poorly visualized on MR images and obliterated throughout the spinal cord.[11] Occasionally a thin and linear, 1 to 2 mm cystic cavity in the center

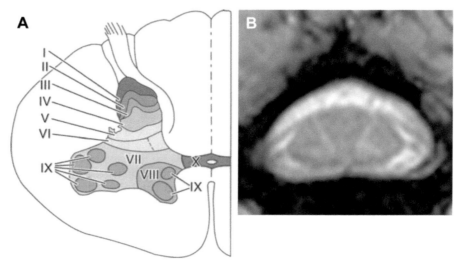

Fig. 6. Axial diagram of spinal cord gray matter, subdivided according to Rexed (*A*), with corresponding axial MEDIC MR image (*B*) at 3T. (*From* Nieuwenhuys R, Voogd J, van Huijzen C. Topography of Spinal Cord, Brain Stem and Cerebellum. In: *The Human Central Nervous System*. 4th ed. Springer, Berlin, Heidelberg; 2008.)

of the spinal cord may be visualized; in the absence of any cause predisposing to syringohydromyelia, this is called a persistent or prominent central canal.[12]

A ventriculus terminalis (or "fifth ventricle") is a CSF-containing ependyma-lined cavity in continuity with the spinal canal involving the terminal cord. It is thought to be due to canalization and is seen in up to 2.6% of neonates and children aged younger than 5 years.[12] It may persist in adults. An example is seen in Fig. 7.

In about 25% of individuals, there is an accessory radicular vein that accompanies the filum terminale or dorsal lumbosacral nerve roots to drain into the epidural venous plexus. They are typically seen as curvilinear enhancement along the conus and the course of the filum terminale. The awareness of normal venous enhancement helps to avoid potential misdiagnosis.[12]

Focal cystic outpouchings are often visualized on MR imaging along the dorsal roots, dorsal root ganglia, and along the spinal nerves. The most common causes for these findings include meningeal diverticula and cysts, perineurial (or perineural) cysts, and dilated nerve root sheaths. Dilated nerve roots sheaths are not challenging to identify because they represent a true anatomic variant and are simply prolongations of the subarachnoid space along the nerve sheath.[5] However, distinguishing meningeal diverticula from perineurial cysts is not easy with noninvasive neuroimaging techniques. However, knowledge of their pathologic condition and location can be useful for making this distinction. Myelography may be useful as well.

Meningeal diverticula are true outpouchings from the meninges. Histologically, they consist of protruding CSF that is lined by arachnoid and overlying dura, termed perineurium and epineurium, respectively. They are located proximal to the dorsal root ganglia, are in free communication with the subarachnoid space, and usually opacify on initial myelography. Meanwhile, perineurial (or Tarlov) cysts are usually extradural, occurring at the junction of the nerve root and the dorsal root ganglion. They contain neural tissue within the cavity or in the wall of the cyst, and they should not immediately fill with contrast on initial myelography. However, they may demonstrate delayed filling, and this feature is useful for distinguishing perineurial cysts from meningeal diverticula.[5] A diagram depicting these relations is seen in Fig. 8 and clinical examples are visualized in Figs. 9 and 10.

IMAGING ARTIFACTS RELATING TO THE SPINAL CORD, COVERINGS, AND NERVES

Artifacts are common in MR imaging, and familiarity with them is important to avoid misinterpretation. For MR imaging of the spinal cord, its coverings, and nerves, motion-related and truncation artifacts are 2 important and common ones to consider.

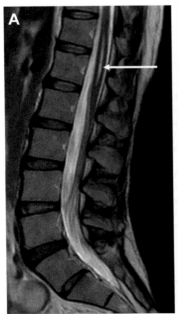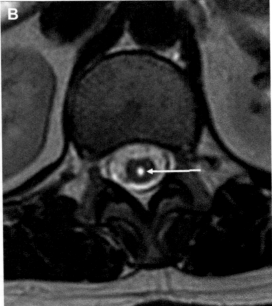

Fig. 7. Sagittal (A) and axial (B) T2-weighted MR images of the lumbar spine at 1.5 T demonstrate mild fusiform enlargement of the terminal central canal of the spinal cord, in keeping with ventriculus terminalis (arrow).

Spinal perineurial and meningeal cysts

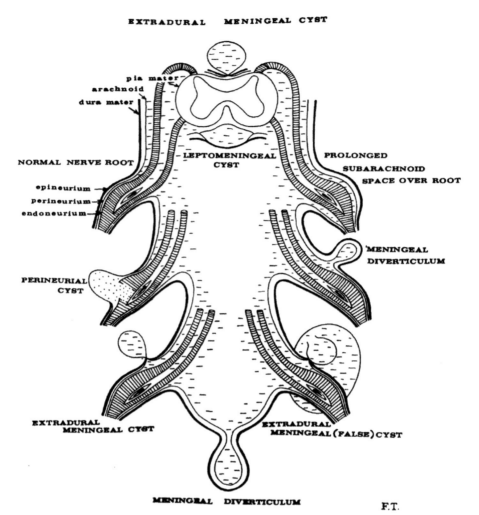

Fig. 8. Diagram demonstrating various spinal perineurial and meningeal cysts. Top: extradural meningeal cyst; leptomeningeal cyst seen below cord figure (composed of arachnoid). Upper left: normal nerve root (note, the arachnoid continuation is perineurium and the subarachnoid space at the root sleeve is continuous with the potential space beneath perineurium, accounting for occasional myelographic filling of perineurial cysts). Middle left: perineurial cyst (note that it lies at the level of the posterior root ganglion and the cyst wall contains neural elements; the space within the cyst may have potential communication with the subarachnoid space, allowing for delayed but not immediate myelographic filling. Lower left: extradural meningeal cyst (this lies proximal to the posterior root ganglion). Bottom: meningeal diverticulum (sealing off neck of diverticulum produces a cyst). Lower right: extradural meningeal (false) cyst (may originate from rupture of extradural meningeal cyst or produced after surgery by nicking the dura). Middle right: meningeal diverticulum (lies proximal to the posterior root ganglion). Upper right: prolongation of subarachnoid space over nerve roots (a frequent finding of no pathologic significance). (*From* Tarlov IM. Spinal perineurial and meningeal cysts. *J Neurol Neurosurg Psychiatry.* 1970;33(6):833-843.)

Motion may result in image blurring (secondary to random patient motion) or ghosting artifacts (from periodic motion). CSF pulsation, respiratory motion, and cardiac motion are the most common sources for periodic motion, with effects mostly visualized in the phase-encoding direction, because this information is acquired over minutes (rather than milliseconds, as in the frequency-encoding direction).[13] CSF flow-related phenomena can be divided into time-of-flight effects, and

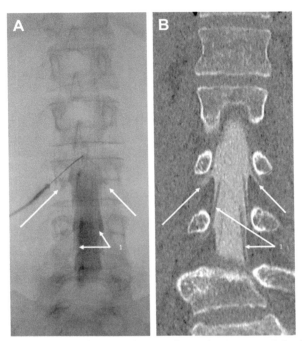

Fig. 9. Fluoroscopic (*A*) and coronal (*B*) reformatted CT-myelographic images of the lumbar spine demonstrate prolonged subarachnoid spaces (*white arrows*) over the L3-4 nerve roots (*red arrow*). Cauda equina nerve roots (1) are outlined by intrathecal contrast.

turbulent flow, which produces a dark signal. These effects occur with spin-echo imaging and are more pronounced with increased proton velocity, thinner slices, and longer time to echo.[13]

Common locations for this artifact are within the cervical and thoracic canal, appearing as a signal void in the dorsal greater than ventral subarachnoid space on sagittal T2-weighted images.[13]

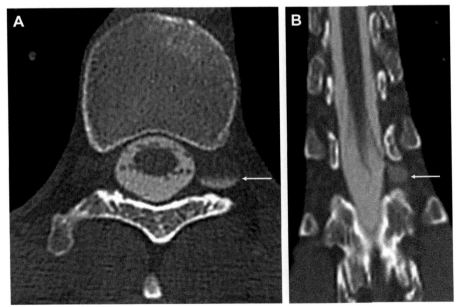

Fig. 10. CT-myelographic axial (*A*) and coronal (*B*) images through the lower thoracic spine demonstrate delayed filling of a cyst in the left T10 to 11 neural foramen (*arrow*), in keeping with a perineurial (Tarlov) cyst.

Truncation, or Gibbs, artifacts seem as alternating bright and dark lines/bands and occur near sharp high-contrast boundaries, such as the spinal cord and CSF interface. Knowledge of this artifact helps avoid misinterpretation of a spinal cord syrinx. Examples of CSF pulsation artifact are seen in Fig. 11.

MYELOGRAPHY

Myelography is a minimally invasive technique where the instillation of intrathecal contrast is used for better evaluation of the spinal canal contents. A lumbar puncture is performed and contrast is injected into the intrathecal subarachnoid space. This technique especially allows for the evaluation of the spinal canal contents in individuals who are unable to obtain an MR image but would otherwise benefit from one.

On injection, the contrast should spread throughout the lumbosacral cistern, outlining the cauda equina nerve roots. The intrathecal contents, as well as the relationship of the thecal sac to the surrounding bone and degenerative changes, are well characterized on a subsequent computerized tomography (CT) of the spine. Emerging techniques, including the use of dual-energy CT, decubitus dynamic CT myelography,

and digital subtraction myelography have increased the clinical utility of this procedure. A CT-myelographic image is seen in Fig. 12.

NORMAL METABOLIC IMAGING OF THE SPINAL CORD, COVERINGS, AND NERVES

Fluorodeoxyglucose (FDG) is a commonly used tracer to assess for cellular glycolysis, with applications for disease evaluation in oncology, differentiating various forms of dementia, and myocardial viability. Physiologic distribution includes high uptake in the brain and liver, urinary excretion, and variable accumulation in the intestines.

Normal spinal cord activation and distribution has been characterized, with mean SUVmax in the cervical and thoracic cord of 2.51 ± 0.5 and 2.33 ± 0.5 in adults.[14] Studies have demonstrated the greatest FDG uptake in areas of focal cord enlargement in the cervical and lower thoracic levels, which correspond to regions innervating the extremities. The presence of increased FDG uptake at these levels may be related to the amount of gray matter, paralleling the increase in cord enlargement and partial volume averaging. These findings are not correlated with age, temperature, or sex, whereas a weak positive

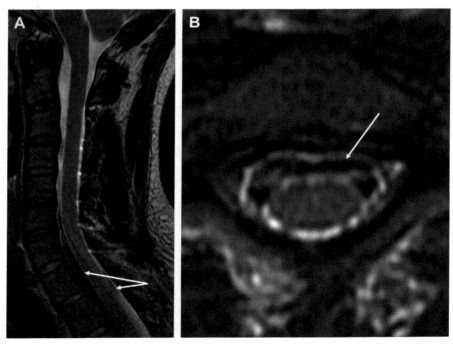

Fig. 11. Sagittal (A) and axial (B) T2-weighted MR images of the cervical spine at 3T demonstrate CSF-pulsation artifact (arrows) in the ventral and dorsal subarachnoid spaces.

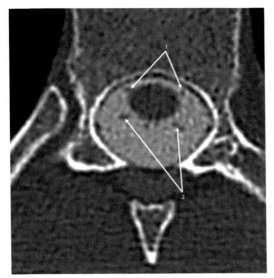

Fig. 12. Axial postcontrast CT-myelographic image of the thoracic cord. Arrows point to ventral (1) and dorsal (2) nerve roots outlined by intrathecal contrast.

correlation with body weight is known.[14] These findings are similar in children.[15]

ADVANCED IMAGING TECHNIQUES OF THE SPINAL CORD, COVERINGS, AND NERVES

There are numerous advanced imaging techniques for assessing the spinal cord, with a complete review beyond the scope of this article. However, we will briefly discuss diffusion tensor imaging and time-resolved contrast-enhanced MR angiography in the spine. Other techniques include diffusion-weighted imaging (DWI), perfusion-weighted imaging, phase contrast MR imaging, functional MR imaging, spinal cord proton MR spectroscopy, myelin-water fraction imaging, and magnetization transfer.

Diffusion tensor imaging (DTI) is an advanced noninvasive technique that enables visualization and quantitative assessment of the integrity of the white matter tracts. It originates from DWI, which is based on the free diffusion of water molecules in the extracellular space. Although DWI visualizes isotropic diffusion (ie, in any direction), DTI evaluates anisotropic diffusion (ie, preferably unidirectional). This is useful for assessing white matter tracts because diffusion is limited in directions perpendicular to the white matter fibers owing to myelinated axons. DTI can therefore detect microstructural variations in white matter tracts, providing a measure of structural integrity and microstructural alterations. DTI indices, including apparent diffusion coefficient, fractional

anisotropy (FA), mean diffusivity, and radial diffusivity can be used to assess for changes following trauma, ischemia, surgery, myelopathy, or in the setting of tumor.[16] Because FA is considered a marker of white matter integrity, its decrease indicates damage, disorganization, and degradation of white matter tracts.[16] An additional application of DTI is diffusion tensor tractography, which can be used to generate a 3-dimensional representation of the white matter tracts.

Time-resolved contrast-enhanced MR angiography (TR-MRA) techniques such as TR imaging of contrast kinetics offer the ability to temporally resolve the arterial and venous phases of an MRA study. This is useful for the evaluation of spinal vascular malformations and is accomplished by variable rate k-space sampling, temporal interpolation, and zero-filling in the slice dimension.[17] This method allows rapid data acquisition and provides dynamic, real-time angiographic information for the clinical area of interest.

SUMMARY

Knowledge of spinal cord anatomy is a requisite for accurate interpretation of diseases affecting the central nervous system. Spinal MR imaging remains the mainstay of accurately evaluating the spinal cord, its coverings, and nerves. Because MR imaging hardware and software will continue to improve, a detailed understanding of spinal anatomy will be useful to delineate normal anatomy from disease processes and artifacts.

CLINICS CARE POINTS

- The spinal cord is focally enlarged at the cervical and lumbar levels secondary to innervation of the extremities.

- A ventriculus terminalis is a CSF-containing ependyma-lined cavity in continuity with the spinal canal involving the terminal cord.

- Meningeal diverticula, perineurial (or perineural) cysts, and dilated nerve root sheaths are focal cystic outpouchings visualized along the dorsal roots, dorsal root ganglia, and along the spinal nerves.

- Truncation, or Gibbs, artifacts seem as alternating bright and dark lines/bands and occur near sharp high-contrast boundaries, such as the spinal cord and CSF interface. Knowledge of this artifact helps avoid misinterpretation of a spinal cord syrinx.

DISCLOSURE

The authors have nothing to disclose.

REFERENCES

1. Goto N, Otsuka N. Development and anatomy of the spinal cord. Neuropathology 1997;17(1):25–31. https://doi.org/10.1111/j.1440-1789.1997.tb00007.x.
2. Miao M, Lin X, Zhang Z, et al. Normal development of the fetal spinal canal and spinal cord at T12 on 3.0-T MRI. Acta Radiol 2019;60(5):623–7. https://doi.org/10.1177/0284185118791197.
3. Nieuwenhuys R, Voogd J, van Huijzen C. Topography of Spinal Cord, Brain Stem and Cerebellum. In: The human central nervous System. 4th ed. Berlin, Heidelberg: Springer; 2008.
4. Nieuwenhuys R, Voogd J, van Huijzen C. Blood Supply, Meninges and Cerebrospinal Fluid Circulation. In: The human central nervous System. 4th ed. Berlin, Heidelberg: Springer; 2008.
5. Tarlov IM. Spinal perineurial and meningeal cysts. J Neurol Neurosurg Psychiatr 1970;33(6):833–43. https://doi.org/10.1136/jnnp.33.6.833.
6. Rexed B. A cytoarchitectonic atlas of the spinal cord in the cat. J Comp Neurol 1954;100:297–379.
7. Frostell A, Hakim R, Thelin EP, et al. A Review of the Segmental Diameter of the Healthy Human Spinal Cord. Front Neurol 2016;7. https://doi.org/10.3389/fneur.2016.00238.
8. Duval T, Saliani A, Nami H, et al. Axons morphometry in the human spinal cord. NeuroImage 2019;185:119–28. https://doi.org/10.1016/j.neuroimage.2018.10.033.
9. Papinutto N, Schlaeger R, Panara V, et al. Age, gender and Normalization Covariates for spinal cord gray matter and total cross-sectional areas at cervical and thoracic levels: a 2D phase sensitive Inversion Recovery imaging Study. PLoS One 2015;10(3):e0118576. https://doi.org/10.1371/journal.pone.0118576. Fehlings M, ed.
10. Morimoto T, Sonohata M, Kitajima M, et al. The termination level of the conus medullaris and lumbosacral transitional vertebrae. J Orthop Sci 2013;18(6):878–84.
11. Jones BV. Cord Cystic Cavities: Syringomyelia and Prominent Central Canal. Semin Ultrasound CT MRI 2017;38(2):98–104. https://doi.org/10.1053/j.sult.2016.07.008.
12. Hiremath SB, Boto J, Regnaud A, et al. Incidentalomas in Spine and Spinal Cord Imaging. Clin Neuroradiol 2019;29(2):191–213. https://doi.org/10.1007/s00062-019-00773-5.
13. Shanechi AM, Kiczek M, Khan M, et al. Spine Anatomy Imaging. Neuroimaging Clin N Am 2019;29(4):461–80. https://doi.org/10.1016/j.nic.2019.08.001.
14. Guner LA, Unal K, Vardareli E, et al. Physiological fluorodeoxyglucose uptake of spinal cord in adults. Nucl Med Commun 2020. https://doi.org/10.1097/MNM.0000000000001188.
15. Taralli S, Leccisotti L, Mattoli MV, et al. Physiological Activity of Spinal Cord in Children: An 18F-FDG PET-CT Study. Spine 2015;40(11):E647–52. https://doi.org/10.1097/BRS.0000000000000895.
16. Shah LM, Ross JS. Imaging of Spine Trauma. Neurosurgery 2016;79(5):626–42. https://doi.org/10.1227/NEU.0000000000001336.
17. Korosec FR, Frayne R, Grist TM, et al. Time-resolved contrast-enhanced 3D MR angiography. Magn Reson Med 1996;36(3):345–51. https://doi.org/10.1002/mrm.1910360304.

UNITED STATES POSTAL SERVICE ®
Statement of Ownership, Management, and Circulation
(All Periodicals Publications Except Requester Publications)

1. Publication Title	2. Publication Number	3. Filing Date
NEUROIMAGING CLINICS OF NORTH AMERICA	010 – 548	9/18/2022

4. Issue Frequency	5. Number of Issues Published Annually	6. Annual Subscription Price
FEB, MAY, AUG, NOV	4	$401.00

7. Complete Mailing Address of Known Office of Publication (Not printer) (Street, city, county, state, and ZIP+4®)

ELSEVIER INC.
230 Park Avenue, Suite 800
New York, NY 10169

Contact Person
Malathi Samayan

Telephone (Include area code)
91-44-4299-4507

8. Complete Mailing Address of Headquarters or General Business Office of Publisher (Not printer)

ELSEVIER INC.
230 Park Avenue, Suite 800
New York, NY 10169

9. Full Names and Complete Mailing Addresses of Publisher, Editor, and Managing Editor (Do not leave blank)

Publisher (Name and complete mailing address)

DOLORES MELONI, ELSEVIER INC.
1600 JOHN F KENNEDY BLVD. SUITE 1800
PHILADELPHIA, PA 19103-2899

Editor (Name and complete mailing address)

JOHN VASSALLO, ELSEVIER INC.
1600 JOHN F KENNEDY BLVD. SUITE 1800
PHILADELPHIA, PA 19103-2899

Managing Editor (Name and complete mailing address)

PATRICK MANLEY ELSEVIER INC.
1600 JOHN F KENNEDY BLVD. SUITE 1800
PHILADELPHIA, PA 19103-2899

10. Owner (Do not leave blank. If the publication is owned by a corporation, give the name and address of the corporation immediately followed by the names and addresses of all stockholders owning or holding 1 percent or more of the total amount of stock. If not owned by a corporation, give the names and addresses of the individual owners. If owned by a partnership or other unincorporated firm, give its name and address as well as those of each individual owner. If the publication is published by a nonprofit organization, give its name and address.)

Full Name	Complete Mailing Address
WHOLLY OWNED SUBSIDIARY OF REED/ELSEVIER, US HOLDINGS	1600 JOHN F KENNEDY BLVD. SUITE 1800 PHILADELPHIA, PA 19103-2899

11. Known Bondholders, Mortgagees, and Other Security Holders Owning or Holding 1 Percent or More of Total Amount of Bonds, Mortgages, or Other Securities. If none, check box ▶ ☐ None

Full Name	Complete Mailing Address
N/A	

12. Tax Status (For completion by nonprofit organizations authorized to mail at nonprofit rates) (Check one)
The purpose, function, and nonprofit status of this organization and the exempt status for federal income tax purposes:
☒ Has Not Changed During Preceding 12 Months
☐ Has Changed During Preceding 12 Months (Publisher must submit explanation of change with this statement)

PS Form 3526, July 2014 [Page 1 of 4 (see instructions page 4)] PSN: 7530-01-000-9931 PRIVACY NOTICE: See our privacy policy on www.usps.com.

13. Publication Title		14. Issue Date for Circulation Data Below
NEUROIMAGING CLINICS OF NORTH AMERICA		MAY 2022

15. Extent and Nature of Circulation			Average No. Copies Each Issue During Preceding 12 Months	No. Copies of Single Issue Published Nearest to Filing Date
a. Total Number of Copies (Net press run)			394	371
b. Paid Circulation (By Mail and Outside the Mail)	(1)	Mailed Outside-County Paid Subscriptions Stated on PS Form 3541 (Include paid distribution above nominal rate, advertiser's proof copies, and exchange copies)	293	276
	(2)	Mailed In-County Paid Subscriptions Stated on PS Form 3541 (Include paid distribution above nominal rate, advertiser's proof copies, and exchange copies)	0	0
	(3)	Paid Distribution Outside the Mails Including Sales Through Dealers and Carriers, Street Vendors, Counter Sales, and Other Paid Distribution Outside USPS®	63	49
	(4)	Paid Distribution by Other Classes of Mail Through the USPS (e.g., First-Class Mail®)	0	0
c. Total Paid Distribution (Sum of 15b (1), (2), (3), and (4))		▶	356	325
d. Free or Nominal Rate Distribution (By Mail and Outside the Mail)	(1)	Free or Nominal Rate Outside-County Copies included on PS Form 3541	22	31
	(2)	Free or Nominal Rate In-County Copies Included on PS Form 3541	0	0
	(3)	Free or Nominal Rate Copies Mailed at Other Classes Through the USPS (e.g., First-Class Mail)	0	0
	(4)	Free or Nominal Rate Distribution Outside the Mail (Carriers or other means)	0	0
e. Total Free or Nominal Rate Distribution (Sum of 15d (1), (2), (3) and (4))		▶	22	31
f. Total Distribution (Sum of 15c and 15e)		▶	378	356
g. Copies not Distributed (See Instructions to Publishers #4 (page #3))		▶	16	15
h. Total (Sum of 15f and g)		▶	394	371
i. Percent Paid (15c divided by 15f times 100)			94.17%	91.29%

* If you are claiming electronic copies, go to line 16 on page 3. If you are not claiming electronic copies, skip to line 17 on page 3.

PS Form 3526, July 2014 (Page 2 of 4)

16. Electronic Copy Circulation		Average No. Copies Each Issue During Preceding 12 Months	No. Copies of Single Issue Published Nearest to Filing Date
a. Paid Electronic Copies	▶		
b. Total Paid Print Copies (Line 15c) + Paid Electronic Copies (Line 16a)	▶		
c. Total Print Distribution (Line 15f) + Paid Electronic Copies (Line 16a)	▶		
d. Percent Paid (Both Print & Electronic Copies) (16b divided by 16c × 100)	▶		

☒ I certify that 50% of all my distributed copies (electronic and print) are paid above a nominal price.

17. Publication of Statement of Ownership

☒ If the publication is a general publication, publication of this statement is required. Will be printed in the NOVEMBER 2022 issue of this publication.   ☐ Publication not required.

18. Signature and Title of Editor, Publisher, Business Manager, or Owner

Malathi Samayan - Distribution Controller   *Malathi Samayan*   Date 9/18/2022

I certify that all information furnished on this form is true and complete. I understand that anyone who furnishes false or misleading information on this form or who omits material or information requested on the form may be subject to criminal sanctions (including fines and imprisonment) and/or civil sanctions (including civil penalties).

PS Form 3526, July 2014 (Page 3 of 4)   PRIVACY NOTICE: See our privacy policy on www.usps.com.

Moving?

Make sure your subscription moves with you!

To notify us of your new address, find your **Clinics Account Number** (located on your mailing label above your name), and contact customer service at:

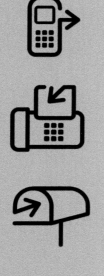

Email: journalscustomerservice-usa@elsevier.com

800-654-2452 (subscribers in the U.S. & Canada)
314-447-8871 (subscribers outside of the U.S. & Canada)

Fax number: 314-447-8029

Elsevier Health Sciences Division
Subscription Customer Service
3251 Riverport Lane
Maryland Heights, MO 63043

*To ensure uninterrupted delivery of your subscription, please notify us at least 4 weeks in advance of move.